THE CONDITION OF EDUCATION IN AMERICA

The Condition of Education in America

Maurice H. Logan
Editor

Nova Science Publishers, Inc.
New York

For permission to use material from this book please contact us:
Telephone 631-231-7269; Fax 631-231-8175
Web Site: http://www.novapublishers.com

LIBRARY OF CONGRESS CATALOGING-IN-PUBLICATION DATA
Available upon request

ISBN: 978-1-60692-298-9

Published by Nova Science Publishers, Inc. ✦ New York

CONTENTS

PREFACE*

To ensure reliable, accurate, and timely data, which are necessary to monitor the progress of U.S. education, Congress has mandated that the National Center for Education Statistics (NCES) produce an annual report, 'The Condition of Education'. This year's report presents indicators of important developments and trends in U.S. education. These indicators focus on participation and persistence in education, student performance and other measures of achievement, the environment for learning, and resources for education.

This book consists of public domain documents which have been located, gathered, combined, reformatted, and enhanced with a subject index, perhaps edited and bound to provide easy access.

Chapter 1 - To ensure reliable, accurate, and timely data, which are necessary to monitor the progress of U.S. education, Congress has mandated that the National Center for Education Statistics (NCES) produce an annual report, *The Condition of Education.* This year's report presents indicators of important developments and trends in U.S. education. These indicators focus on participation and persistence in education, student performance and other measures of achievement, the environment for learning, and resources for education.

This statement summarizes the main findings of the 43 indicators that appear in the five following sections. Each indicator discussed is referenced by its number (e.g., *indicator 1*) in the volume.

Chapter 2 - *The Condition of Education* is available in two forms: this print volume for 2008 and a Web version on the National Center for Education Statistics (NCES) website (http://nces.ed.gov/ programs/coe). The Web version includes the following: the 2008 Commissioner's statement, a user's guide, special analyses from 2000 through 2007, all indicators from this edition, and selected indicators from earlier editions of *The Condition of Education.* (See page xxiv for a list of all the indicators that appear on *The Condition of Education* website.)

Chapter 3 - This volume of *The Condition of Education* was authored by a team of analysts under the general direction of Michael Planty and Thomas Snyder of NCES with technical review by Marilyn Seastrom (Chief Statistician of NCES) and many others. Val Plisko (Associate Commissioner of NCES) provided overall guidance in the volume's development and reviewed the indicators. Barbara Kridl of MPR Associates, Inc. (MPR) was

---

* This is an edited, excerpted and augmented edition of a National Center for Education Statistics publication, dated June 2008.

the managing editor of the publication. Andrea Livingston (MPR) wrote the style guide for this publication, edited the final volume, and assisted in writing and editing the Commissioner's Statement.

Chapter 5 - The indicators in this section of *The Condition of Education* report trends in enrollments across all levels of education. There are 14 indicators in this section: 11, prepared for this year's volume, appear on the following pages, and all 14, including indicators from previous years, appear on the Web (see Website Contents on the facing page for a full list of the indicators). Enrollment is a key indicator of the scope of and access to educational opportunities and is a basic descriptor of American education. Changes in enrollment have implications for the demand for educational resources, such as qualified teachers, physical facilities, and funding levels, which are required to provide a high- quality education for our nation's students.

Chapter 6 - The indicators in this section of *The Condition of Education* examine student achievement and other outcomes of education among students in elementary and secondary education and among adults in the larger society. There are 27 indicators in this section: 9, prepared for this year's volume, appear on the following pages, and all 27, including indicators from previous years, appear on the Web (see Web- site Contents on the facing page for a full list of the indicators). The indicators on student achievement show how students are performing on assessments in reading, mathematics, science, and other academic subject areas; trends over time in student achievement; and gaps in achievement. The indicators in this section are organized into five subsections.

Chapter 7 - The indicators in this section of *The Condition of Education* examine student achievement and other outcomes of education among students in elementary and secondary education and among adults in the larger society. There are 27 indicators in this section: 9, prepared for this year's volume, appear on the following pages, and all 27, including indicators from previous years, appear on the Web (see Website Contents on the facing page for a full list of the indicators). The indicators on student achievement show how students are performing on assessments in reading, mathematics, science, and other academic subject areas; trends over time in student achievement; and gaps in achievement. The indicators in this section are organized into five subsections.

Chapter 8 - The indicators in this section of The Condition of Education report on the progress students make through the education system. There are 24 indicators in this section: 7, prepared for this year's volume, appear on the following pages, and all 24, including indicators from previous volumes, appear on the Web (see Website Contents on the facing page for a full list of the indicators). Particular attention is paid to how various subgroups in the population proceed through school and attain different levels of education as well as the factors that are associated with their success along the way.

Chapter 9 - The indicators in this section of *The Condition of Education* measure features of the context of learning in elementary and secondary schools. This includes the content of learning and expectations for student performance; processes of instruction; mechanisms of choice in education; characteristics of teachers and the teaching profession; the climate for learning and other organizational aspects of schools; and financial resources. There are 35 indicators in this section: 11, prepared for this year's volume, appear on the following pages, and all 35, including indicators from previous years, appear on the Web (see Website Contents on the facing page for a full list of the indicators).

Chapter 10 - The indicators in this section of *The Condition of Education* examine features of postsecondary education, many of which parallel those presented in the previous section on elementary and secondary education. There are 21 indicators in this section: 5, prepared for this year's volume, appear on the following pages, and all 21, including indicators from previous years, are on the Web (see Website Contents on the facing page for a full list of the indicators).

ACKNOWLEDGMENTS

This volume of *The Condition of Education* was authored by a team of analysts under the general direction of Michael Planty and Thomas Snyder of NCES with technical review by Marilyn Seastrom (Chief Statistician of NCES) and many others. Val Plisko (Associate Commissioner of NCES) provided overall guidance in the volume's development and reviewed the indicators. Barbara Kridl of MPR Associates, Inc. (MPR) was the managing editor of the publication. Andrea Livingston (MPR) wrote the style guide for this publication, edited the final volume, and assisted in writing and editing the Commissioner's Statement.

The key contributors to *The Condition of Education* are the authors of the indicators. As a matter of practice, the authorship of individual indicators is not given in the volume because each indicator reflects the joint effort of many analysts. Nonetheless, substantial expertise and analytical ability are required to craft an indicator from the survey data to tell an important story in a compelling manner using text, graphs, and tables economically and to perform the necessary statistical tests. Some indicators in this volume were originally conceived for *The Condition of Education* and involved extensive analyses of data. The rest were adapted from existing NCES reports or analyses authored by others.

A large team of analysts—including those from NCES and staff at the Education Statistics Services Institute (ESSI), which is funded by NCES and composed of staff from the American Institutes for Research (AIR) and a number of partner organizations—authored individual indicators. Authors include Michael Planty, William Hussar, Thomas Snyder, Stephen Provasnik, Peter Tice, and Patrick Gonzales (NCES); Grace Kena, Rachel Dinkes, Angelina KewalRamani, and Mary Ann Fox (ESSI-AIR); Jana Kemp and Kristen Darling (ESSI-Child Trends); and Kevin Bianco and Lauren Drake (ESSI-MacroSys); and Xiaojie Li (MPR). Grace Kena (ESSI-AIR), Jana Kemp (ESSI-Child Trends), Kevin Bianco (ESSI-MacroSys), and Mary Ann Fox (ESSI-AIR) updated and revised other sections of the report, helped with planning and the development of the production schedule, coordinated with the authors and reviewers, and circulated the indicator drafts and reviews.

Programming and other analytical assistance was provided by William Sonnenberg (NCES), Qingshu Xie (ESSI-MacroSys), Nancy Collins (ESSI), and Elizabeth Jacinto (ESSI-AIR). Technical and copyedit reviews were conducted by Kevin Bromer (formerly ESSI-AIR), Ben Kaplan (ESSI-AIR), Jason Murray (ESSI-AIR), Alexandra Henning (ESSI-QIP), Stephen Hocker (formerly ESSI-MacroSys), Alison Slade (ESSI-AIR), Aparna Sundaram (ESSIAIR), Jed Tank (formerly ESSI-AIR), Xiaolei Wang (ESSI-NISS), Siri Warkentien

(ESSIChild Trends), Zeyu Xu (formerly ESSI-AIR), Thomas Nachazel, Sandra Eyster, and Kristin Flanagan (ESSI-AIR).

Alicia Broadway (MPR) and contractor Goura Fotadar McCarty proofread the text and checked the numbers against their original sources. Natesh Daniel and Patti Gildersleeve (MPR) did the desktop publishing of the publication with help from contractors Rebecca Chapman-Winter and Martha Hoeper and prepared it for printing. Helen Jang (MPR) headed the team responsible for updating and revising the Web version of *The Condition of Education*. She was assisted by Nick Branigan, David Jimenez, Stephanie Nevill, and Leslie Retallick (MPR). These Web materials were reviewed by a team of reviewers led by Jennifer Young (Kforce). Julia Marshall prepared the index. Natesh Daniel (MPR) designed this year's cover.

The efforts of many people who reviewed individual indicators and the entire volume, often under tight deadlines, are greatly appreciated. Each indicator was assigned to at least two NCES staff members, who followed it through all phases of development from initial plans to final review. Stephen Broughman, Susan Broyles, Jacquelyn Buckley, Kathryn Chandler, Chris Chapman, Arnold Goldstein, James Griffith, Kerry Gruber, Lee Hoffman, Lisa Hudson, Frank Johnson, Andrew Kolstad, Laura LoGerfo, Andrew Mary, Edith McArthur, Dan McGrath, Frank Morgan, Gail Mulligan, Sabrina Ratchford, John Sietsema, Emmanuel Sikali, William Sonnenberg, and Peter Tice (NCES) provided detailed and helpful reviews of the indicators or other parts of the volume.

A number of individuals from academia served as external reviewers: Sandy Baum, Jeremy Finn, Frederick Hess, Jeremy Kilpatrick, and Leanna Stiefel.

In: The Condition of Education in America
Editor: Maurice H. Logan
ISBN: 978-1-60692-298-9

COMMISSIONER'S STATEMENT

INTRODUCTION

To ensure reliable, accurate, and timely data, which are necessary to monitor the progress of U.S. education, Congress has mandated that the National Center for Education Statistics (NCES) produce an annual report, *The Condition of Education*. This year's report presents indicators of important developments and trends in U.S. education. These indicators focus on participation and persistence in education, student performance and other measures of achievement, the environment for learning, and resources for education.

This statement summarizes the main findings of the 43 indicators that appear in the five following sections. Each indicator discussed is referenced by its number (e.g., *indicator 1*) in the volume.

PARTICIPATION IN EDUCATION

As the U.S. population increases in size, so does enrollment at all levels of education. At the elementary and secondary levels, growth is due largely to the increase in the size of the school-age population. At the postsecondary level, both population growth and increasing enrollment rates help account for rising enrollments in undergraduate, graduate, and first-professional programs. The cohorts of learners have become more diverse, with students who are members of racial/ethnic minorities or who speak a language other than English at home making up an increasing proportion of the school-age population over time.

- Between 1970 and 2006, children ages 3–4 (typically preschool ages) experienced the largest increase in enrollment rates, from 20 to 56 percent, of any age group. Notable growth was also seen in the enrollment rates for those ages 18–24, the period when young adults are typically enrolled in or transitioning into postsecondary education. For example, the overall enrollment rate increased from 48 to 65 percent for those ages 18–19, from 32 to 48 percent for those ages 20–21, and from 15 to 27 percent for those ages 22–24 (*indicator 1*).
- A greater percentage of children who were about 4 years old in 2005–06 were in a center-based setting as their primary type of early education and care (57percent) than in other arrangements such as regular parental care (20 percent), home-based

relative care (13 percent), home-based nonrelative care (8 percent), or multiple arrangements (2 percent). A smaller percentage of Hispanic children (49 percent) were in a center- based setting as their primary type of early education and care than their White, Black, Asian, or American Indian/Alaska Native peers (60 to 62 percent each). The percentage of children in a center-based setting increased as parents' highest level of education increased (*indicator 2*).

- In 2008, public elementary and secondary school enrollment in the United States is expected to approach about 49.8 million students: 34.9 million in prekindergarten through 8th grade and 14.9 million in grades 9 through 12. Total public elementary and secondary school enrollment is projected to set new enrollment records each year from 2008 through 2017, at which time it is expected to reach an estimated high of 54.1 million students. According to projections, the South is expected to experience the largest increase in enrollment of all regions in the country (*indicator 3*).
- From 1989 to 2001, private school enrollment in kindergarten through grade 12 increased from 4.8 to 5.3 million students; by 2005, enrollment had declined to 5.1 million students. Overall, while the number of students enrolled in private schools was higher in 2005 than in 1989, the percentage of all students attending private schools declined from 11 to 9 percent. Along with the changing level of private school enrollment, the distribution of students across different types of private schools changed during this period. Roman Catholic schools continued to have the largest percentage of total private school enrollment, but the distribution of students shifted from Roman Catholic to other religious and nonsectarian private schools at both the elementary and secondary levels (*indicator 4*).
- The percentage of racial/ethnic minority students enrolled in the nation's public schools increased from 22 percent in 1972 to 31 percent in 1986 to 43 percent in 2006. This increase in minority enrollment largely reflects the growth in the percentage of students who were Hispanic. In 2006, Hispanic students represented 20 percent of public school enrollment, up from 6 percent in 1972 and 11 percent in 1986. The distribution of minority students in public schools differed across regions of the country, with minority public school enrollment (55 percent) exceeding White enrollment (45 percent) in the West in 2006 (*indicator 5*).
- The percentage of school-age children (ages 5–17) whose parents had completed a bachelor's degree or higher increased from 19 to 35 percent between 1979 and 2006. During this period, the percentage of parents with a bachelor's degree or higher increased for White children (from 22 to 44 percent), Black children (from 5 to 21 percent), and Hispanic children (from 7 to 15 percent). In 2006, some 67 percent of school-age children were living in two-parent households, representing a decrease since 1979, although this percentage has remained relatively stable since 1995. A larger percentage of school-age children were living in poor households in 2006 than in 1979 (17 vs. 15 percent), but both percentages were lower than the high of 21 percent in 1995 (*indicator 6*).
- Between 1979 and 2006, the number of school-age children (ages 5–17) who spoke a language other than English at home increased from 3.8 to 10.8 million, or from 9 to 20 percent of the population in this age range. Among these children, the percentage who spoke English with difficulty increased from 3 to 6 percent between 1979 and 2000, but this percentage did not change measurably between 2000 and 2006

(remained between 5 and 6 percent). In 2006, about 72 percent of the school-age children who spoke a language other than English at home spoke Spanish (*indicator 7*).

- Since the enactment of the Individuals with Disabilities Education Act (IDEA) in the mid-1970s, the number and percentage of children and youth ages 3–21 receiving special education services increased nearly every year until 2004–05. In 1976–77, some 3.7 million children and youth in this age group were served under IDEA (5 percent), and by 2006–07, some 6.7 million received services (about 9 percent). The percentage receiving special education services for a specific learning disability was 3 percentage points higher in 2006–07 than in 1976–77 (5 vs. 2 percent). In comparison, the prevalence of speech or language impairments remained fairly constant (*indicator 8*).
- Total undergraduate enrollment in degree- granting postsecondary institutions has generally increased since 1970 and is projected to reach 15.6 million students in 2008. From 1970 to 2006, women's undergraduate enrollment increased over three times as fast as men's, surpassing men's enrollment in 1978. Women are projected to make up 57 percent of undergraduate enrollment through 2017. In addition, over the next 10 years, full- time undergraduate enrollment is expected to continue to exceed part-time enrollment, and enrollment at 4-year institutions is expected to continue to surpass that at 2-year institutions (*indicator 9*).
- In 2006, three-quarters of 4-year college freshmen who had graduated from high school in the previous 12 months attended an in-state college. The percentage of such freshmen who attended an in-state college ranged from 28 percent in the District of Columbia and 40 percent in New Jersey to 89 percent in Louisiana and 90 percent in Utah. Many of the southern states had relatively high percentages of in-state college attendance among college freshmen who had graduated from high school in the previous 12 months: 8 southern states had more than 85 percent of such freshmen attending in-state colleges *(indicator 10*).
- Graduate and first-professional enroll ments in degree-granting institutions increased between 2000 and 2006. According to projections, increases in enrollment in both types of programs will continue, with graduate enrollment ex ceeding 2.6 million and first-professional enrollment reaching 418,000 by 2017. Over the past 30 years, female enrollment has increased by a larger percentage than male enrollment in both types of programs. Between 2000 and 2006, total minority enrollment increased by a larger percentage than did White enrollment (44 vs. 15 percent in graduate programs and 20 vs. 10 percent in first- professional programs) (*indicator 11*).

LEARNER OUTCOMES

How well does the American educational system—and its students—perform? Data from national and international assessments of students' academic achievement can help address this question, as can data on adults' educational and work experiences, literacy levels, and earnings. In some areas, such as mathematics and science, the performance of elementary and secondary students has shown some improvement over the past decade. However, such progress has not been seen on all assessments, in all grades assessed, or equally for all groups of students.

- Reading scores of 4th- and 8th-graders assessed by the National Assessment of Educational Progress (NAEP) were higher in 2007 than in 1992, by 4 and 3 points, respectively. The average reading score of 12th-graders, however, was 6 points lower in 2005 than in 1992. The percentage of 4th-graders performing at or above *Basic* was higher in 2007 than in 1992, as was the percentage at or above *Proficient*. The percentage of 8th-graders at or above *Basic* was higher in 2007 than in 1992, while there was no measurable difference in the percentage at or above *Proficient*. The percentage of 12th-graders at or above *Basic* was lower in 2005 than in 1992, as was the percentage at or above *Proficient* (*indicator 12*).
- Average NAEP mathematics scores increased 27 points for 4th-graders and 19 points for 8th-graders between 1990 and 2007. Increases in scores were seen by sex and across racial/ethnic groups. The percentages of 4th- and 8th-graders performing at or above *Basic*, at or above *Proficient*, and at *Advanced* were higher in 2007 than in all previous mathematics assessments. The percentage of4th-graders at or above *Proficient* tripled from 1990 to 2007 and increased by 3 percentage points from 2005 to 2007. At the 8th- grade level, the percentage doubled since 1990 and increased by 2 percentage points from the 2005 assessment (*indicator 13*).
- Reported on a scale of 0 to 300, average NAEP writing scores of 8th- and 12th-graders were higher in 2007 than in either 1998 or2002. The percentage of 8th-graders performing at or above *Basic* was higher in 2007 than in 1998, as was the percentage at or above *Proficient*. The percentage of 8th- graders at or above *Basic* was also higher in 2007 than in 2002, but no measurable difference was found in the percentage at or above *Proficient* between these two years. The percentage of 12th-graders at or above *Basic* increased from 2002 to 2007 and was also higher in 2007 than in 1998. For all assessment years, females at each grade level outscored males (*indicator 14*).
- In 2006, NAEP conducted its first assessment of economics, which evaluated 12th-graders' knowledge about markets, the national economy, and international trade. About 79 percent of 12th-graders performed at or above the *Basic* level on this assessment, and 42 percent performed at or above *Proficient*, including 3 percent at the *Advanced* level. Students who reported higher levels of parental education outperformed those who reported lower levels. For example, 54 percent of students whose parents were college graduates performed at or above *Proficient,* compared with 17 percent of students whose parents did not finish high school (*indicator 15*).
- NAEP reading and mathematics assessments indicate that the achievement gap between Whites and Blacks at the 4th-grade level was smaller in 2007 than in the early 1990s. On a 0 to 500 scale, the 4th-grade White-Black achievement gap in reading decreased from 32 points in 1992 to 27 points in 2007, while in mathematics it decreased from 32 points in 1990 to 26 points in 2007. At the 8th-grade level, however, the White- Black achievement gap in 2007 was not measurably different in reading from the gap in 1992 or in mathematics from the gap in 1990. For these same years, there also was no measurable difference in the achievement gap in mathematics between Whites and Hispanics at either grade level (*indicator 16*).

- NAEP long-term trend results indicate that the achievement of 9- and 13-yearolds in reading and mathematics improved between the early 1970s and 2004. In reading, 9-year-olds scored higher in 2004 than in previous assessments, with an increase of 7 points between 1999 and 2004. In mathematics, the achievement of 9- and 13-year-olds in 2004 was the highest of any assessment year. Though the overall performance of 17-year-olds on both NAEP assessments was not measurably different from their performance in prior years, scores for Black and Hispanic students improved from the early 1970s (*indicator 17*).
- According to the Progress in International Reading Literacy Study (PIRLS), which assessed the reading literacy of 4th-graders in 45 educational jurisdictions around the world, U.S. 4th-graders performed abovethe international average of these jurisdictions in 2006. Students in 10 jurisdictions scored higher than U.S. students, on average, and U.S. students scored higher, on average, than their peers in 22 jurisdictions. No differences were detected between the U.S. average scores in 2001 and 2006 on the combined reading literacy scale or on the two subscales, reading for literary purposes and reading for informational purposes (*indicator 18*).
- The 2006 Program for International StudentAssessment (PISA2006) reports on the scientific literacy of 15-year-olds in 57 educational jurisdictions, including the 30 member countries of the Organization for Economic Cooperation and Development (OECD) and 27 non-OECD countries and subnational education systems. According to the results of PISA 2006, the average U.S. scientific literacy score was 489, which was below the average of the 30 OECD countries (500). U.S. students had a lower average score than students in 16 OECD-member countries and a higher average score than students in 5 OECD countries (*indicator 19*).
- Full-time, full-year workers ages 25–34 with greater educational attainment earned higher salaries than those with less education in each year between 1995 and 2006. For example, young adults with a bachelor's degree as their highest degree consistently had higher median earnings than those with less education. This pattern held for male, female, White, Black, Hispanic, and Asian subgroups. In 2006, young adults with a bachelor's degree earned 28 percent more than those with an associate's degree, 50 percent more than those who had completed high school, and 98 percent more than those who did not earn a high school diploma (*indicator 20*).

Student Effort and Educational Progress

Many factors are associated with school success, persistence, and progress toward a high school diploma or a college or advanced degree. These include students' motivation and effort, learning experiences, and expectations for further education, as well as various family characteristics, such as parents' educational attainment and family income. Monitoring these factors and tracking educational attainment provide key indicators for describing the progress of students and schooling in the United States.

- Among public high school students in the class of 2004–05, about three-fourths graduated on time, based on an estimate of the incoming freshman class and the number of diplomas awarded 4 years later. Nebraska had the highest *averaged freshman graduation rate* in 2004–05, at 87.8 percent. Sixteen other states had graduation rates above 80 percent, and 10 other states and the District of Columbia had rates below 70 percent. The overall averaged freshman graduation rate increased from 71.7 percent in 2000–01 to 74.7 percent in 2004–05 (*indicator 21*).

- Between 1996–97 and 2005–06, the percentage of students with a disability exiting school with a regular high school diploma increased from 43 to 57 percent. About 94 percent of these students were ages 17–19. In addition, the percentage of students with disabilities exiting with a certificate of attendance increased from 9 to 15 percent, while the percentage who dropped out without a credential decreased from 46 to 26 percent. Among students with disabilities, the two groups with the highest percentages exiting with a regular high school diploma were those with visual impairments and those with hearing impairments (*indicator 22*).
- The *status dropout rate* represents the percentage of persons in an age group who are not enrolled in school and have not earned a high school diploma or equivalent credential, such as a General Educational Development (GED) certificate. Status dropout rates for Whites, Blacks, and Hispanics ages 16–24 have each generally declined between 1972 and2006. However, during this period, status dropout rates for Whites remained lower than rates for Hispanics and Blacks (*indicator 23*).
- The rate at which high school completers enrolled in college in the fall immediately after high school increased from 49 percent in 1972 to 67 percent in 1997. Since then, the rate has fluctuated between 62 and 69 percent. Though immediate college enrollment rates increased overall between 1972 and 2006 for both Whites and Blacks, there has been no overall change in the White-Black gap. For Hispanics, the rate has fluctuated over time but increased overall between 1972 and 2006. Nonetheless, the White-Hispanic gap has widened over this period. Since 1972, the immediate college enrollment rate for high school completers has increased faster for females than for males (*indicator 24*).
- Some 87 percent of 25- to 29-year-olds had received a high school diploma or equivalency certificate by 2007. This rate has remained between 85 and 88 percent over the last 30 years. The percentage of students in this age group who had completed at least some college education increased from 34 to 58 percent between 1971 and 2007, though increases were not consistent throughout this period. In most years during this period, the percentage completing a bachelor's degree or higher was roughly half that for completing at least some college. While the percentage of 25- to 29-year-olds with a bachelor's degree or higher increased for all three racial/ethnic groups, the gaps between Whites and their Black and Hispanic peers widened between 1971 and 2007 (*indicator 25*).
- Between 1995–96 and 2005–06, the number of associate's degrees earned by minority students grew at a faster rate than for White students and accounted for over 60 percent of the increase in the total number of associate's degrees awarded. While the number of bachelor's degrees earned by White students rose by 19 percent, the number of bachelor's degrees earned by minority students rose by 64 percent and accounted for 44 percent of the total increase during this period (*indicator 26*).
- Women have earned a larger number and percentage of bachelor's and master's degrees overall than men have since the early 1980s, but their share in various fields

has varied. For example, though women earned over 75 percent of bachelor's and master's degrees awarded in health professions, education, and psychology in 2005–06, they earned less than 30 percent of degrees awarded in computer and information sciences and in engineering at both levels. In addition, women have made gains at the doctoral level: in 2005–06, they earned 49 percent of doctoral degrees awarded (up from 40 percent in 1995–96), and during this period, the number of doctoral degrees earned by women increased by 54 percent (*indicator 27*).

CONTEXTS OF ELEMENTARY AND SECONDARY EDUCATION

The school environment is described by a number of features, including the characteristics of teachers and staff, student/teacher ratios, and the climate for learning. Monitoring these and other factors provides a fuller picture of the conditions in schools that can influence education. Society also influences and provides support for education through means including learning activities that take place outside school, as well as financial support for education.

- During the 2005–06 school year, 86 percent of public schools indicated that one or more incidents—including violent ones (serious violent incidents, physical attack or fight without a weapon, and threat of physical attack without a weapon), thefts of items over $10, and other incidents— had taken place at school. That year, 61 percent of public schools reported at least one incident to the police. Some 38 percent of public schools reported at least one violent incident, 13 percent reported at least one serious violent incident, 28 percent reported at least one theft, and 51 percent reported at least one of the other specified incidents. The percentage of schools experiencing at least one violent incident was lower in 2005–06 than in 2003–04, but was lowest in 1999–2000 (*indicator 28*).
- In 2005–06, larger percentages of Black, Hispanic, and American Indian/Alaska Native students attended high-poverty schools—defined as public schools with more than 75 percent of students eligible for free or reduced-price lunch—than did White or Asian/Pacific Islander students, and higher percentages of Asian/Pacific Islander than White students did so. Overall, a similar pattern was found among racial/ethnic groups within different school locales: in each locale (cities, suburban areas, towns, and rural areas), higher percentages of Black, Hispanic, and American Indian/Alaska Native students attended high-poverty schools than did their White and Asian/Pacific Islander peers (*indicator 29*).
- Public schools with high minority enrollments (defined as schools in which 75 percent or more of the students were Black, Hispanic, Asian/Pacific Islander, or American Indian/Alaska Native) enrolled 23 percent of all public elementary and secondary students in 2005–06. However, about half of all Hispanic and Black public school students attended such schools—larger percentages than Asian/ Pacific Islander, American Indian/Alaska Native, or White public school students at such schools. A larger percentage of public school students in schools with high minority

enrollments were found in cities than in suburban areas, towns, or rural areas (*indicator 30*).

- At the end of the 20 03–04 school year, 17 percent of the elementary and secondary teachers left the public and private schools where they had been teaching. Almost half of this teacher turnover was due to transferring to a different school: 8 percent did so. The remainder (9 percent of the teacher workforce) was due to teachers who left teaching to take a job in another field, pursue further education, leave for family reasons, retire, or leave for other reasons. In 2003–04, the turnover rate for high-poverty public schools (where 75 percent or more of their students were eligible for free or reduced-price lunch) was greater than for low-poverty public schools (where less than 15 percent of their students were eligible) (*indicator 31*).
- In 2003–04, public schools employed over 5.5 million staff: 2.8 million were employed by elementary schools, 950,000 by middle schools, and 1.4 million by secondary schools. Professional instructional staff— including principals, teachers, instructional coordinators and supervisors, librarians/ library media specialists, and school counselors—accounted for 64 percent of public school staff, with teachers making up the majority (57 percent) of all staff. Schools in rural areas generally had lower average numbers of students per staff member than did schools in other locales for most professional instructional and student services professional staff (*indicator 32*).
- The ratio of students to teachers, which is sometimes used as a proxy measure for class size, declined between 1990 and 2005 from 17.6 to 16.1 students per teacher for all regular public elementary, secondary, and combined schools. In every year during this period, the student/teacher ratios tended to be higher in public schools with larger enrollments than in public schools with smaller enrollments. For example, in 2005, regular secondary schools with 1,500 students or more enrolled 6.6 more students per teacher, on average, than regular secondary schools with enrollments under 300 (*indicator 33*).
- Total elementary and secondary public school revenues increased 55 percent in constant dollars from 1989–90 to 2004–05. Federal and state revenues increased at a faster rate than all local revenues (both property tax revenue and other local revenue). During this period, the percentage of total revenue for public elementary and secondary education from local sources declined (from 47 to 44 percent), while the proportion of total revenue flowing to public schools from federal sources increased (from 6 to 9 percent) and the proportion from state sources stayed the same (47 percent) (*indicator 34*).
- Between 1989–90 and 2004–05, total expenditures per student in public elementary and secondary schools rose 29 percent in constant 2006–07 dollars, from $8,437 to $10,892. Among the functions of current expenditures, spending on student and staff support increased the most (48 percent), followed by instruction (26 percent) and transportation (20 percent). Although the amount of current expenditures spent on salaries increased by 16 percent during this period, the percentage of current expenditures spent on salaries declined 4 percentage points, from 66 to 62 percent. The percentage spent on employee benefits increased almost 3 percentage points (*indicator 35*).

- Differences between states accounted for a greater percentage of the variation in instruction expenditures per student among unified public school districts than did differences within states from 1997–98 to 2004–05. The between-state differences increased during this period, while the within-state differences remained largely unchanged. In the 1997–98 school year, 57 percent of the variation in instruction expenditures per student was due to the between-state differences, and 43 percent was due to the within-state differences. In the 2004–05 school year, the corresponding percentages were 66 and 34 percent (*indicator 36*).
- In 2004–05, current expenditures per student, which include instructional, administrative, and operation and maintenance expenditures, were highest in high-poverty districts ($9,892), next highest in low-poverty districts ($9,263), and lowest in middle-poverty districts ($8,536). Between 1997–98 and 2004–05, current expenditures per student increased by 20 percent in constant 2006–07 dollars, from $7,602 to $9,094. Current expenditures per student increased the most for the high-poverty districts (26 percent) and the least for the middle-poverty districts (16 percent) (*indicator 37*).
- In 2004, U.S. expenditures per student at the combined elementary and secondary levelwere $9,368—higherthantheaverage of $6,604 for the member countries of the Organization for Economic Cooperation and Development (OECD) reporting data. At the postsecondary level, U.S. expenditures per student were $22,476, higher than the OECD average of $11,418 (*indicator 38*).

Contexts of Postsecondary Education

The postsecondary education system encompasses various types of institutions under public, private not-for-profit, and private for-profit control. Important indicators of this context include student fields of study; the price of attending college; the availability of financial aid; the instructional responsibilities of faculty and staff; and the ways in which colleges and universities attract and compensate faculty.

- Overall, 158,000 more associate's degrees were awarded in 2005–06 than in 1995–96 (a 28 percent increase). About 85 percent of this growth was attributable to the increases in the number of associate's degrees awarded in liberal arts and sciences, general studies, and humanities; health professions; business; and computer and information sciences. Overall 320,000 more bachelor's degrees were awarded in 2005–06 than in 1995–96 (a 28 percent increase). Degrees in the field of business made up 21 percent of degrees awarded at the bachelor's degree level in 2005–0 6, with over 318,000 bachelor's degrees awarded in business that year (*indicator 39*).
- Overall, 188,000 more master's degrees were awarded in 2005–06 than in 1995–96 (a 46 percent increase). Of the 594,000 master's degrees awarded in 2005–06, over 50 percent were in the fields of education (29 percent) and business (25 percent). Overall, 11,400 more doctoral degrees were awarded in 2005–06 than in 1995–96 (a 26 percent increase). Of the 56,000 doctoral degrees awarded in 2005–06, some 13 to 14 percent each were in the fields of education, engineering, and health professions.

The number of first- professional degrees awarded increased by 11,000 (a 14 percent increase) between 1995–9 6 and 2005–06. The increase in the number of degrees awarded in pharmacy (264 percent) accounted for 62 percent of this overall growth (*indicator 40*).

- Although the number of degrees conferred by public and private institutions increased between 1995–9 6 and 2005–06, the percentage increase varied among types of institutions. During this period, the number of associate's, bachelor's, master's, and doctoral degrees conferred by private for-profit institutions increased by a larger percentage than did the number conferred by private not-for-profit and public institutions. Despite relatively large percentage increases in the number of degrees conferred by private for-profit institutions, the number of degrees awarded remained substantially lower than at public or private not-for-profit institutions, with the exception of associate's degrees (*indicator 41*).
- Average inflation-adjusted salaries for full-time instructional faculty in colleges and universities increased by 20 percent overall between 1979–80 and 2006–07. The average salary increased at all types of institutions as well, ranging from 8 percent at public 2-year colleges to 37 percent at private doctoral universities. However, after increasing during the 1980s and 1990s, recent increases in faculty salaries have been relatively small (1 percent between 1999–2000 and 200 6–07). The percentage of faculty compensation received in the form of benefits rose from 16 percent in 1979–80 to 21 percent in 2006–07 (*indicator 42*).
- The percentage of full-time college students ages 16–24 who were employed increased from 34 to 52 percent between 1970 and 2000 and fluctuated between 46 and 49 percent after that. In addition, the number of hours these students worked per week has increased since 1970. In contrast to the increase among full-time college students, there was no measurable change between 1970 and 2006 in the percentage of part-time college students who were employed. In 2006, approximately 81 percent of part-time college students were employed, but these students worked fewer hours in 2006 than they did in 1970 (*indicator 43*).

CONCLUSION

Over the long-term, there has been improvement in the scores of 9- and 13-year-olds on national reading and mathematics assessments since the early 1970s, but the scores of 17-yearolds have remained flat. In the short-term, progress on national assessments in reading and mathematics has been made among 4th- and 8th-graders since the early 1990s, but reading scores for 12th-graders have declined. In other subject areas, such as writing, scores for 8th- and 12th-graders have improved. However, significant achievement gaps among racial/ethnic groups remain. International assessments show that U.S. students are in the top third of 4th- graders in reading, but below the international averages in science and mathematics at age 15. Other measures of progress show an increase in the high school graduation rate since 2000 and a decline in the status dropout rate.

The U.S. education system also shows signs of continued growth for years to come. In elementary and secondary education, enrollments have followed population shifts and are projected to increase each year through 2017 to an all-time high of 54 million, with the South expected to experience the largest increase in enrollments. Rates of enrollment in degree-granting postsecondary education at both the undergraduate and graduate levels have increased and are projected to continue to do so throughout the next 10 years. The number of school-age children who spoke a language other than English at home more than doubled between 1979 and 2006, and the number and percentage of children receiving special education services in our elementary and secondary schools have increased nearly every year up until 2004–05.

NCES produces an array of reports each year that present findings about the U.S. education system. *The Condition of Education 2008* is the culmination of a yearlong project. It includes data that were available by early April 2008. In the coming months, other reports and surveys informing the nation about education will be released. Along with the indicators in this volume, NCES intends these surveys and reports to help inform policymakers and the American public about trends and conditions in U.S. education.

Mark Schneider
Commissioner
National Center for Education Statistics

In: The Condition of Education in America
Editor: Maurice H. Logan
ISBN: 978-1-60692-298-9

READER'S GUIDE

The Condition of Education is available in two forms: this print volume for 2008 and a Web version on the National Center for Education Statistics (NCES) website (http://nces.ed.gov/ programs/coe). The Web version includes the following: the 2008 Commissioner's statement, a user's guide, special analyses from 2000 through 2007, all indicators from this edition, and selected indicators from earlier editions of *The Condition of Education*. (See page xxiv for a list of all the indicators that appear on *The Condition of Education* website.)

The print volume of *The Condition of Education 2008* includes five sections of indicators. Each section begins with a summary of the general topic areas covered by the indicators in the section. Each indicator contains a discussion along with a graph or table on the main indicator page(s), and one or more supplemental tables found in *appendix 1*. The supplemental tables feature the estimates used in the indicator discussion as well as additional estimates related to the indicator. Where applicable, tables of standard errors for estimate tables are available on the Web (http:// nces.ed.gov/programs/coe). Additional information on data sources, analyses conducted, and definitions of variables and measures can be found in the supplemental notes in *appendix 2*. Finally, a glossary of key terms, bibliography, and index are provided at the end of the volume.

The "eye" icon on the main indicator page is located to the side of the graph or table and provides references for supplemental notes, supplemental tables, or other sources for more information relating to the indicator.

Indicators use the most recent national data available from either NCES or other sources serving the purposes of the indicator. When the source is an NCES publication, such as the *Digest of Education Statistics, 2007* (NCES 200 8-022), the publication can be viewed at the NCES website (http://nces.ed.gov/pubsearch).

DATA SOURCES AND ESTIMATES

The data in this report were obtained from many different sources, including state education agencies, local schools, and colleges and universities using surveys and compilations of administrative records. Users of *The Condition of Education* should be cautious when comparing data from different sources. Differences in procedures, timing, question phrasing, interviewer training, and so forth can all affect the comparability of results across data sources.

Most indicators in *The Condition of Education* summarize data from surveys conducted by NCES or by the Census Bureau with support from NCES. Brief explanations of the major NCES surveys used in this edition of *The Condition of Educatio*n can be found in *supplemental notes 3* and *4* of this volume. More detailed explanations can be obtained at the NCES website (http://nces.ed.gov) under "Surveys and Programs." Information about the Current Population Survey (CPS), another frequent source of survey data used in *The Condition of Education*, can be obtained in *supplemental note 2* as well as at http://www.census.gov/cps/.

Data for indicators reported in this volume are obtained primarily from two types of surveys: universe surveys and sample surveys. Some indicators report data taken from entire populations (universe surveys), such as *indicator 37* (Public Elementary and Secondary Expenditures by District Poverty). With this type of survey, information is collected from every member of the population. For example, data for *indicator 37* were obtained for each school district (approximately 17,000) in the United States. When data from an entire population are available, estimates of the total population or a subpopulation are made by simply summing the units in the population or subpopulation. A universe survey is usually expensive and time consuming, so researchers often opt to collect data from a sample of the population of interest (sample survey). Other indicators report data from such sample surveys, such as *indicator 16* (Trends in the Achievement Gaps in Reading and Mathematics). *Indicator 16* reports information from the National Assessment of Educational Progress (NAEP), which assesses a representative sample of students each year, rather than the entire population of students. When a sample survey is used, the statistical uncertainty introduced from having data from only a portion of the entire population must be considered in reporting estimates and making comparisons.

Various types of estimates are reported in *The Condition of Education* using universe and sample surveys. Many indicators report the size of a population or a subpopulation, and often the size of a subpopulation is expressed as a percentage of the total population. In addition, the average (or *mean*) values of some characteristic of the population or subpopulation may be reported. The average is obtained by summing the values for all members of the population and dividing the sum by the size of the population. An example is the annual average salaries of full-time instructional faculty at degree-granting institutions (*indicator 42*). Another population measure that is sometimes used is the *median*. The median is the value of a population characteristic at or above which 50 percent of the population is estimated to fall and at or below which 50 percent of the population is estimated to fall. An example is the median annual earnings of young adults who are full-time, full-year wage and salary workers (*indicator 20*).

Estimates based on universe and sample survey data may be affected by a wide range of potential data collection errors, such as coverage errors, response errors, data coding errors, and data entry errors. Estimates of the size of these types of errors are typically not available.

Using estimates calculated from data based on a sample of the population requires consideration of several factors before the estimates become meaningful. However conscientious an organization may be in collecting data from a sample of a population, some margin of error will always be present in estimations of the size of the actual total population or subpopulation because the data are available from only a portion of the total population.

Consequently, data from samples can provide only an approximation of the true or actual value. The margin of error, or the range, of an estimate depends on several factors, such as the amount of variation in the responses, the size and representativeness of the sample, and the size of the subgroup for which the estimate is computed. The magnitude of this margin of error is measured by what statisticians call the "standard error" of an estimate.

STANDARD ERRORS

When data from samples are reported, as is the case with most of the indicators in *The Condition of Education*, the standard error is calculated for each estimate. The standard errors for all estimated totals, means, medians, or percentages reported in the supplemental tables of *The Condition of Education* can be viewed at the NCES website (http://nces.ed.gov/programs/coe).

The standard errors of the estimates for different subpopulations in an indicator can vary considerably. As an illustration, *indicator 19* reports on the average combined science literacy scores of 15-year-old students in 2006. In Australia, the average combined science literacy scores of male and female students were each 527 (see supplemental table 19-2). In contrast to the similarity of these scores, the standard errors for these estimates were 3.2 and 2.7, respectively (see table S 19-2 at http://nces.ed.gov/programs/coe/2008/section2/table.asp?tableID=971). The average score with the smaller standard error provides a more reliable approximation of the true value than does the average score with a higher standard error. In addition, standard errors tend to diminish in size as the size of the sample (or subsample) increases. Consequently, for the same kinds of data, such as reading, mathematics, writing, and economics scores on the National Assessment of Educational Progress (*indicators 12, 13, 14, 15,* and *16*), standard errors will almost always be larger for Blacks and Hispanics than for Whites, who represent a larger proportion of the population.

For *indicator 20*, which reports median annual earnings, special procedures are followed for computing the standard errors for these medians. See *appendix G* of the source and accuracy statement for the Current Population Study (CPS) 2006 Annual Social and Economic supplement (ASEC) for information on how to calculate the standard errors (http://www. census.gov/apsd/techdoc/cps/cpsmar06.pdf).

DATA ANALYSIS AND INTERPRETATION

Due to standard errors, caution is warranted when drawing conclusions about the size of one population estimate in comparison to another or about whether a time series of population estimates is increasing, decreasing, or staying about the same. Although one estimate may be larger than another, a statistical test may find that there is no measurable difference between the two estimates because of a large standard error associated with one or both of the estimates. Whether differences in means or percentages are statistically significant can be determined using the standard errors of the estimates.

Readers who wish to compare two sample estimates to see if there is a statistical difference will need to estimate the precision of the difference between the two sample estimates. This would be necessary if one wanted to compare, for example, the mean proficiency scores between groups assessed in the National Assessment of Educational Progress. To estimate the precision of the difference between two sample estimates, one must find the standard error of the difference between the two sample estimates (sample estimate A, or E_A, and sample estimate B, or E_B). Expressed mathematically, the difference between the two estimates E_A and E_B is $E_A – E_B$.

The standard error of the difference (or $seA–B$) can be calculated by taking the square root of the sum of the two standard errors associated with each of the two sample estimates (se_A and se_B) after each has been squared. This relationship can be expressed as

$$se_{A-B} = \sqrt{se_A^2 + se_B^2}$$

After finding the standard error of the difference, one divides the difference between the two sample estimates by this standard error to determine the "t value," or "t statistic," of the difference between the two estimates. This t statistic measures the precision of the difference between two independent sample estimates. The formula for calculating this ratio is expressed mathematically as

$$t = \frac{E_A - E_B}{se_{A-B}}$$

The next step is to compare this t statistic to 1.96, the statistically determined value for making a decision at a 95 percent confidence level as to whether there is a difference between two estimates. If the t statistic is greater than 1.96, then there is evidence that a difference exists between the two populations because this means that if a test is conducted 100 times, only 5 times out of 100 would it be expected that the difference between the two sample estimates (E_A and E_B) is due to chance alone. If the t statistic is equal to or less than 1.96, then there is less certainty that the observed difference is a real difference, it may be simply due to sampling error. This level of certitude, or significance, is commonly referred to as the ".05 level of (statistical) significance."

As an example of a comparison between two sample estimates to determine whether there is a statistically significant difference between the two, consider the data on the performance of 12th-grade students in the reading assessment of the 1992 and 2005 National Assessment of Educational Progress (see supplemental table 12-1). The average scale score in 1992 was 292, and the average scale score in 2005 was 286. Is the difference of 6 scale points between these two different samples statistically significant? The standard errors of these estimates are 0.6 and 0.6, respectively (see table S12-1 at http://nces.ed.gov/programs/coe/2008/section2/table. asp?tableID=953). Using the formula above, the standard error of the difference is 0.85. The t statistic of the estimated difference of 6 scale points to the standard error of the difference is 7.07. This value is greater than 1.96—the critical value of the t

distribution for a .05 level of significance with a large sample. Thus, one can conclude that there was a statistically significant difference in the performance of 12th-graders between 1992 and 2005 in reading and that the reading score for 12th-graders in 2005 was lower than the reading score for 12th-graders in 1992.

For all indicators reporting estimates based on samples in *The Condition of Education*, differences between estimates (including increases or decreases) are stated only when they are statistically significant. To determine whether differences reported are statistically significant, two-tailed t tests, at the 0.05 level, are typically used. The t test formula for determining statistical significance is adjusted when the samples being compared are dependent. When the difference between estimates is not statistically significant, tests of equivalence are often conducted. An equivalence test determines the probability (generally at the 0.15 level) that the estimates are statistically equivalent, that is, within the margin of error that the two estimates are not substantively different. When the difference is found to be equivalent, language such as "x" and "y" "were similar" or "about the same" has been used; otherwise, the data will be described as having "no measurable difference."

When the variables to be tested are postulated to form a trend, the relationship may be tested using linear regression, logistic regression, or ANOVA trend analysis instead of a series of t tests. These other methods of analysis test for specific relationships (e.g., linear, quadratic, or cubic) among variables.

A number of considerations influence the ultimate selection of data years to feature in *The Condition of Education*. To make analyses as timely as possible, the latest year of data is shown if available during report production. The choice of comparison years is also based on the need to show the earliest available survey year, as in the case of the National Assessment of Educational Progress and the international assessment surveys. In the case of surveys with long time frames, such as for enrollment, the decade's beginning year (e.g., 1980 or 1990) starts the trend line. Intervening years are selected in increments to show the general trend in the figures and tables. The narrative for the indicators typically compares the most current year's data with those from the initial year and then with those from a more recent period. The narrative may also note years in which the data begin to diverge from previous trends where applicable.

Variations in Populations

In considering the estimates in the tables and figures shown in this volume and on the NCES website, it is important to keep in mind that there may be considerable variation among the members of a population in the characteristic or variable represented by the population estimate. For example, the estimated average combined reading literacy score of 4th-graders in the United States in 2006 was 540 (see supplemental table 18-1). In reality, many U.S. students scored above 540 points, and many scored below 540 points. Likewise, not all faculty salaries, benefits, and total compensation at postsecondary institutions were the same at each type of institution in 2006–07 (*indicator 42*). Because of this variation, there may be considerable overlap among the members of two populations that are being compared. Although the difference in the estimated means of the two populations may be statistically significant, many members of the population with the lower estimated mean may be above the estimated mean of the other population, and vice versa. For example, some percentage of young adults with a high school diploma or equivalent have higher earnings than young adults with a bachelor's degree or higher (*indicator 20*). The extent of such overlap is not generally considered in the indicators in this volume. Estimates of the extent of variation in such population characteristics can be computed from the NCES survey datasets or are available in published reports. For example, estimates of the variation in students' assessment scores can be found using the NAEP Data Explorer at http://nces.ed.gov/nationsreportcard/nde/ or in the appendixes to most NAEP reports.

ROUNDING AND OTHER CONSIDERATIONS

All calculations within *The Condition of Education* are based on unrounded estimates. Therefore, the reader may find that a calculation, such as a difference or a percentage change, cited in the text or figure may not be identical to the calculation obtained by using the rounded values shown in the accompanying tables. Although values reported in the supplemental tables are generally rounded to one decimal place (e.g., 76.5 percent), values reported in each indicator are generally rounded to whole numbers (with any value of 0.50 or above rounded to the next highest whole number). Due to rounding, cumulative percentages may sometimes equal 99 or 101 percent, rather than 100 percent.

Indicators in this volume that use the Current Price Index (CPI) use a base academic year of 2006–07 and a base calendar year of 2006 for constant dollar calculations.

In accordance with the NCES Statistical Standards, many tables in this volume use a series of symbols to alert the reader to special statistical notes. These symbols, and their meanings, are as follows:

— Not available. Data were not collected or not reported.
† Not applicable. Category does not exist.
# Rounds to zero. The estimate rounds to zero.
! Interpret data with caution. Estimates are unstable.
‡ Reporting standards not met. Did not meet reporting standards.
* $p < .05$ Significance level.[1]

[1] This level of signifi cance means that the chance is less than 5 out of 100 that a difference was found between two estimates when no real difference exists.

In: The Condition of Education in America
Editor: Maurice H. Logan
ISBN: 978-1-60692-298-9

LIST OF INDICATORS ON THE CONDITION OF EDUCATION WEBSITE (2000–2008)

This List of Indicators includes all the indicators that appear on *The Condition of Education* website (http://nces.ed.gov/programs/coe), drawn from the 2000–2008 print vol umes. The list is organized first by section and then by subject area. Thus, the indicator num bers and the years in which the indicators were published are not sequential.

Special Analyses	Indicator–Year
Entering Kindergarten: A Portrait of American Children When They Begin School	2000
Students Whose Parents Did Not Go to College: Postsecondary Access, Persistence, and Attainment	2001
Private Schools: A Brief Portrait	2002
Nontraditional Undergraduates	2002
Reading—Young Children's Achievement and Classroom Experiences	2003
Paying for College: Changes Between 1990 and 2000 for Full-Time Dependent Undergraduates	2004
Mobility in the Teacher Workforce	2005
U.S. Student and Adult Performance on International Assessments of Educational Achievement	2006
High School Coursetaking	2007
Community Colleges	Summer 2008
Section 1—Participation in Education	
Al Ages Enrollment Trends by Age	1–2008
Preprimary Education Early Education and Child Care Arrangements of Young Children	2–2008
Elementary/Secondary Education	
Trends in Full- and Half-Day Kindergarten	3–2004
Past and Projected Public School Enrollments	3–2008
Trends in Private School Enrollments	4–2008
Homeschooled Students	3–2005
Racial/Ethnic Distribution of Public School Students	5–2008
Family Characteristics of 5- to 17-Year-Olds	6–2008
Language Minority School-Age Children	7–2008
Children and Youth With Disabilities in Public Schools	8–2008
Undergraduate Education	
Past and Projected Undergraduate Enrollments	9–2008
Mobility of College Students	10–2008

Continued.

Special Analyses	Indicator–Year
Postsecondary Persistence and Progress	
Remediation and Degree Completion	18–2004
Transfers From Community Colleges to 4-Year Institutions	19–2003
Institutional Retention and Student Persistence at 4-Year Institutions	20–2003
Trends in Undergraduate Persistence and Completion	19–2004
Postsecondary Participation and Attainment Among Traditional-Age Students	22–2005
Completions	
Educational Attainment	25–2008
Degrees Earned	26–2008
Degrees Earned by Women	27–2008
Time to Bachelor's Degree Completion	21–2003
Postsecondary Attainment of 1988 8th-Graders	22–2003
Advanced Degree Completion Among Bachelor's Degree Recipients	32–2006
Persistence and Attainment of Students With Pell Grants	23–2003
Section 4—Contexts of Elementary and Secondary Education *School Characteristics and Climate*	
Size of High Schools	30–2003
Student Perceptions of Their School's Social and Learning Environment	29–2005
Parents' Attitudes Toward Schools	38–2006
Rates of School Crime	36–2007
School Violence and Safety	28–2008
Poverty Concentration in Public Schools by Locale and Race/Ethnicity	29–2008
Concentration of Public School Enrollment by Locale and Race/Ethnicity	30–2008
Teachers and Staff	
Characteristics of School Principals	34–2007
Characteristics of Full-Time School Teachers	33–2007
Beginning Teachers	29–2003
Elementary/Secondary School Teaching Among Recent College Graduates	37–2006
Teacher Turnover	31–2008
Public School Staff	32–2008
Student Support Staff in Public Schools	35–2007
High School Guidance Counseling	27–2004
Learning Opportunities	
Early Development of Children	35–2005
Early Literacy Activities	33–2006
Care Arrangements for Children After School	33–2004
Afterschool Activities	29–2007
Availability of Advanced Courses in High Schools	25–2005
Student/Teacher Ratios in Public Elementary and Secondary Schools	33–2008
Out-of-Field Teaching in Middle and High School Grades	28–2003
Out-of-Field Teaching by Poverty Concentration and Minority Enrollment	24–2004
Special Programs	
Public Alternative Schools for At-Risk Students	27–2003
Inclusion of Students With Disabilities in General Classrooms	31–2007
School Choice	
Charter Schools	32–2007
Parental Choice of Schools	36–2006
Profile and Demographic Characteristics of Public Charter Schools	28–2005
Finance	Indicator–Year
Changes in Sources of Public School Revenue	34–2008
Public Elementary and Secondary Expenditures by Type and Function	35–2008
Variations in Instruction Expenditures per Student	36–2008
Public Elementary and Secondary Expenditures by District Poverty	37–2008
Public Elementary and Secondary Expenditures by District Location	35–2004
Public Effort to Fund Elementary and Secondary Education	39–2005
International Comparisons of Expenditures for Education	38–2008

Continued.

Special Analyses	Indicator–Year
Section 5—Contexts of Postsecondary Education	
Characteristics of Postsecondary Students	
Minority Student Enrollments	3 1–2005
Programs and Courses	
Undergraduate Fields of Study	39–2008
Graduate Fields of Study	40–2008
Degrees Conferred by Public and Private Institutions	41 –2008
Top 30 Postsecondary Courses	30–2004
International Comparisons of Degrees by Field	43–2007
Learning Opportunities	
Remedial Coursetaking	3 1–2004
Instructional Faculty and Staff Who Teach Undergraduates	46–2006
Distance Education by Postsecondary Faculty	47–2006
Distance Education at Postsecondary Institutions	32–2004
Special Programs	
Services and Accommodations for Students With Disabilities	34–2003
Faculty and Staff	
Faculty Salary, Benefits, and Total Compensation	42–2008
Colege Resources	
Electronic Services in Academic Libraries	33–2005
State Policy	
State Transfer and Articulation Policies	34–2005
Finance	
Institutional Aid at 4-Year Colleges and Universities	37–2004
Total and Net Access Price of Attending a Postsecondary Institution	47–2007
Total and Net Access Price for Graduate and First-Professional Students	48–2007
Debt Burden of College Graduates	38–2004
Employment of College Students	43–2008
Federal Grants and Loans to Undergraduate Students	46–2007
Public Effort to Fund Postsecondary Education	40–2005

SECTION 1. PARTICIPATION IN EDUCATION

In: The Condition of Education in America
Editor: Maurice H. Logan
ISBN: 978-1-60692-298-9

Chapter 1

INTRODUCTION

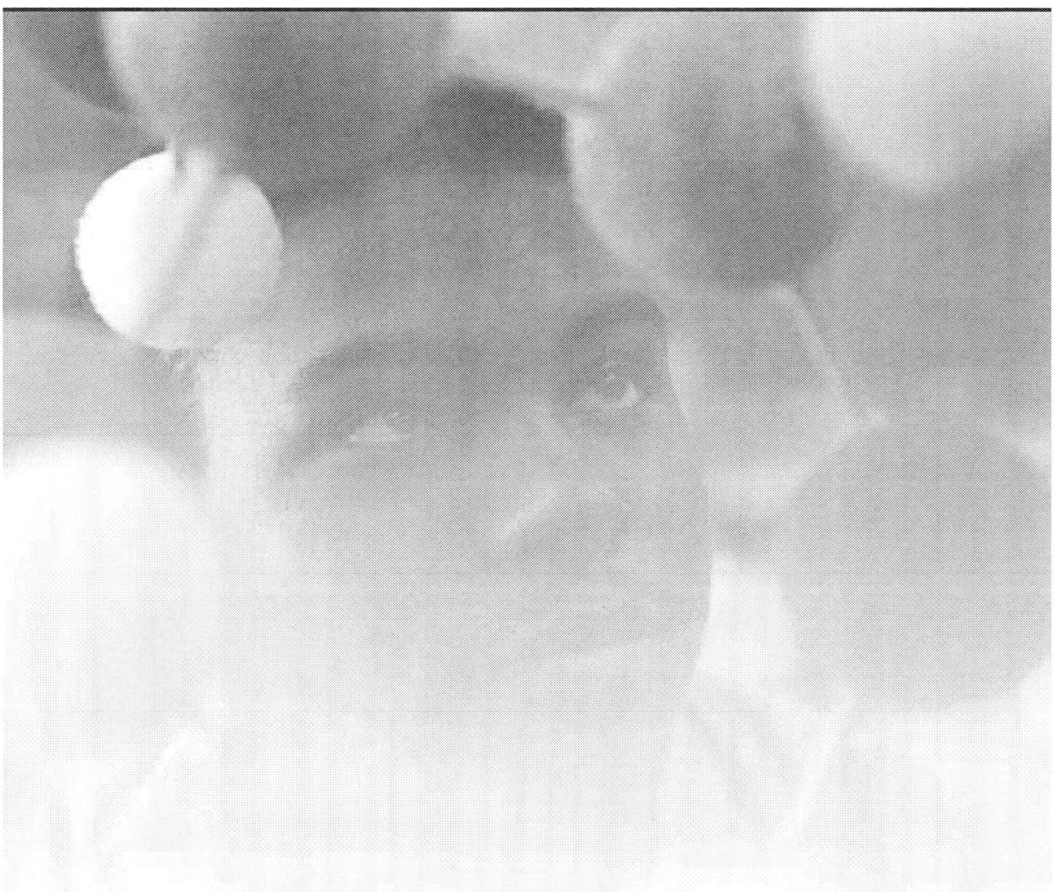

The indicators in this section of *The Condition of Education* report trends in enrollments across all levels of education. There are 14 indicators in this section: 11, prepared for this year's volume, appear on the following pages, and all 14, including indicators from previous years, appear on the Web (see Website Contents on the facing page for a full list of the indicators). Enrollment is a key indicator of the scope of and access to educational opportunities and is a basic descriptor of American education. Changes in enrollment have implications for the demand for educational resources, such as qualified teachers, physical facilities, and funding levels, which are required to provide a high- quality education for our nation's students.

	Indicator–Year
All Ages	
Enrollment Trends by Age	1–2008
Preprimary Education	
Early Education and Child Care Arrangements of Young Children	2–2008
Elementary/Secondary Education	
Trends in Full- and Half-Day Kindergarten	
Past and Projected Public School Enrollments	
Trends in Private School Enrollments	3–2004
Homeschooled Students	3–2008
Racial/Ethnic Distribution of Public School Students	4–2008
Family Characteristics of 5- to 17-Year-Olds	3–2005
Language Minority School-Age Children	5–2008
Children and Youth With Disabilities in Public Schools	6–2008
Undergraduate Education	
Past and Projected Undergraduate Enrollments	9–2008
Mobility of College Students	10–2008
Graduate and Professional Education	
Trends in Graduate and First-Professional Enrollments	11–2008
Adult Learning	
Participation in Adult Education	10–2007

The indicators in this section are organized into an overview subsection, which is made up of an indicator on enrollment rates reported by age group, and a series of subsections organized by level of the education system. These levels are preprimary education, elementary and secondary education, undergraduate education, graduate and professional education, and adult education.

The indicator in the first subsection compares rates of enrollment in formal education programs across age groups in the population. Looking at trends in the enrollment rates of individuals provides a perspective on the education of the U.S. population at different points in the life cycle and over time.

Participation in center-based early childhood care and education programs, such as Head Start, nursery school, and prekindergarten, helps to prepare children for elementary school or serves as child care for parents. Elementary and secondary education provides knowledge and skills that prepare students for further learning and productive membership in society. Because enrollment at the elementary and secondary levels is mandatory in most states until at least age 16, and in a number of states until age 17 or 18, changes in enrollment are driven primarily by shifts in the size and composition of the school-age population, as well as by shifts in the type of schools students attend, for example, between public schools, private schools, and homeschooling. Postsecondary education offers students opportunities to gain advanced knowledge and skills either immediately after high school or later in life. Because postsecondary education is voluntary, changes in total undergraduate enrollments reflect fluctuations in enrollment rates and the perceived availability and value of postsecondary education, as well as the size of college-age populations. Graduate and professional enrollments form an important segment of postsecondary education, allowing students to pursue advanced coursework in a variety of areas. Adult education includes formal education activities in which adults participate to upgrade their work skills, to change careers, or to expand personal interests.

Some of the indicators in the subsections provide information about the characteristics of the students who are enrolled and, in some cases, how these students are distributed across schools. For example, one indicator in this volume describes the number and prevalence of children with disabilities, and a second shows the distributions of select family characteristics of 5- to 17-year-olds.

The indicators on participation in education from previous editions of *The Condition of Education*, which are not included in this volume, are available at http://nces.ed.gov/programs/coe/list/index.asp.

In: The Condition of Education in America
Editor: Maurice H. Logan

ISBN: 978-1-60692-298-9

Chapter 2

ALL AGES

ENROLLMENT TRENDS BY AGE

Between 1970 and 2006, children ages 3–4 saw the largest increase in enrollment rates. There was also notable growth in enrollment rates for those ages 18–19 and 20–24, the period when individuals are typically enrolled in postsecondary education.

Changes in enrollment patterns may reflect changes in attendance requirements, the perceived value or cost of education, as well as the time taken to complete degrees. Between 1970 and 2006, the enrollment rate of children ages 3–4 (typically nursery school ages) increased from 20 to 56 percent. This rate is up from 52 percent of students in this age group 5 years earlier in 2001. Some of this increase may reflect changes in the data collection method in 1994;[2] however, the rate of nursery school attendance had already doubled before that year (see supplemental table 1-1). The enrollment rate of children ages 5–6 (typically kindergarten[3] or 1st-grade ages) increased from 90 percent in 1970 to 96 percent in 1976 and has since remained roughly stable.

The enrollment rate for youth ages 7–13 has remained high over the past 35 years (between 98 and 99 percent), reflecting state school attendance requirements. The maximum compulsory age of school attendance varies by state between ages 16 and 18; this fact may account for the lower enrollment rates for youth ages 14–17 (between 93 and 97 percent) compared with those for youth ages 7–13 (Education Commission of the States 2006).

No measurable differences have been found in the enrollment rates for these age groups since 2001.

Youth ages 18–19 are typically transitioning into postsecondary education or the workforce. Between 1970 and 2006, the enrollment rates for these youth increased at the elementary/ secondary level (from 10 to 19 percent) and at the postsecondary level (from 37 to 46 percent), raising the overall enrollment rate of those ages 18–19 from 48 to 65 percent. This overall rate is up from 61 percent of students in this age group 5 years earlier in 2001.

---

[2] Beginning in 1994, new procedures were used to collect preprimary enrollment data. As a result, pre-1994 data may not be comparable to data from 1994 or later.

[3] As of April 2005, of the 50 states and the District of Columbia, there were 36 states or jurisdictions that did not require kindergarten attendance; however, most mandate that school districts offer kindergarten programs (Education Commission of the States 2005).

Adults ages 20–34 who are enrolled in school are usually enrolled in postsecondary education. Between 1970 and 2006, the enrollment rate of young adults ages 20–21 increased from 32 to 48 percent, and the rate of those ages 22–24 increased from 15 to 27 percent. Among older adults, the enrollment rate increased from 8 to 12 percent for those ages 25–29 during this period, and from 4 percent in 1970 to 7 percent in 2006 for those ages 30–34. Despite this pattern of increase from 1970 to 2006, there was no measurable change in the enrollment rates for those ages 20–34 between 2001 and 2006.

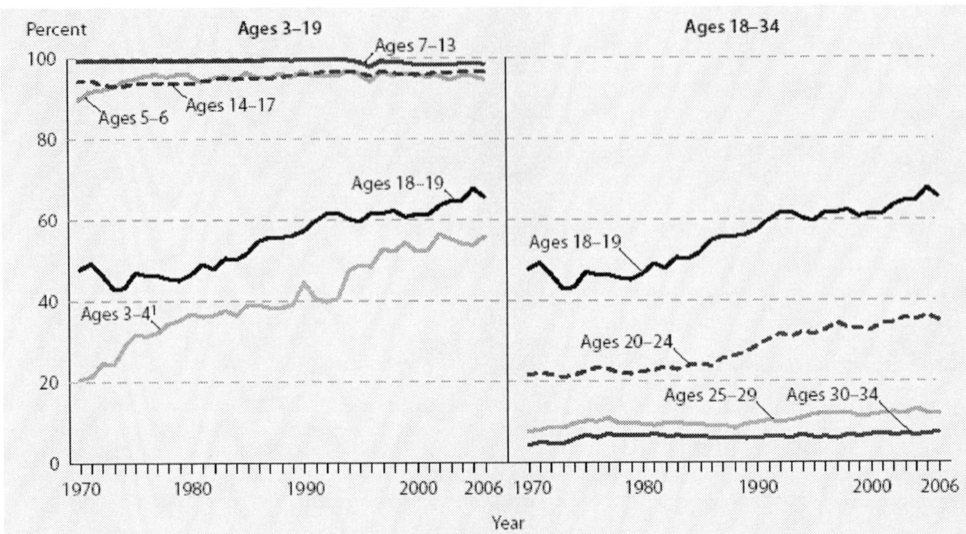

NOTE: Includes enrollment in any type of graded public, parochial, or other private schools. Includes nursery schools, kindergartens, elementary schools, high schools, colleges, universities, and professional schools. Attendance may be on either a full-time or part-time basis and during the day or night. Excludes homeschooled students and enrollments in less-than-2-year postsecondary institutions and enrollments in "special" schools, such as trade schools, business colleges, or correspondence schools. The age breakouts used in this indicator reflect the different schooling stages that are typical for students given their age. For example, students at ages 18–19 are typically transitioning from elementary/secondary education into postsecondary education or the workforce. See *supplemental note 2* for more information on the Current Population Survey (CPS).

Source: U.S. Department of Education, National Center for Education Statistics, *Digest of Education Statistics, 2007* (NCES 2008-022), table 7, data from U.S. Department of Commerce, Census Bureau, Current Population Survey (CPS), October, 1970–2006.

NT RATES: Percentage of the population ages 3–34 enrolled in school, by age group: October 1970–2006.

In: The Condition of Education in America
Editor: Maurice H. Logan
ISBN: 978-1-60692-298-9

Chapter 3

Preprimary Education

Early Education and Child Care Arrangements of Young Children

A greater percentage of 4-year-olds from the 2001 birth cohort were in a center-based setting (including Head Start) as their primary type of early education and care (57 percent) than in other arrangements.

The Early Childhood Longitudinal Study, Birth Cohort of 2001 (ECLS-B) has followed a nationally representative cohort of children from birth through preschool age. This indicator presents findings on these children's early education and child care arrangements in 2005–06, when most of the children were about 4 years old.[4]

A greater percentage of 4-year-olds from the 2001 birth cohort were in a center-based setting (including Head Start) as their primary type of early education and care (57 percent) than in other arrangements such as home-based relative care[5] (13 percent), home-based nonrelative care (8 percent), or multiple arrangements (2 percent) (see supplemental table 2-1). The overall percentage of children in center-based settings includes children in Head Start (13 percent) as well as those in other center-based settings (45 percent). Twenty percent of children had no nonparental care and education arrangements.

Differences in the percentage of children who were in a center-based setting as their primary type of early education and care were observed by race/ethnicity. A smaller percentage of Pacific Islander children (20 percent) and Hispanic children (49 percent) were in a center-based setting as their primary type of early education and care than their White, Black, Asian, or American Indian/Alaska Native peers (60 to 62 percent).

Racial and ethnic differences in the use of Head Start as the primary type of early education and child care were observed. A larger percentage of Black children (25 percent) and American Indian children (31 percent) were in Head Start as their primary type of early education and care than their White (7 percent) and Asian peers (5 percent).

---

[4] Findings are based on all children who participated in the ECLS-B. Although most of the children in the sample were about 4 years old during the 2005–06 interview (74.6 percent were between 48 and 57.9 months), some 16 percent were younger than 4 years old (between 44 and 48 months), and 9 percent were between 58 and 65 months. Findings are representative of the approximately 4 million children born in the United States in 2001.

[5] Care provided in the child's home or in another private home by a relative (excluding parents).

The percentage of children who were in a center-based setting increased as parents' highest level of education increased. For example, 43 percent of children about 4 years old whose parents' highest level of education was less than high school were enrolled in a center-based setting, compared with 71 percent of their peers whose parents' highest level of education was any graduate or professional school.

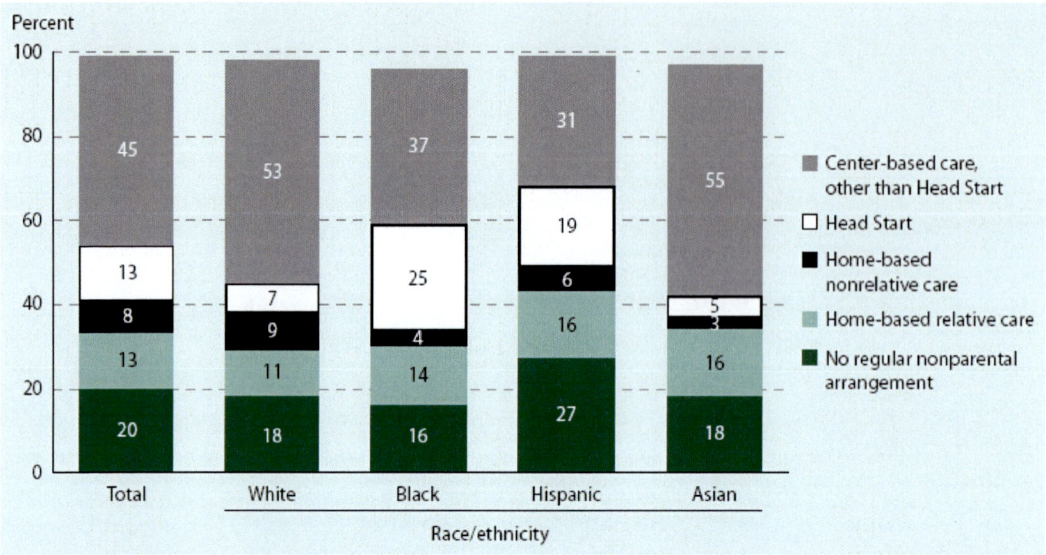

Note: Race categories exclude persons of Hispanic ethnicity. Not all racial/ethnic groups are shown in the figure due to small sample sizes and relatively large standard errors. Detail may not sum to totals because of rounding and suppression of care arrangement cells that do not meet standards. Children who were in multiple arrangements are not included in the figure. *Center-based care* includes day care, preschool, and prekindergarten programs. *Nonrelative care* in a private home includes family day care. Estimates weighted by W3R0. Primary type of care arrangement is the type of nonparental care in which the child spent the most hours each week. See *supplemental note 3* for more information about the Early Childhood Longitudinal Study, Birth Cohort (ECLS-B).

Source: U.S. Department of Education, National Center for Education Statistics, Early Childhood Longitudinal Study, Birth Cohort, Longitudinal 9-Month–Preschool Restricted-Use Data File.

CHILD CARE ARRANGEMENTS: Percentage distribution of the early education and child care arrangements of the 2001 birth cohort at about 4 years old, by race/ethnicity: 2005–06.

In: The Condition of Education in America
Editor: Maurice H. Logan
ISBN: 978-1-60692-298-9

Chapter 4

ELEMENTARY/SECONDARY EDUCATION

PAST AND PROJECTED PUBLIC SCHOOL ENROLLMENTS

Public elementary and secondary enrollment is projected to increase to 54 million in 2017. The South is projected to experience the largest increase in the number of students enrolled.

In 2008, about 49.8 million students are expected to be enrolled in public elementary and secondary schools. Of these students, 34.9 million will be enrolled in prekindergarten (preK) through 8th grade and 14.9 million will be enrolled in grades 9 through 12.

Public school enrollment declined during the 1970s and early 1980s and increased in the latter part of the 1980s. Enrollment continued to increase throughout the 1990s and early 2000s. Between 2000 and 2008, public school enrollment is expected to increase by 2.6 million students, reaching 49.8 million students in 2008 (see supplemental table 3-1). Total public school enrollment is projected to set new enrollment records each year from 2008 through 2017, reaching an estimated high of 54.1 million students.

Enrollment trends in grades preK–8 and 9–12 have differed over time as students move through the public school system. For example, enrollment in grades preK–8 decreased throughout the 1970s and early 1980s, while enrollment in grades 9–12 decreased in the late 1970s and throughout the 1980s. Public school enrollment in grades preK–8 is projected to increase to 34.9 million in 2008 and to reach 38.4 million in 2017. Enrollment in grades 9–12 is projected to decrease from 15 million in 2007 to 14.6 million in 2011 and then increase to 15.7 million in 2017.

Between 2000 and 2008, total enrollment is expected to increase by over 1.8 million students in the South and by 1.0 million students in the West, and to decrease slightly in both the Midwest and Northeast. Since 1965, the South has had the largest share of public school enrollment in the United States. Projections indicate that, by 2008, the share for the South will have increased from 33 percent in 1965 to 38 percent by 2008 and to 40 percent by 2017. The share for the West is projected to increase from 18 percent in 1965 to 25 percent by 2008, and to remain at 25 percent in 2017. In contrast, the share of enrollment in the Midwest is projected to decrease from 28 percent in 1965 to 22 percent by 2008, and to reach 20 percent in 2017. Enrollment in the Northeast is projected to decrease from 21 percent in 1965 to 16 percent by 2008, and to reach 15 percent in 2017.

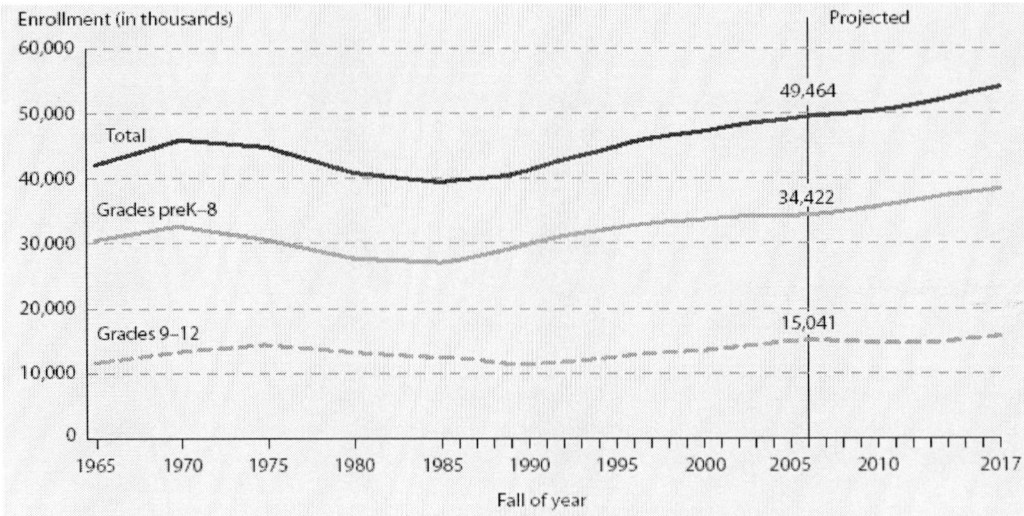

Note: Data are fall enrollment counts or estimates for the referenced year. Some data have been revised from previously published figures. See *supplemental note 1* for states in each region.

Source: U.S. Department of Education, National Center for Education Statistics (NCES). *Digest of Education Statistics, 2007* (NCES 2008-022), table 33; Hussar, W. (forthcoming). *Projections of Education Statistics to 2017* (NCES 2008-078), table 1; Snyder, T., and Hoffman, C.M. (1995). *State Comparisons of Education Statistics: 1969–70 to 1993–94* (NCES 95-122), table 10, retrieved December 4, 2007, from http://nces.ed.gov/ pubsearch/pubsinfo.asp?pubid=95122; and table ESE65, retrieved December 4, 2007, from http:// www.nces.ed.gov/surveys/AnnualReports/ historicaltables.asp.

SCHOOL ENROLLMENT: Public school enrollment in prekindergarten through grade 12, with projections, by grade level: Various years, fall 1965–2017.

Trends in Private School Enrollments

From 1989 to 2005, the percentage of students enrolled in private schools declined from 11 to 9 percent. The number of private school students enrolled in kindergarten through grade 12 increased from 1989 to 2001 and then declined through 2005.

From 1989 to 2001, private school enrollment in kindergarten through grade 12 increased from 4.8 million to 5.3 million students. By 2005, enrollment had declined to 5.1 million students (see supplemental table 4-1).

In addition to the changing level of enrollment in private schools, the distribution of students across different types of private schools changed between 1989 and 2005. Although Roman Catholic schools maintained the largest share of total private school enrollment, the percentage of all private school students enrolled in Roman Catholic schools decreased from 55 to 44 percent. This decrease stemmed from the decline in the percentage of these students enrolled in parochial schools (those run by a parish, not by a diocese or independently). On the other hand, the percentage of students enrolled in Conservative Christian schools increased from 11 to 16 percent during this period. In addition, there was an increase in the percentage of students enrolled in nonsectarian private schools, from 13 to 18 percent. This shift in private school enrollment, from Roman Catholic to other religious and nonsectarian private schools, occurred at both the elementary and secondary levels.

Overall, while the number of students enrolled in private schools was higher in 2005 than in 1989, the percentage of all students attending private schools declined from 11 to 9 percent (see supplemental table 4-2). Enrollment of private school students as a percentage of total enrollment differed by region. In 2005, the percentage of students in private schools was higher in the Northeast (13 percent) than in the Midwest (10 percent), the South, and the West (8 percent each).

The student composition of private schools differed from that of public schools. In 2005, Whites made up a greater share of private than of public school enrollment (75 vs. 58 percent), while the opposite was true for Blacks (10 vs. 16 percent) and Hispanics (9 vs. 20 percent; see supplemental table 4-3 and *indicator 5*). In addition, the student composition in private schools differed by locale. Within cities, 32 percent of private school students enrolled were minorities, compared with 23 percent in suburban areas, 12 percent in towns, and 14 percent in rural areas.

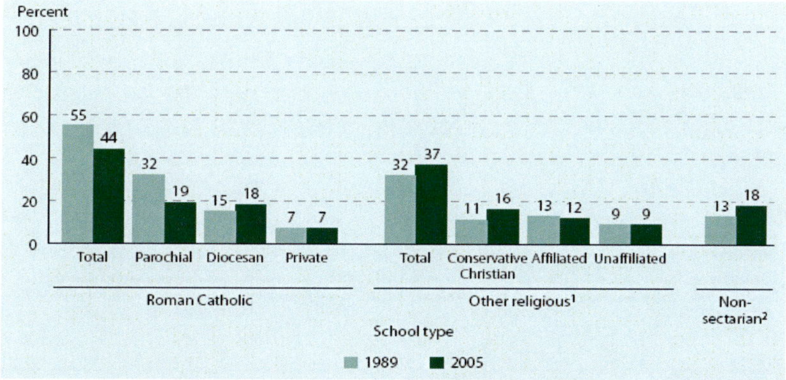

Note: Detail may not sum to totals because of rounding. Race categories exclude persons of Hispanic ethnicity. *Supplemental note 1* identifies the states in each region.

Source: U.S. Department of Education, National Center for Education Statistics, Private School Universe Survey (PSS), 1989–90 and 2005–06.

[1] Other religious schools have a religious orientation or purpose, but are not Roman Catholic. Conservative Christian schools are those with membership in at least one of four associations: Accelerated Christian Education, American Association of Christian Schools, Association of Christian Schools International, or Oral Roberts University Education Fellowship. Affiliated schools are those with membership in 1 of 12 associations—Association of Christian Teachers and Schools, Christian Schools International, Council of Islamic Schools in North America, Evangelical Lutheran Education Association, Friends Council on Education, General Conference of the Seventh-Day Adventist Church, Islamic School League of America, National Association of Episcopal Schools, National Christian School Association, National Society for Hebrew Day Schools, Solomon Schechter Day Schools, or Southern Baptist Association of Christian Schools—or indicating membership in "other religious school associations." Unaffiliated schools are those that have a religious orientation or purpose, but are not classified as Conservative Christian or affiliated.

[2] Nonsectarian schools do not have a religious orientation or purpose.

PRIVATE SCHOOL ENROLLMENT: Percentage distribution of private school students in kindergarten through grade 12, by school type: Fall 1989 and fall 2005.

RACIAL/ETHNIC DISTRIBUTION OF PUBLIC SCHOOL STUDENTS

The percentage of racial/ethnic minority students enrolled in the nation's public schools increased between 1986 and 2006, primarily due to an increase in the proportion of Hispanic students.

The shifting racial and ethnic distribution of public school students enrolled in kindergarten through 12th grade is one aspect of change in the composition of school enrollment. The percentage of public school students who were considered to be part of a racial or ethnic minority group increased from 22 percent in 1972 to 31 percent in 1986 to 43 percent in 2006 (see supplemental table 5-1). Between 1972 and 2006, the percentage of public school students who were White decreased from 78 to 57 percent. The minority increase largely reflected the growth in the proportion of students who were Hispanic. In 2006, Hispanic students represented 20 percent of public school enrollment, up from 6 percent in 1972 and 11 percent in 1986. Since 1986, the proportion of public school students who were Hispanic has increased more than the proportion who were Black or members of other[1] minority groups. For example, in 2006, Black students made up 16 percent of public school enrollment, compared with 17 percent in 1986. Hispanic enrollment measurably surpassed Black enrollment for the first time in 2002. Together, Asian (3.8 percent), Pacific Islander (0.2 percent), and American Indian/Alaskan Native (0.7 percent) students and students of more than one race (2.7 percent) made up about 7.3 percent of public school enrollment in 2006.

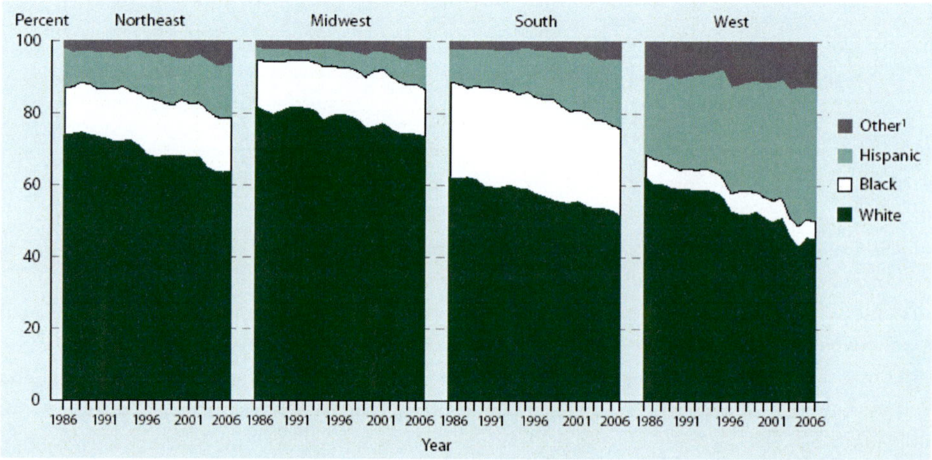

Note: Race categories exclude persons of Hispanic ethnicity. Estimates include all public school students enrolled in kindergarten through 12th grade. See *supplemental note 2* for more information on the Current Population Survey. See *supplemental note 1* for the states in each region.

Source: U.S. Department of Commerce, Census Bureau, Current Population Survey (CPS), October Supplement, 1986–2006.

[1] "Other" includes all students who did not identify themselves as White, Black, or Hispanic.

MINORITY ENROLLMENT: Percentage distribution of the race/ethnicity of public school students enrolled in kindergarten through 12th grade, by region: October 1986–2006.

The distribution of minority students in public schools differed by region, though minority enrollment generally grew in all regions between 1986 and 2006 and during the broader period of 1972 and 2006 (see supplemental table 5-2). Between 1972 and 2006, the South and West had larger minority enrollments than the Northeast and Midwest, and the Midwest had the smallest minority enrollment of any region. In the West, beginning in 2003, minority enrollment exceeded White enrollment, and by 2006, minority students made up 55 percent of public school enrollment, compared with 45 percent for White students. In 2006, as in all years since 1972, the percentage of Hispanic students exceeded the percentage of Black students in the West, while in the South and Midwest, the percentage of Black enrollment continued to exceed that of Hispanic enrollment.

Family Characteristics of 5- to 17-Year-Olds

The percentage of 5- to 17-year-olds whose parents had completed a bachelor's degree or higher increased from 19 percent in 1979 to 35 percent in 2006.

The percentage of school-age children (ages 5–17) whose parents had completed a bachelor's degree or higher increased from 19 percent in 1979 to 35 percent in 2006 (see supplemental table 6-1); this same measure increased for White children (from 22 to 44 percent), Black children (from 5 to 21 percent), and Hispanic children (from 7 to 15 percent). In 2006, a higher percentage of parents of White children had completed a bachelor's degree or higher than did parents of Black or Hispanic children.

The percentage of school-age children living in two-parent households decreased from 75 percent in 1979 to 67 percent in 2006; however, this percentage has remained between 67 and 69 percent since 1995. Another 23 percent of children lived only with their mother and 5 percent were in father-only households in 2006. Higher percentages of White (75 percent) and Hispanic (65 percent) children lived in two-parent households than did their Black (35 percent) peers in 2006. One-half of Black children lived in mother-only households, compared with about one-fourth of Hispanic children and 16 percent of White children.

The percentage of school-age children living in families below the poverty threshold increased from 15 percent in 1979 to 21 percent in 1995, and then decreased to 16 percent in 2002. In 2006, a larger percentage of children were living in poor households than in 1979 (17 vs. 15 percent), but both were lower than the high in 1995 of 21 percent. This same general pattern was evident across racial/ethnic groups. The percentage of White children in poor households increased from 9 percent in 1979 to 12 percent in 1995, and then decreased to 10 percent in 2006. The percentage of Black children in poor households increased from 41 percent in 1979 to 44 percent in 1992, and then decreased to 33 percent in 2006. Among Hispanics, this percentage increased from 27 percent in 1979 to 40 percent in 1995, and then decreased to 26 percent in 2006.

In 2006, some 95 percent of school-age children were born in the United States, not measurably different from the percentage in 1995 (when citizenship data were first collected). A higher percentage of Hispanics (86 percent) were born in the United States in 2006 than in 1995 (81 percent), but no measurable differences were detected for Whites or Blacks over this same period.

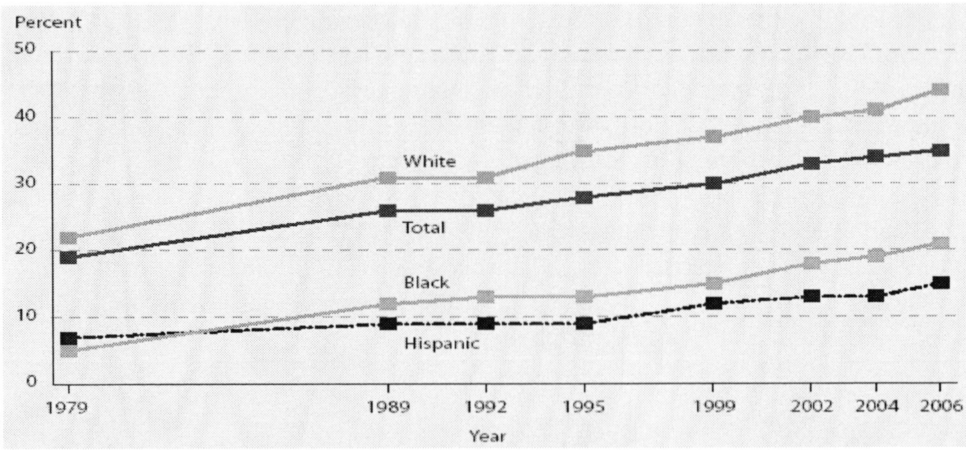

Note: Included in the totals but not shown separately are estimates for those from other racial/ethnic categories. In 1994, the survey instrument for the Current Population Survey (CPS) was changed and weights were adjusted. See *supplemental note 2* for further discussion. See *supplemental note 1* for more information on poverty levels. Some estimates are revised from previous publications. Detail may not sum to totals because of rounding. Race categories exclude persons of Hispanic ethnicity.

Source: U.S. Department of Commerce, Census Bureau, Current Population Survey (CPS), March Supplement, selected years, 1979–2006.

FAMILY CHARACTERISTICS: Percentage of 5- to 17-year-olds whose parents had attained a bachelor's degree or higher, by race/ethnicity: Selected years, 1979–2006.

Language Minority School-Age Children

In 2006, about 20 percent of children ages 5–17 spoke a language other than English at home, and 5 percent spoke English with difficulty.

Between 1979 and 2006, the number of school-age children (children ages 5–17) who spoke a language other than English at home increased from 3.8 to 10.8 million, or from 9 to 20 percent of the population in this age range (see supplemental table 7-1). An increase was also evident during the more recent period of 2000 to 2006 (from 18 to 20 percent). The percentage of 5- to 17-year-old children who spoke English with difficulty increased from 3 to 6 percent between 1979 and 2000, but this percentage did not change measurably between 2000 and 2006 (it remained between 5 and 6 percent). The number of children who spoke English with difficulty as a proportion of children who spoke another language at home has continued to decrease over time. For example, of the children who spoke a language other than English at home, 34 percent spoke English with difficulty in 1979, compared with 31 percent in 2000 and 25 percent in 2006.

In 2006, about 72 percent (7.8 million) of the school-age children who spoke a language other than English at home spoke Spanish (see supplemental table 7-2). The next largest number of children who spoke a non-English language at home spoke other Indo-European[6] languages, followed by those who spoke Asian/ Pacific Islande[7] languages, and then by those

[6] An Indo-European language other than Spanish (e.g., French, German, Portuguese, etc.).

[7] Any native language spoken by Asians or Pacifi c Islanders, which linguists classify variously as Sino-Tibetan, Austroasiatic, or Austronesian languages.

who spoke other languages. Higher percentages of children who spoke Spanish or an Asian/ Pacific Islander language at home spoke English with difficulty (27 and 28 percent, respectively) than did those who spoke other Indo-European languages (19 percent) or other languages (18 percent) at home.

The percentages of school-age children speaking a language other than English at home and who spoke English with difficulty varied by race/ ethnicity and poverty status in 2006. Among school-age children, 18 percent of Hispanics and 17 percent of Asians spoke a language other than English at home and spoke English with difficulty, compared with 6 percent of Pacific Islanders, 3 percent of American Indians/ Alaska Natives, and 1 percent each of Whites, Blacks, and children of more than one race. In terms of poverty status, higher percentages of poor (10 percent) and near-poor (8 percent) 5- to 17-year-olds spoke a non-English language at home and spoke English with difficulty than did nonpoor 5- to 17-year-olds (3 percent).

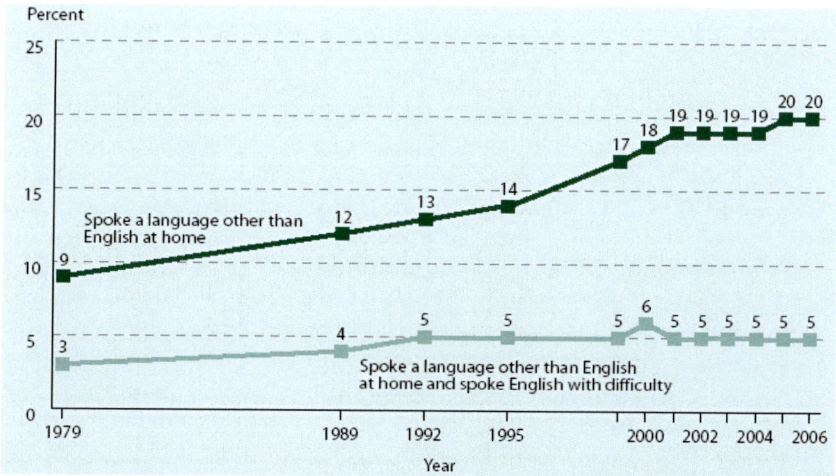

Note: Data on language spoken at home and difficulty speaking English were obtained from household respondents. Respondents were asked if each child in the household spoke a language other than English at home. If they answered "yes," they were asked how well each child could speak English. Categories used for reporting were "very well," "well," "not well," and "not at all." All those who reported speaking English less than "very well" were considered to have difficulty speaking English. Since the American Community Survey (ACS) does not ask whether household children speak English at home, these data cannot be used to determine whether English or another language is the primary language spoken at home. In 1994, the survey methodology for the Current Population Survey (CPS) was changed and weights were adjusted. Spanish-language versions of both the CPS and the ACS were available to respondents. *Poor* is defined to include families below the poverty threshold, *near-poor* is defined to include families at 100–199 percent of the poverty threshold, and *nonpoor* is defined to include families at 200 percent or more than the poverty threshold. See *supplemental note 1* for more information. Race categories exclude persons of Hispanic ethnicity.

Source: U.S. Department of Commerce, Census Bureau, Current Population Survey (CPS), 1979 and 1989 November Supplement and 1992, 1995, and 1999 October Supplement, and American Community Survey (ACS), 2000–06.

LANGUAGE MINORITY: Percentage of 5- to 17-year-olds who spoke a language other than English at home and who spoke English with difficulty: Selected years, 1979–2006.

CHILDREN AND YOUTH WITH DISABILITIES IN PUBLIC SCHOOLS

The Individuals with Disabilities Education Act (IDEA), first enacted in 1975, mandates that children and youth ages 3–21 with disabilities be provided a free and appropriate public school education. Data collection activities to monitor compliance with IDEA began in 1976.

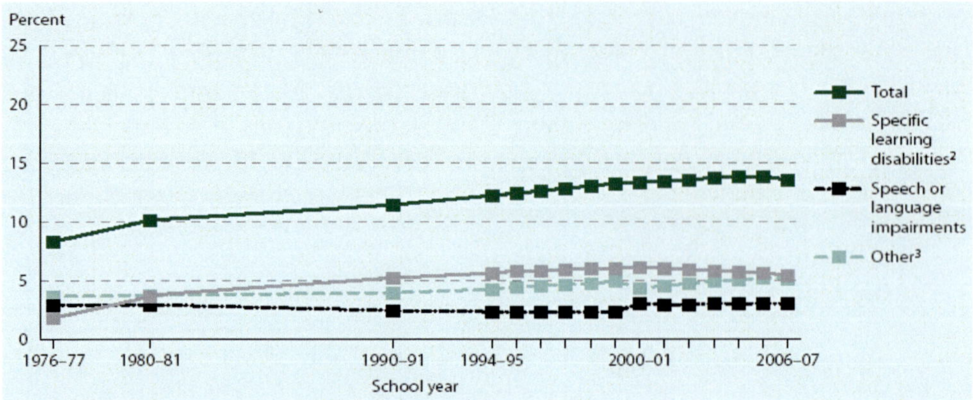

Note: Special education services through the Individuals with Disabilities Education Act (IDEA) are available for eligible children and youth identified by a team of qualified professionals as having a disability that adversely affects their academic performance and as in need of special education and related services. The total is the number and percentage of children and youth receiving special education services through IDEA in early education centers and public schools in the 50 states and the District of Columbia and in Bureau of Indian Affairs (BIA) schools through 1993–94. Beginning in 1994–95, estimates exclude BIA schools. See *supplemental note 8* for more information about the student disabilities presented here.

Source: U.S. Department of Education, Office of Special Education and Rehabilitative Services (OSERS), Office of Special Education Programs (OSEP). (2006a, b). *26th Annual (2004) Report to Congress on the Implementation of the Individuals with Disabilities Education Act*, vols. 1 and 2, data from OSERS, OSEP, Data Analysis System (DANS), 1976–2006. Retrieved November 29, 2007 from http://www.ed.gov/about/reports/annual/osep/2004/introduction.html and https://www.ideadata.org/index.html.

[1] A disorder in one or more of the basic psychological processes involved in understanding or in using language, spoken or written, that may manifest itself in an imperfect ability to listen, think, speak, read, write, spell, or to do mathematical calculations, including conditions such as perceptual disabilities, brain injury, minimal brain dysfunction, dyslexia, and developmental aphasia.

[2] "Other" disability types include mental retardation, emotional disturbance, hearing impairments, orthopedic impairments, other health impairments, visual impairments, multiple disabilities, deaf-blindness, autism, traumatic brain injury, and developmental delay. There is a wide range of disabilities included in this category; they are included together here to represent cases contributing to the total not otherwise presented in this graph due to their relatively low prevalence in the population.

STUDENTS WITH DISABILITIES: Percentage of children and youth ages 3–21 in early education centers or public schools receiving services under the Individuals with Disabilities Education Act (IDEA), by primary disability type: Selected years, 1976–77 through 2006–07.

The number and percentage of children and youth ages 3–21 receiving special education services increased nearly every year since the inception of IDEA until 2004–05 (see supplemental table 8-1). However, the number and percentage declined between 2004–05 and 2006–07. In 1976–77, some 3.7 million children and youth were served under IDEA, representing 5 percent of all children and youth ages 3–21. By 2006–07, some 6.7 million children and youth received IDEA services, corresponding to about 9 percent of all children and youth ages 3–21. Among students served under IDEA in 2006–07, about 1 percent were American Indian/Alaska Native, 2 percent were Asian/Pacific Islander, 17 percent were Hispanic, 20 percent were Black, and 59 percent were White.[8]

Since 1980–81 a larger percentage of children and youth ages 3–21 have received special education services for specific learning disabilities than for any other disabilities (see supplemental table 8-2). A specific learning disability is a disorder of one or more of the basic psychological processes involved in understanding or in using language, spoken or written, that may manifest itself in an imperfect ability to listen, think, speak, read, write, spell, or to do mathematical calculations. This includes conditions such as perceptual disabilities, brain injury, minimal brain dysfunction, dyslexia, and developmental aphasia. The percentage of children and youth ages 3–21 receiving special education services for a specific learning disability was 3 percentage points higher in 2006–07 than in 1976–77 (5 versus 2 percent). In comparison, the prevalence of speech or language impairments remained fairly constant, with variations of less than 1 percentage point during this period.

[8] Race categories exclude persons of Hispanic ethnicity. Data from reference below.

In: The Condition of Education in America
Editor: Maurice H. Logan
ISBN: 978-1-60692-298-9

Chapter 5

UNDERGRADUATE EDUCATION

PAST AND PROJECTED UNDERGRADUATE ENROLLMENTS

Women are projected to make up 57 percent of undergraduate enrollment in 2008.

Total undergraduate enrollment in degree- granting postsecondary institutions has generally increased since 1970. This increase has been accompanied by changes in the proportions of students who are female, students who attend full time, students who attend 4-year institutions, and students who attend public institutions. Overall enrollment is projected to reach 15.6 million students in 2008 and 17.0 million in 2017 (see supplemental table 9-1). The number of students enrolled part and full time, the number at 2- and 4-year institutions, the number at public and private institutions, and the number of male and female undergraduates are all projected to reach a new high each year from 2007 to 2017.

From 1970 to 2006, women's undergraduate enrollment increased over three times as fast as men's, surpassing men's enrollment in 1978. In this period, women's enrollment rose from 3.2 to 8.7 million (an increase of 178 percent), while men's rose from 4.3 to 6.5 million (an increase of 53 percent). From 2007 to 2017, both men's and women's undergraduate enrollments are projected to increase, with women maintaining 57 percent of total enrollment.

Though full-time enrollment was higher than part-time enrollment from 1970 to 2006, part- time enrollment increased over five times as fast as full-time enrollment in the 1970s (from 28 to 40 percent), before stabilizing from 1980 to 1999. From 2000 to 2006, full-time enrollment grew almost three times as fast as part-time enrollment, from 60 to 63 percent, where it is expected to remain from 2007 to 2017.

Undergraduate enrollment has been larger at 4-year institutions than at 2-year institutions since 1970, yet 2-year enrollment increased more rapidly than 4-year enrollment in the 1970s (from 31 to 42 percent), before leveling off from 1980 to 1999. From 2000 to 2006, 4-year enrollment grew over twice as fast as 2-year enrollment, from 55 to 57 percent, where it is expected to remain from 2007 to 2017.

Enrollment at public institutions has been higher than at private institutions from 1970 to 2006. Public enrollment increased almost four times as fast as private enrollment in the 1970s (from 76 to 80 percent), before stabilizing from 1980 to 1999. From 2000 to 2006, private enrollment grew over twice as fast as public enrollment (from 20 to 22 percent). Public enrollment is expected to remain at 78 percent from 2007 to 2017.

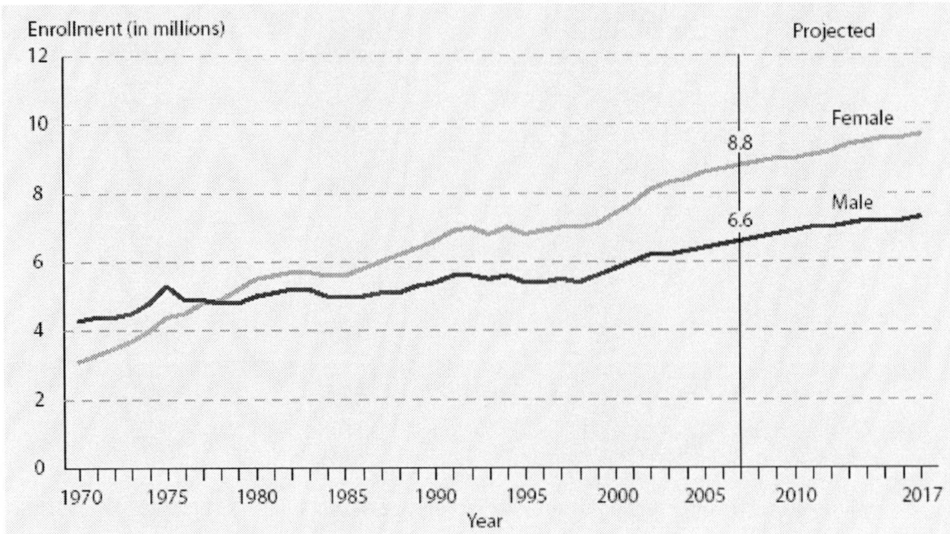

Note: Projections are based on data through 2006 and middle alternative assumptions concerning the economy. For more information, see NCES 2008-078. Data for 1999 were imputed using alternative procedures. For more information, see NCES 2001-083, *appendix E*. See *supplemental note 3* for more information on the Integrated Postsecondary Education Data System (IPEDS). See *supplemental note 9* for more information about the classification of postsecondary education institutions.

Source: U.S. Department of Education, National Center for Education Statistics (NCES). *Digest of Education Statistics, 2007* (NCES 2008-022), table 196, and Hussar, W. (forthcoming). *Projections of Education Statistics to 2017* (NCES 2008-078), table 1 8, data from U.S. Department of Education, NCES, Higher Education General Information Survey (HEGIS), "Fall Enrollment in Colleges and Universities" surveys, 1970–1985, and 1986–2006 Integrated Postsecondary Education Data System, "Fall Enrollment Survey" (IPEDS-EF:86–99), and Spring 2001 through Spring 2007.

UNDERGRADUATE ENROLLMENT: Total undergraduate enrollment in degree-granting 2- and 4-year postsecondary institutions with projections, by sex: Fall 1970–2017.

MOBILITY OF COLLEGE STUDENTS

In 2006, three-fourths of 4-year college freshmen who had graduated from high school in the previous 12 months attended an in-state college, and one-fourth attended an out-of-state college.

The majority of college freshmen attend colleges in the same state in which they graduate from high school; however, many freshmen, particularly those attending 4-year institutions, attend out-of-state colleges. This indicator compares the percentage of college freshmen who had graduated from high school in the previous 12 months and who attended an in-state public or private not-for-profit 4-year college or university (hereafter referred to as the *freshman in-state attendance percentage*) in 2006 and 1996.[9] In 2006, the national freshman

[9] Freshmen who attended private for-profit 4-year colleges are not included because some large institutions enroll distance education students only.

in-state attendance percentage was about 75 percent, which was similar to the percentage for 1996 (74 percent; see supplemental tables 10-1 and 10-2).

In 2006, the freshman in-state attendance percentage ranged from 28 percent in the District of Columbia and 40 percent in New Jersey to 89 percent in Louisiana and 90 percent in Utah. Altogether, there were 11 states in which the freshman in-state attendance percentage was 85 percent or more, and 12 states and the District of Columbia in which it was 60 percent or less. There were some regional patterns, with many of the southern states having relatively high freshman in-state attendance percentages.

For example, 8 of the 11 states with freshman in-state attendance percentages over 85 percent were southern states. Seven of the 13 jurisdictions with freshman in-state attendance percentages below 60 percent were Northeastern states. Although classified as southern areas, Maryland, Delaware, and the District of Columbia also had freshman in-state attendance percentages below 60 percent. The other states with freshman instate attendance percentages below 60 percent were Alaska, Hawaii, and Wyoming.

In Massachusetts, Delaware, New Hampshire, Vermont, Rhode Island, and the District of Columbia, 50 percent or more of the freshmen enrolled in their 4-year colleges were from out-of-state.

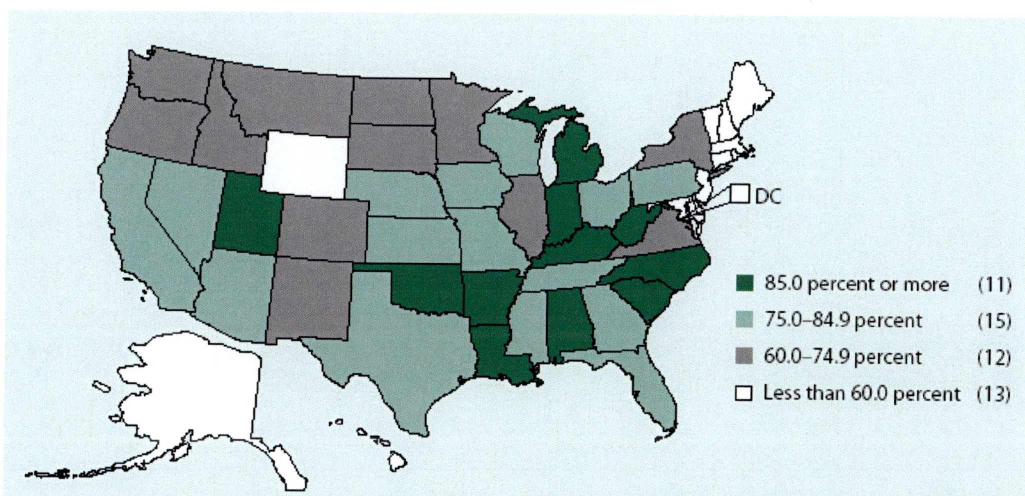

Note: Includes first-time postsecondary students who were enrolled at public and private notfor-profit 4-year degree-granting institutions that participated in Title IV federal financial aid programs. See *supplemental note 9* for more information. Foreign students studying in the United States are included as out-of-state students. See *supplemental note 1* for a list of states in each region.

Source: U.S. Department of Education, National Center for Education Statistics, Fall 2006 Integrated Postsecondary Education Data System (IPEDS), Spring 2007.

MOBILITY OF COLLEGE STUDENTS: Percentage of freshmen who had graduated from high school in the previous 12 months attending a public or private not-for-profit 4-year college in their home state: Fall 2006.

Between 1996 and 2006, there was a relatively large increase in the freshman in-state attendance percentage in some states. In Alaska, it increased 15 percentage points (from 44 to 59 percent), and in Nevada, Florida, and New Mexico, it increased more than 10 percentage points. In contrast, the freshman in-state attendance percentage decreased by 11 percentage points in Delaware and by 15 percentage points in the District of Columbia.

In: The Condition of Education in America
Editor: Maurice H. Logan
ISBN: 978-1-60692-298-9

Chapter 6

GRADUATE AND PROFESSIONAL EDUCATION

TRENDS IN GRADUATE AND FIRST-PROFESSIONAL ENROLLMENTS

Enrollment in graduate and first-professional programs each increased from 2000 to 2006. For both program types, total minority enrollment increased by a larger percentage than did White enrollment.

Enrollment in graduate programs increased from 1.3 to 2.2 million (67 percent) between 1976 and 2006 and is expected to reach 2.3 million in 2008 (see supplemental table 11-1). First- professional program enrollment increased from 244,000 to 343,000 (41 percent) between 1976 and 2006 and is expected to reach 354,000 in 2008. According to projections, increases in both graduate and first-professional enrollment will continue, with graduate enrollment exceeding 2.6 million and first-professional enrollment reaching 418,000 by 2017.

Enrollment trends in both graduate and first- professional programs differ by sex. More men than women attended both types of programs in 1976. By 2006, female enrollment in graduate programs had increased from 619,000 to 1.3 million (117 percent), while male enrollment fluctuated but increased overall from 714,000 to 887,000 (24 percent). Women represented 46 percent of total graduate enrollment in 1976, some 50 percent in 1984, and 60 percent in 2006. In 2008, graduate enrollment is projected to reach 1.4 million for women and 919,000 for men. In first-professional programs, between 1976 and 2006, female enrollment rose from 54,000 to 170,000 (211 percent), while male enrollment fluctuated but decreased overall from 190,000 to 174,000 (8 percent). By 2008, first- professional enrollment is expected to reach 171,000 for women and 183,000 for men.

Minorities experienced enrollment gains between 2000 and 2006. In 2006, minorities represented 23 percent of total graduate enrollment, compared with 19 percent in 2000 (see supplemental table 11-2). Minority enrollment in graduate programs increased from 359,000 to 519,000 (44 percent) during this period, while White enrollment increased from 1.3 to 1.4 million (15 percent). Among minorities, the greatest relative growth in graduate enrollment was seen for Blacks (57 percent), Hispanics (42 percent), and American Indians/Alaska Natives (40 percent). In first-professional programs, minority enrollment grew from 78,000 to 93,000 (20 percent) during this period, while White enrollment rose from 220,000 to 242,000 (10 percent). Among minorities, relative growth in first-professional enrollment was greatest for Asians/Pacific Islanders (24 percent) and Hispanics (19 percent).

[Enrollment in thousands]

Characteristic	Graduate enrollment 2000	Graduate enrollment 2006	Graduate enrollment Percent change	First-professional enrollment 2000	First-professional enrollment 2006	First-professional enrollment Percent change
Total	**1,850**	**2,231**	**21**	**307**	**343**	**12**
Sex						
Male	780	887	14	164	174	6
Female	1,071	1,344	26	143	170	19
Race/ethnicity[1]						
White	1,259	1,445	15	220	242	10
Total minority	359	519	44	78	93	20
Black	158	247	57	24	27	14
Hispanic	95	136	42	15	18	19
Asian/Pacific Islander	96	122	27	37	46	24
American Indian/ Alaska Native	10	14	40	2	3	9
Nonresident alien	232	266	15	8	8	0

[1] Because of underreporting and nonreporting of racial/ethnic data, some figures are slightly lower than corresponding data in other published tables. Race categories exclude persons of Hispanic ethnicity.

Note: See *supplemental note 3* for more information on the Integrated Postsecondary Education Data System (IPEDS). See the glossary for definitions of minority and first-professional degree. Detail may not sum to totals because of rounding. Percent changes for figures are based on unrounded numbers.

Source: U.S. Department of Education, National Center for Education Statistics (NCES). *Digest of Education Statistics, 2008* (forthcoming), table 216, data from U.S. Department of Education, NCES, Integrated Postsecondary Education Data System (IPEDS), "Fall Enrollment Survey," Spring 2001 and Spring 2007.

GRADUATE AND FIRST-PROFESSIONAL ENROLLMENT: Graduate and first-professional enrollment in degree-granting institutions and percent change in enrollment, by sex and race/ethnicity: 2000 and 2006.

SECTION 2. LEARNER OUTCOMES

In: The Condition of Education in America
Editor: Maurice H. Logan
ISBN: 978-1-60692-298-9

Chapter 7

INTRODUCTION

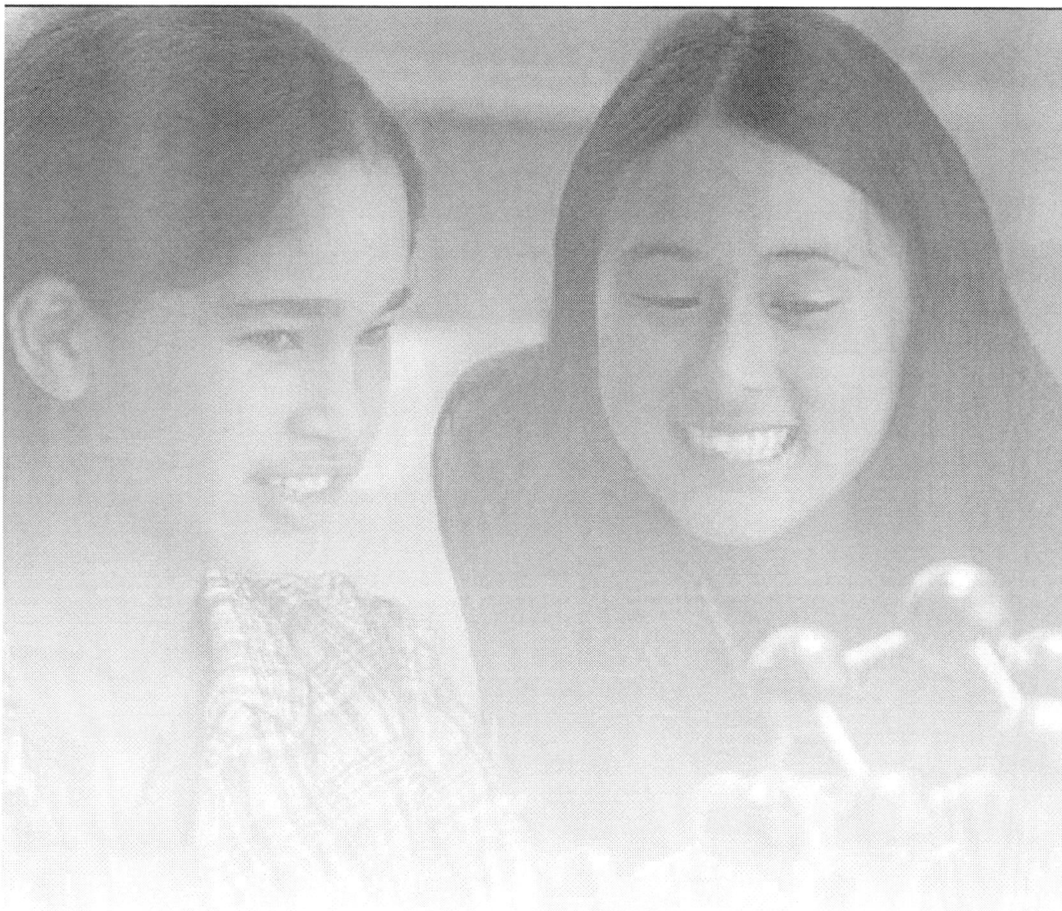

Indicator–Year	
Early Childhood Outcomes	
Students' Reading and Mathematics Achievement Through 3rd Grade	8–2004
Children's Skills and Proficiency in Reading and Mathematics Through Grade 3	8–2005
Academic Outcomes	
Reading Performance of Students in Grades 4, 8, and 12	12–2008
Mathematics Performance of Students in Grades 4 and 8	13–2008
Writing Performance of Students in Grades 8 and 12	14–2008
Economics Performance of Students in Grade 12	15–2008
Trends in the Achievement Gaps in Reading and Mathematics	16–2008
International Comparison of 4th- and 8th-Grade Performance in Mathematics	11–2005
Poverty and Student Mathematics Achievement	15–2006
Reading and Mathematics Score Trends by Age	17–2008
Reading and Mathematics Achievement at 5th Grade	16–2007
Student Reading and Mathematics Performance in Public Schools by Urbanicity	14–2005
International Comparisons of Reading Literacy in Grade 4	18–2008
International Comparisons of Mathematics Literacy	17–2006
International Comparisons of Mathematics Cognitive Domains of 4th- and 8th-Graders	17–2007
International Comparisons of Science Literacy	19–2008
Science Performance of Students in Grades 4, 8, and 12	13–2007
International Comparison of 4th- and 8th-Grade Performance in Science	12–2005
U.S. History Performance of Students in Grades 4, 8, and 12	14–2003
Geography Performance of Students in Grades 4, 8, and 12	13–2003
Adult Literacy	
Trends in Adult Literacy	18–2007
Trends in Adult Literary Reading Habits	15–2005
Adult Reading Habits	20–2006
Social and Cultural Outcomes	
Education and Health	12–2004
Youth Neither in School nor Working	19–2007
Economic Outcomes	
Annual Earnings of Young Adults	20–2008
Employment Outcomes of Young Adults by Race/Ethnicity	17–2005

The indicators in this section of *The Condition of Education* examine student achievement and other outcomes of education among students in elementary and secondary education and among adults in the larger society. There are 27 indicators in this section: 9, prepared for this year's volume, appear on the following pages, and all 27, including indicators from previous years, appear on the Web (see Web- site Contents on the facing page for a full list of the indicators). The indicators on student achievement show how students are performing on assessments in reading, mathematics, science, and other academic subject areas; trends over time in student achievement; and gaps in achievement. The indicators in this section are organized into five subsections.

The indicators in the first subsection trace the gains in achievement and specific reading and mathematics skills of children through the early years of elementary education. Children enter school with varying levels of knowledge and skill. Measures of these early childhood competencies represent important indicators of students' future prospects both inside and outside of the classroom. Two indicators available on the website highlight changes in student achievement for a cohort of children who began kindergarten in fall 1998 as they progressed through 3rd grade in 2001–02.

The indicators in the second subsection report trends in student performance by age or grade in the later years of elementary education through high school. As students progress through school, it is important to know the extent to which they are acquiring necessary skills and becoming proficient in challenging subject matter. Academic outcomes are basically measured in three ways: as the change in students' average performance over time, as the change in the percentage of students achieving predetermined levels of achievement, and through international comparisons of national averages. Several indicators in this section show the achievement of students in reading at grades 4, 8, and 12 and in mathematics at grades 4 and 8. Another indicator that appears on the Web highlights achievement in science for students in these grades. Two new indicators feature writing and economics scores. Also, several indicators examine skills in reading, mathematics, and science at the international level. Together, indicators in the first two subsections help to create a composite picture of academic achievement in U.S. schools.

In addition to academic achievement, there are adult literacy measures in the third subsection and socially and culturally desirable outcomes of education in the fourth subsection. These outcomes, which are measured here by adult literacy, adult reading habits, and the health status of individuals, contribute to an educated, capable, and engaged citizenry.

The fifth subsection looks specifically at the economic outcomes of education. Economic outcomes include the likelihood of being employed, the salaries paid to individuals with varying levels of educational attainment, the job and career satisfaction of employees, and other measures of economic well being and productivity.

The indicators on learner outcomes from previous editions of *The Condition of Education*, which are not included in this volume, are available at http://nces.ed.gov/ programs/coe/ list/i2.asp.

In: The Condition of Education in America
Editor: Maurice H. Logan
ISBN: 978-1-60692-298-9

Chapter 8

ACADEMIC OUTCOMES

READING PERFORMANCE OF STUDENTS IN GRADES 4, 8, AND 12

National average reading scores of 4th- and 8th-graders were higher in 2007 than in 1992, by 4 and 3 points, respectively. However, the reading score of 12th-graders was 6 points lower in 2005 than in 1992.

The percentage of 4th-graders performing at or above the Basic achievement level on the National Assessment of Educational Progress (NAEP) reading assessment was higher in 2007 than in 1992 (67 vs. 62 percent), as was the percentage performing at or above the Proficient achievement level (33 vs. 29 percent).[1] Percentages at both of these achievement levels were higher in 2007 than in 2005 (see supplemental table 12-1). The percentage of 8th-graders performing at or above Basic was higher in 2007 than in 1992 (74 vs. 69 percent), while there was no measurable difference in the percentage performing at or above Proficient. In 2007, the percentage of 8th-graders at or above Basic was higher than that in 2005, but the percentages at or above Proficient for these two years were not measurably different. The percentage of 12th- graders performing at or above Basic was lower in 2005[2] than in 1992 (73 vs. 80 percent), as was the percentage of 12th-graders performing at or above Proficient (35 vs. 40 percent).

Reported on a scale of 0 to 500, national average reading scores of 4th- and 8th-graders were higher in 2007 than in 1992, by 4 and 3 points, respectively (see supplemental table 12-2). These 2007 scores were higher than 2005 scores. The reading score of 12th-graders was 6 points lower in 2005 than in 1992. In the most recent assessment, females at each grade level outscored their male counterparts. For example, 12th-grade females scored 13 points higher than males in 2005. Average scores were higher in 2007 than in 1992 for White, Black, Hispanic, and Asian/Pacific Islander 4th-graders (ranging from 6 to 16 points) and for White, Black, and Hispanic 8th-graders (ranging from 5 to 7 points), while scores were lower in 2005 than in 1992 for White, Black, and Hispanic 12th- graders (ranging from 5 to 7 points).

NAEP results also permit state-level comparisons of the abilities of 4th- and 8th-graders in public schools.[3] The percentage of 4th-grade students performing at or above Basic was higher in 2007 than in 1992 in 24 of the 42 states that participated in both assessment years (see supplemental table 12-3). Of the 38 states that participated in the grade 8 assessment in both years, the percentage of students performing at or above Basic was higher in 2007 than in 1998 in 5 states and lower in 2007 than in 1998 in 7 states.

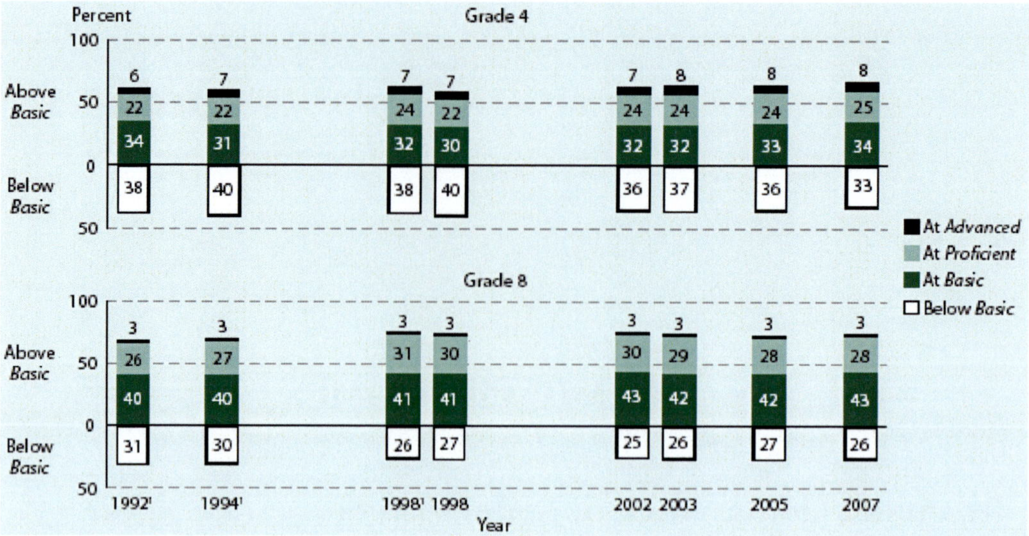

[1] Testing accommodations (e.g., extended time, small group testing) for children with disabilities and limited-English-proficient students were not permitted in 1992 and 1 994, and students were tested with and without accommodations in 1998.

[2] The 2003 and 2007 National Assessment of Educational Progress (NAEP) Reading Assessments were not administered to 12th-grade students.

[3] State samples were not collected for grade 12; therefore, state results for grade 12 are not available.

Note: The National Assessment of Educational Progress (NAEP) has assessed the reading abilities of students in grades 4, 8, and 12 in public and private schools since 1992. NAEP reading scores range from 0 to 500. The achievement levels define what students should know and be able to do: *Basic* indicates partial mastery of fundamental skills; *Proficient* indicates demonstrated competency over challenging subject matter; and *Advanced* indicates superior performance. The percentage of students at or above *Proficient* includes students at the *Advanced* achievement level. Similarly, the percentage of students at or above *Basic* includes students at the *Basic*, those at the *Proficient*, and those at the *Advanced* achievement levels. Beginning in 2002, the NAEP national sample for grades 4 and 8 was obtained by aggregating the samples from each state and the District of Columbia, rather than by obtaining an independently selected national sample. As a consequence, the size of the national samples for grades 4 and 8 increased, and smaller differences between years or between types of students were found to be statistically significant than would have been detected in previous assessments. Calculations are based on unrounded numbers. See *supplemental note 4* for more information on NAEP. Detail may not sum to totals because of rounding.

Source: U.S. Department of Education, National Center for Education Statistics, National Assessment of Educational Progress (NAEP), selected years, 1992–2007 Reading Assessments, NAEP Data Explorer.

READING PERFORMANCE: Percentage distribution of 4th- and 8th-grade students across NAEP reading achievement levels: Selected years, 1992–2007

Mathematics Performance of Students in Grades 4 and 8

In 2007, students in grades 4 and 8 showed improvements from all previous assessments at all mathematics achievement levels.

The percentages of 4th- and 8th-grade students at or above Basic, at or above Proficient, and at Advanced achievement levels were higher in 2007 than the percentages for all previous mathematics assessments[10] (see supplemental table 13-1). For example, the percentage of 4th-grade students at or above Proficient increased by 3 percentage points from 2005 to 2007 and tripled from 1990 to 2007 (13 vs. 39 percent). For 8th-grade students, the percentage scoring at or above Proficient increased by 2 percentage points from 2005 to 2007 and doubled from 1990 to 2007 (15 vs. 32 percent).

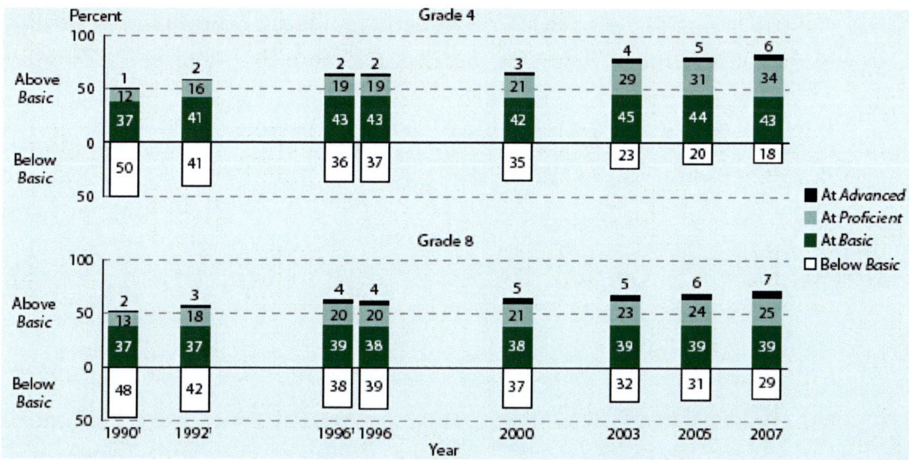

Note: The National Assessment of Educational Progress (NAEP) has assessed the mathematical abilities of students in grades 4 and 8 in public and private schools since 1990. NAEP mathematics scores range from 0 to 500. The achievement levels define what students should know and be able to do: *Basic* indicates partial mastery of fundamental skills; *Proficient* indicates demonstrated competency over challenging subject matter; and *Advanced* indicates superior performance. The percentage of students at or above *Proficient* includes students at the *Advanced* achievement level. Similarly, the percentage of students at or above *Basic* includes students at the *Basic*, those at the *Proficient*, and those at the *Advanced* achievement levels. See *supplemental note 4* for more information on NAEP. Calculations are based on unrounded numbers. Detail may not sum to totals because of rounding.

Source: U.S. Department of Education, National Center for Education Statistics, National Assessment of Educational Progress (NAEP), selected years, 1990–2007 Mathematics Assessments, NAEP Data Explorer.

MATHEMATICS PERFORMANCE: Percentage distribution of 4th- and 8th-grade students across NAEP mathematics achievement levels: Selected years, 1990–2007.

From 1990 to 2007, the average NAEP mathematics scores increased 27 points for 4th-graders and 19 points for 8th-graders. Increases in scores were seen for both males and females and for most racial/ethnic groups. Both male and female 4th- and 8th-graders scored higher in 2007 than in any of the previous assessments (see supplemental table 13-2). In 2007, at each grade, males outscored females by 2 points; these score gaps were not measurably different from the gaps in either 2005 or 1990. For grade 4, average scores in 2007 for White, Black, Hispanic, and Asian/Pacific Islander students were higher than the

[10] Testing accommodations (e.g., extended time, small group testing) for children with disabilities and limited-English-proficient students were not permitted in 1990 and 1992, and students were tested with and without

scores in any of the previous assessments. Although the score for American Indian/Alaska Native 4th-graders increased over time, there was no measurable difference between their 2005 and 2007 scores. For grade 8, average scores in 2007 for White, Black, and Hispanic students were higher than in any of the previous assessments. The average score for 8th-grade Asian/Pacific Islander students was higher in 2007 than in 1990, but not measurably different from their 2005 score. No measurable differences were detected in the scores for American Indian/Alaska Native 8th-graders over the assessment years.

NAEP results also permit state-level comparisons of the abilities of 4th- and 8th-graders in public schools. There were 42 states that participated in both the 1992 and 2007 assessments for 4th grade and 38 states that participated in both the 1990 and 2007 assessments for 8th grade. For each of these participating states and at each grade level, there was an increase in the average score as well as in the percentages of students scoring at or above Basic and at or above Proficient (see supplemental table 13-3).

Writing Performance of Students in Grades 8 and 12

Average writing scores of 8th- and 12th-graders were higher in 2007 than in previous years.

The National Assessment of Educational Progress (NAEP) has assessed trends in the writing abilities of students in grades 8 and 12 in both public and private schools since 1998. Reported on a scale of 0 to 300, average writing scores of 8th- and 12th-graders were higher in 2007 than in either 1998 or 2002 (see supplemental table 14-1). Eighth-graders scored 3 points higher in 2007 than in 2002 and 6 points higher than in 1998. The average writing score for 12thgraders was 5 points higher in 2007 than in 2002 and 3 points higher than in 1998.

The percentage of 8th-graders performing at or above the Basic achievement level was higher in 2007 than in 1998 (88 vs. 84 percent), as was the percentage performing at or above the Proficient achievement level (33 vs. 27 percent).[11]

The percentage of students at or above the Basic achievement level was also higher in 2007 than in 2002, but no measurable difference was detected in the percentage of students at or above Proficient between these two years. The percentage of 12th-graders performing at or above Basic increased from 74 percent in 2002 to 82 percent in 2007 and was higher in 2007 than in 1998. There was no measurable difference in the percentage performing at or above Proficient between 2002 and 2007, but there has been a 2 percentage point increase since 1998.

For all assessment years, females at each grade level outscored their male counterparts (see supplemental table 14-2). For example, 12th-grade females scored 18 points higher than their male peers in 2007. White, Black, and Hispanic 8thgraders had higher average scores in 2007 than in 1998 and 2002. Asian/Pacific Islander 8th-grade students scored higher in 2007 than in 2002, but the apparent change was not measurably different from 1998. Overall gains

accommodations in 1996.

[11] The percentage of students at or above Profi cient includes students at the Advanced achievement level. Similarly, the percentage of students at or above Basic includes students at the Basic, those at the Proficient, and those at the Advanced achievement levels.

made by 12th-graders in 2007 were not consistent across all racial/ethnic groups. White students scored higher in 2007 than in either previous assessment year. Black and Asian/Pacific Islander students scored higher in 2007 than in 2002, but apparent differences were not measurably different from 1998. Writing scores in 2007 for Hispanic and American Indian/ Alaska Native 12th-graders were not measurably different from those in previous assessments. For all assessment years, White students at each grade level outscored their Black and Hispanic peers.

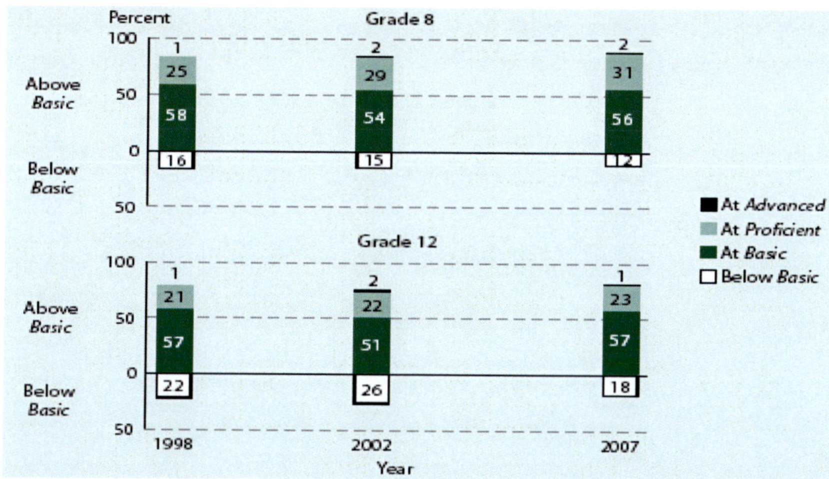

Note: The National Assessment of Educational Progress (NAEP) assessed the writing abilities of students in grades 8 and 12 in public and private schools in 1998, 2002, and 2007. As a result of larger 8th-grade sample sizes beginning in 2002, smaller differences can be found to be statistically significant than would have been detected with the smaller samples sizes used in 1998 or in the 12th-grade samples. NAEP writing scores range from 0 to 300. The achievement levels define what students should know and be able to do: *Basic* indicates partial mastery of fundamental skills; *Proficient* indicates demonstrated competency over challenging subject matter; and *Advanced* indicates superior performance. Calculations are based on unrounded numbers. Detail may not sum to totals because of rounding. See *supplemental note 4* for more information on NAEP.

Source: U.S. Department of Education, National Center for Education Statistics, National Assessment of Educational Progress (NAEP), 1998, 2002, and 2007 Writing Assessments, NAEP Data Explorer.

WRITING PERFORMANCE: Percentage distribution of students across NAEP writing achievement levels, by grade: 1998, 2002, and 2007.

Economics Performance of Students in Grade 12

On the 2006 12th-grade economics assessment, students who reported higher levels of parental education outperformed their peers who reported lower levels of parental education.

The National Assessment of Educational Progress (NAEP) conducted its first assessment of economics in 2006. The assessment evaluated 12th-grade students' understanding of economies and markets, the benefits and costs of economic interaction and interdependence, and choices made because of limited resources in three areas: market, national, and international economics.[12]

About 79 percent of 12th -graders performed at or above the *Basic* level[13] on this assessment, and 42 percent performed at or above the *Proficient* level (indicating solid academic achievement), including 3 percent at the *Advanced* level (indicating superior performance; see supplemental table 15-1). Reported on a scale of 0 to 300, the average score of 12th-graders was set at 150; this score fell within the *Basic* achievement level (indicating partial mastery of fundamental skills).[14]

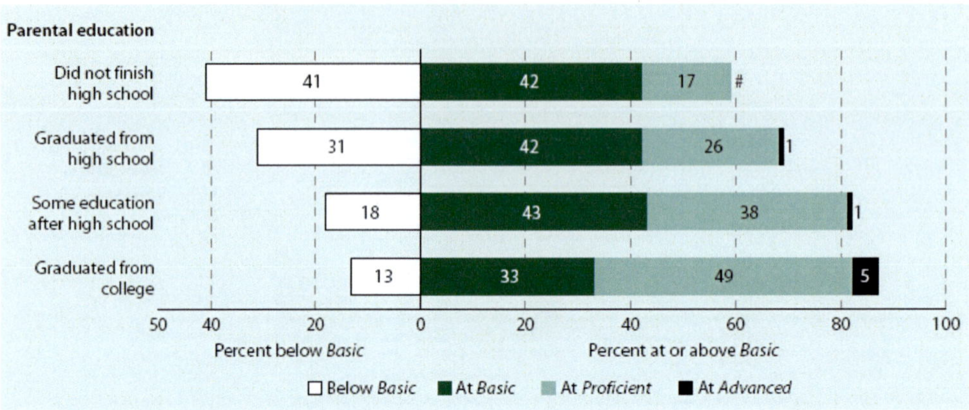

Note: Detail may not sum to totals because of rounding. See *supplemental note 4* for more information on the NAEP and NAEP achievement levels.

Source: Mead, N., and Sandene, B. (2007). *The Nation's Report Card: Economics 2006* (NCES 2007-475), data from U.S. Department of Education, National Center for Education Statistics, NAEP Data Explorer. ECONOMICS PERFORMANCE: Percentage distribution of 12th-grade students across NAEP economics achievement levels, by highest level of parental education: 2006.

ECONOMICS PERFORMANCE: Percentage distribution of 12th-grade students across NAEP economics achievement levels, by highest level of parental education: 2006

Results from the assessment varied by student characteristics, including parental education and sex. Students who reported higher levels of parental education outperformed those who reported lower levels of parental education. For example, 54 percent of students whose parents were college graduates performed at or above the *Proficient* level, compared with 17 percent of students whose parents did not finish high school. In addition, males outperformed females on the assessment overall. About 45 percent of male students performed at or above the *Proficient* level, compared with 38 percent of female students.

---

[12] Market economy—traditionally described as "microeconomics"—covers how individuals, businesses, and institutions make decisions about allocating resources in the marketplace. National economy—traditionally described as "macroeconomics"—encompasses the sum of decisions made by individuals, businesses, and government. International economy concentrates on international trade—that is, how individuals and businesses interact in foreign markets.

[13] The percentage of students at or above *Profi cient* includes students at the *Advanced* achievement level. Similarly, the percentage of students at or above *Basic* includes students at the *Basic*, those at the *Proficient*, and those at the *Advanced* achievement levels.

[14] The cutoff scores for economics achievement levels were as follows: *Basic* (123), *Profi cient* (160), and *Advanced* (208).

Student performance in the three content areas also followed the above patterns for parental education and sex (see supplemental table 15-2).

Student exposure to economics in the classroom was also highlighted in the assessment. Previous findings show that economic content in the high school curriculum has increased in recent decades: in 2005, some 66 percent of graduates reported that they had taken an economics course, compared with 49 percent in 1982 (NCES 2007-475).[15] In the 2006 NAEP assessment, most 12th-graders reported exposure to economics content: 16 percent had taken an advanced economics course,[16] and 49 percent had taken general economics. Twenty-three percent indicated that they had taken a business or personal finance course, or a course that combined economics with another subject. Thirteen percent said that they had not had any economics instruction.

Trends in the Achievement Gaps in Reading and Mathematics

In 2007, the achievement gap between White and Black scores in reading and mathematics at the 4th grade was smaller than in 1992, while not measurably different at the 8th grade or between Whites and Hispanics in either grade.

The main National Assessment of Educational Progress (NAEP) program has assessed student reading and mathematics performance since the early 1990s. NAEP thus provides a picture of the extent to which student performance in each subject has changed over time, including the achievement gaps between White and Black and White and Hispanic students.

In reading, the achievement gap between White-Black 4th-graders was smaller in 2007 than in any previous assessment. However, the gap between White-Hispanic 4th-graders was not measurably different in 2007 compared with 1992. In 2007, at the 4th-grade level, Blacks scored, on average, 27 points lower than Whites (on a 0–500 scale), and Hispanics scored, on average, 26 points lower than Whites (see supplemental table 16-1). At 8th grade, there was no measurable difference in the White-Black or White-Hispanic reading achievement gaps in 2007 compared with 1992 or 2005. In 2007, at the 8th-grade level, Blacks scored, on average, 27 points lower on the reading assessment than Whites, and Hispanics scored, on average, 25 points lower than Whites.

In mathematics, the achievement gap between White-Black 4th-graders was lower in 2007 than in 1990 (26 vs. 32 points), but there was no measurable change over the last two years. The gap between White-Hispanic 4th-graders increased in the 1990s before decreasing in the first half of the 2000s, but the gap in 2007 (21 points) was not measurably different from that in 1990. Among 8th-graders, a similar trend existed in both the White-Black and White-Hispanic score gaps: increases occurred in the 1990s before decreasing to the current levels, which are not measurably different from those in 1990. The White-Black 8th-grade mathematics gap was lower in 2007 than in 2005, but there was no measurable change in the White- Hispanic gap. In 2007, among 8th-graders, the White-Black mathematics gap was 32 points, and the White-Hispanic gap was 26 points.

---

[15] These estimates are taken from the National Assessment of Educational Progress (NAEP) High School Transcript Study.

[16] For example, Advanced Placement economics.

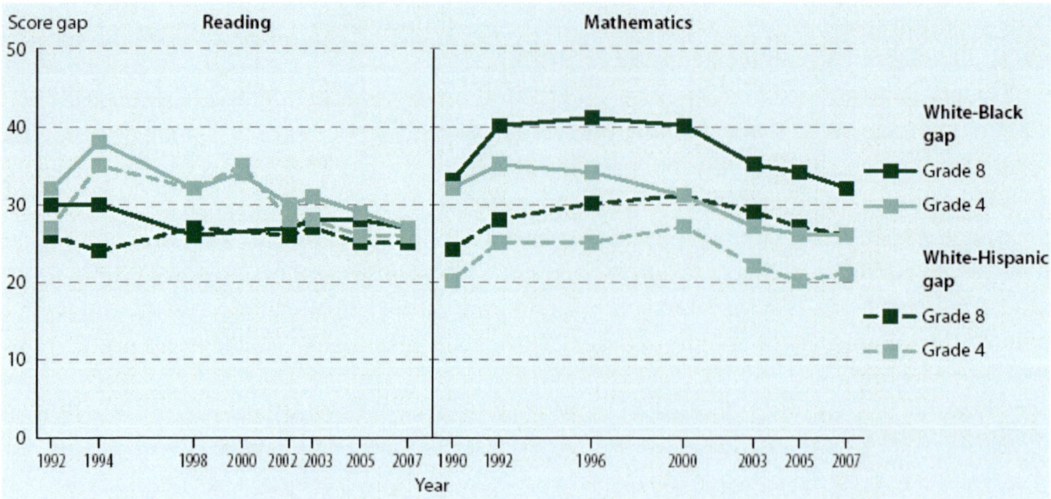

Note: NAEP scores are calculated on a 0 to 500 scale. Student assessments are not designed to permit comparisons across subjects or grades. Race categories exclude persons of Hispanic ethnicity. The score gap is determined by subtracting the average Black and Hispanic score, respectively, from the average White score. Testing accommodations (e.g., extended time, small group testing) for children with disabilities and limited-English-proficient students were not permitted from 1990 through 1994. Beginning in 2002, the NAEP national sample for grades 4 and 8 was obtained by aggregating samples from each state, rather than by obtaining an independently selected national sample. See *supplemental note 4* for more information on NAEP.

Source: U.S. Department of Education, National Center for Education Statistics, National Assessment of Educational Progress (NAEP), various years, 1990–2007 Reading and Mathematics Assessments, NAEP Data Explorer.

ACHIEVEMENT GAP: Differences in White-Black and White-Hispanic 4th- and 8th-grade average reading and mathematics scale scores: Various years, 1990–2007.

Reading and Mathematics Score Trends by Age

The average reading and mathematics scores on the long-term trend National Assessment of Educational Progress were higher in 2004 than in the early 1970s for 9- and 13-year-olds.

The long-term trend National Assessment of Educational Progress (NAEP) has provided information on the reading and mathematics achievement of 9-, 13-, and 17-year-olds in the United States since the early 1970s and is used as a measure of progress over time. These results may differ from the main NAEP results presented in *indicators 12*, *13, 14, 15*, and *16* as the content of the long-term trend assessment has remained consistent over time, while the main NAEP undergoes changes periodically (see *supplemental note 4*).

NAEP long-term trend results indicate that the reading and mathematics achievement of 9- and 13-year-olds improved between the early 1970s and 2004. In reading, 9-year-olds scored higher in 2004 than in any previous assessment year, with an increase of 7 points between 1999 and 2004. The 2004 average score for 13-year-olds was not measurably different from the 1999 average score, but still was higher than the scores in 1971 and 1975. In mathematics, the achievement of 9- and 13-yearolds in 2004 was the highest of any assessment year. The performance of 17-year-olds on the 2004 reading and mathematics assessments, however, was not measurably different from their performance on either the first reading and mathematics assessments (in 1971 and 1973, respectively) or the 1999 reading and mathematics assessments.

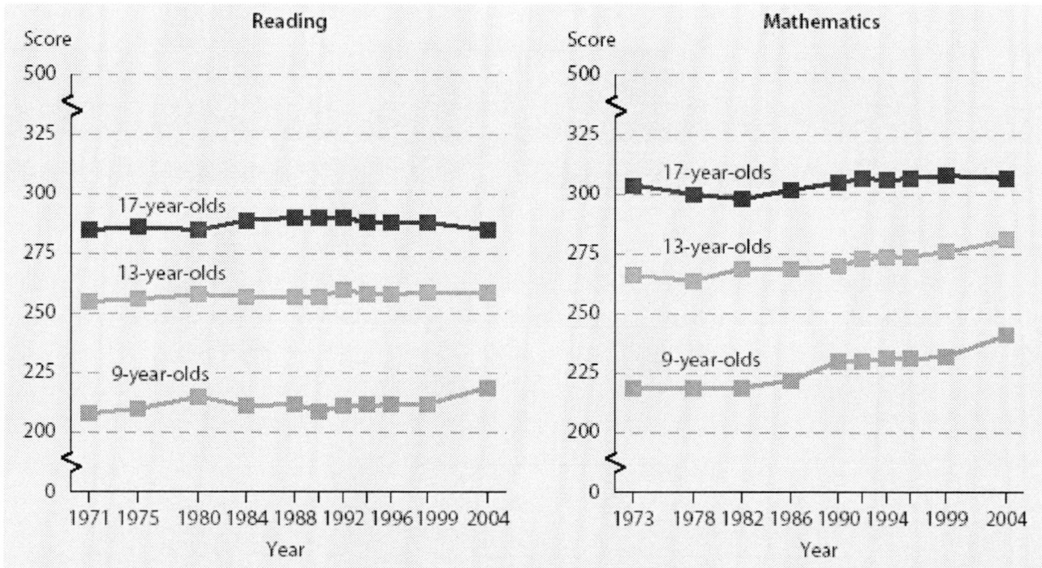

Note: NAEP has two distinct assessment programs: the long-term trend assessment program and the main assessment program. Data from the long-term trend program, presented in this indicator, come from subject assessments that have remained substantially the same since the early 1970s in order to measure and compare student achievement over time. In contrast, data from the main NAEP assessment program, presented in *indicators 12, 13, 14, 15,* and *16*, come from subject assessments that are periodically adapted to employ the latest advances in assessment methodology and to reflect changes in educational objectives and curricula. Because the instruments and methodologies of the two assessment programs are different, it is not possible to compare long-term trend results with the main assessment results (see *supplemental note 4* for more information on the two NAEP programs). NAEP scores range from 0 to 500.

Source: Perie, M., Moran, R., and Lutkus, A.D. (2005). *NAEP 2004 Trends in Academic Progress: Three Decades of Student Performance in Reading and Mathematics* (NCES 2005-464), figures 2-1 and 2-4, data from U.S. Department of Education, National Center for Education Statistics, National Assessment of Educational Progress (NAEP), various years, 1971–2004 Long-Term Trend Reading and Mathematics Assessments.

NAEP SCORES: Average reading and mathematics scale scores on the long-term trend National Assessment of Educational Progress (NAEP), by age: Various years, 1971 through 2004.

The performance of subgroups of students generally mirrored the overall national patterns; however, there were some notable differences. The average reading and mathematics scores of Black and Hispanic 9-year-olds in 2004 were the highest of any assessment year (see supplemental tables 17-1 and 17-2). For Black 13-year-olds, reading and mathematics scores were higher in 2004 than the scores in the early 1970s, and the 2004 mathematics score was higher than in any previous assessment year. For Hispanic 13-yearolds, mathematics scores were higher in 2004 than in any previous assessment year. In contrast to the overall national results, the average scores of Black and Hispanic 17-year-olds were higher in 2004 than in the early 1970s. Black 17-yearolds improved 25 points in reading between 1971 and 2004, and 15 points in mathematics between 1973 and 2004 on a 0–500 point scale. Hispanic 17-year-olds improved 12 points in reading between 1975 (the first year the reading achievement of Hispanics was specifically measured) and 2004, and 12 points in mathematics between 1973 and 2004.

INTERNATIONAL COMPARISONS OF READING LITERACY IN GRADE 4

In 2006, U.S. 4th-graders performed above the international average and above 22 of the 45 educational jurisdictions. There were no differences detected between the U.S. average scores from 2001 to 2006.

The 2006 Progress in International Reading Literacy Study (PIRLS) assessed the reading literacy of 4th-graders in 45 educational jurisdictions around the globe. The average U.S. 4th-grade score on the combined reading literacy scale was 540, above the PIRLS international average of 500. Students in 10 jurisdictions scored above U.S. students, on average. U.S. students scored higher, on average, than their peers in 22 jurisdictions. No differences were detected between the average score in the United States and those in 12 jurisdictions.

Average score relative to the U.S. average score	Educational jurisdiction and score					
Significantly higher	Russian Federation	565	Singapore	558	Italy	551
	Hong Kong, SAR[1]	564	Luxembourg	557	Sweden	549
	Alberta, Canada	560	Ontario, Canada	555		
	British Columbia, Canada	558	Hungary	551		
Not significantly different	Germany	548	Nova Scotia, Canada	542	Lithuania	537
	Belgium (Flemish)[2]	547	Latvia	541	Chinese Taipei	535
	Bulgaria	547	**United States[2]**	**540**	Quebec, Canada	533
	Netherlands[2]	547	England	539		
	Denmark	546	Austria	538		
Significantly lower	New Zealand	532	Iceland	511	Trinidad and Tobago	436
	Slovak Republic	531	Belgium (French)	500	Iran, Islamic Republic of	421
	Scotland[2]	527	Moldova	500	Indonesia	405
	France	522	*International average*	*500*	Qatar	353
	Slovenia	522	Norway[3]	498	Kuwait	330
	Poland	519	Romania	489	Morocco	323
	Spain	513	Georgia	471	South Africa	302
	Israel	512	Macedonia	442		

[1] Hong Kong SAR is a Special Administrative Region (SAR) of the People's Republic of China.
[2] Met guidelines for sample participation rates only after replacement schools were included.
[3] Did not meet guidelines for sample participation rates after replacement schools were included.

Note: Jurisdictions were required to assess students who were in the grade that represented 4 years of formal schooling, counting from the first year of primary or basic education. In the United States and most educational jurisdictions, this corresponds to grade 4. See *supplemental note 5* for more information on the Progress in International Reading Literacy Study (PIRLS). The PIRLS international scale average is set at 500 with a standard deviation of 100.

Source: Baer, J., Baldi, S., Ayotte, K., and Green, P. (2007). *The Reading Literacy of U.S. Fourth-Grade Students in an International Context: Results From the 2001 and 2006 Progress in International Reading Literacy Study (PIRLS)* (NCES 2008-017), data from the International Association for the Evaluation of Educational Achievement (IEA), Progress in International Reading Literacy Study (PIRLS), 2006.

INTERNATIONAL READING PERFORMANCE: Average combined reading literacy scale scores of 4th-graders, by educational jurisdiction: 2006.

In addition to a combined reading literacy score, PIRLS provides two subscales: reading for literary purposes and for informational purposes. In 2006, U.S. 4th-graders' average scores on the two subscales were above the international averages (see supplemental table 18-1).

The United States was among 29 educational jurisdictions that participated in both the 2001 and 2006 PIRLS assessments. No differences were detected between the U.S. average scores in 2001 and 2006 on the combined reading literacy scale or on the two subscales (see supplemental table 18-2). Students in 8 jurisdictions showed measurable gains on the combined reading literacy scale between 2001 and 2006, while students in 7 jurisdictions showed measurable declines.

With few exceptions, in almost all participating jurisdictions, including the United States, 4th-grade girls scored higher than 4th-grade boys, on average, on the combined reading literacy scale. In most countries, 4th-grade girls also scored higher than 4th-grade boys on the two subscales in 2006 (see supplemental table 18-3). Within the United States, White 4thgraders had higher average scores than their Black, Hispanic, and American Indian/Alaska Native peers on the combined reading literacy scale (see supplemental table 18-4).

International Comparisons of Science Literacy

The 2006 Program for International Student Assessment (PISA 2006) reports on the science literacy of 15-year-olds in 57 educational jurisdictions, including the 30 member countries of the Organization for Economic Cooperation and Development (OECD) and 27 non-OECD countries and subnational education systems. PISA 2006 provides scores on three subscales of scientific competencies in addition to a combined scientific literacy score. The average U.S. science literacy score was 489, which was below the average of the 30 OECD countries (500). U.S. students had a lower average score than students in 16 OECD-member countries and a higher average score than students in 5 OECD countries. U.S. students also scored lower than their peers in 6 non-OECD jurisdictions and higher than their peers in 17 non-OECD-member jurisdictions.

On specific scientific skill subscales measured in PISA 2006, the average score of U.S. students was below the OECD average in explaining phenomena scientifically and in using scientific evidence. No measurable difference was found between U.S. students' average score and the OECD average in identifying scientific issues (see supplemental table 19-1).

In a majority of participating jurisdictions (37 out of 57), including the United States, no measurable differences were found between the average combined science literacy scores of males and females (see supplemental table 19-2). Among jurisdictions where significant score differences were found by sex, 8 showed males outperforming females and 12 showed females outperforming males. In two of the three scientific skill subscales measured in PISA 2006, most jurisdictions showed a significant difference in the scores of males and females: in identifying scientific issues, females outperformed males; in explaining phenomena scientifically, males generally outperformed females.

Within the United States, the combined science literacy scores of U.S. 15-year-old Hispanic, Black, and American Indian/Alaska Native students were below the OECD average (see supplemental table 19-3). The average score of U.S. White students was above the

OECD average, while the average scores of U.S. Asian, Native Hawaiian/Other Pacific Islander, and students of more than one race were not measurably different from the OECD average.

INTERNATIONAL SCIENCE LITERACY PERFORMANCE: Average combined science literacy scale scores of 15-year-old students, by country or jurisdiction: 2006

Average score relative to U.S. average score	OECD-member country and average score							
Significantly higher	Finland	563	Netherlands	525	Switzerland	512	Sweden	503
	Canada	534	Korea, Republic of	522	Austria	511	*OECD average*	500
	Japan	531	Germany	516	Belgium	510		
	New Zealand	530	United Kingdom	515	Ireland	508		
	Australia	527	Czech Republic	513	Hungary	504		
Not significantly different	Poland	498	Iceland	491	Spain	488		
	Denmark	496	United States	489	Norway	487		
	France	495	Slovak Republic	488	Luxembourg	486		
Significantly lower	Italy	475	Greece	473	Mexico	410		
	Portugal	474	Turkey	424				
	Non-OECD-member jurisdiction and average score							
Significantly higher	Hong Kong-China	542	Estonia	531	Slovenia	519		
	Chinese Taipei	532	Liechtenstein	522	Macao-China	511		
Not significantly different	Croatia	493	Lithuania	488				
	Latvia	490	Russian Federation	479				
Significantly lower	Israel	454	Jordan	422	Indonesia	393	Azerbaijan	382
	Chile	438	Thailand	421	Argentina	391	Qatar	349
	Serbia, Republic of	436	Romania	418	Brazil	390	Kyrgyz Republic	322
	Bulgaria	434	Montenegro,		Colombia	388		
	Uruguay	428	Republic of	412	Tunisia	386		

Note: The Organization for Economic Cooperation and Development (OECD) is an intergovernmental organization of 30 industrialized nations. The OECD average represents the average of the 30 member nations where each country is counted equally regardless of population size. The OECD average was set to 500 with a standard deviation of 100.

Source: Baldi, S., Jin, Y., Skewer, M., Green, P. J., and Herget, D. (2007). *Highlights From PISA 2006: Performance of U.S. 15-Year-Old Students in Science and Mathematics Literacy in an International Context* (NCES 2008-016), table 2a, data from the Organization for Economic Cooperation and Development (OECD), Program for International Student Assessment (PISA), 2006.

INTERNATIONAL SCIENCE LITERACY PERFORMANCE: Average combined science literacy scale scores of 15-year-old students, by country or jurisdiction: 2006.

In: The Condition of Education in America
Editor: Maurice H. Logan
ISBN: 978-1-60692-298-9

Chapter 9

Economic Outcomes

Annual Earnings of Young Adults

In 2006, young adults ages 25–34 with a bachelor's degree earned 28 percent more than young adults with an associate's degree and 50 percent more than young adult high school completers.

Measured in constant 2006 dollars, median earnings for young adults ages 25–34 who worked full time throughout a full year increased as education level increased for each year shown between 1995 and 2006 (see supplemental tables 20-1 and 20-2). For example, young adults with a bachelor's degree as their highest degree consistently had higher median earnings than those with less education. This pattern held for male, female, White, Black, Hispanic, and Asian subgroups.

In 2006, the median earnings of young adults with a bachelor's degree were $43,500, while the median earnings were $34,000 for those with an associate's degree, $29,000 for high school completers,[17] and $22,000 for those who did not earn a high school diploma. In other words, in 2006, young adults with a bachelor's degree earned 28 percent more than young adults with an associate's degree, 50 percent more than young adult high school completers, and 98 percent more than those who did not earn a high school diploma (see supplemental table 20-1). In 2006, the median earnings of young adults with a master's degree or higher were $50,000, or 15 percent more than young adults with a bachelor's degree.

The earnings difference between those with at least a bachelor's degree and those with less education increased between the longer period of 1980 and 2006. However, between 2000 and 2006, there was generally no measurable change in the earnings difference between these groups. For example, in 1980, young adults with a bachelor's degree or higher earned $14,600 more than those who did not earn a high school diploma or its equivalent. In 2000, this difference increased to $23,400 and was $23,000 in 2006.

In 2006, Asian young adults with a master's degree or higher had higher earnings than their White, Black, and Hispanic counterparts (see supplemental table 20-2). Unlike in earlier years, there were no measurable differences in earnings among White, Black, and Hispanic

---

[17] Includes those who earned a high school diploma or its equivalent (e.g., a General Educational Development [GED] certifi cate).

young adults with a master's degree or higher in 2006. In 2006, the average median earnings of Asian young adults with a master's degree or higher were $60,000, while the average median earnings for their White, Black, and Hispanic peers were between $48,000 and $50,000.

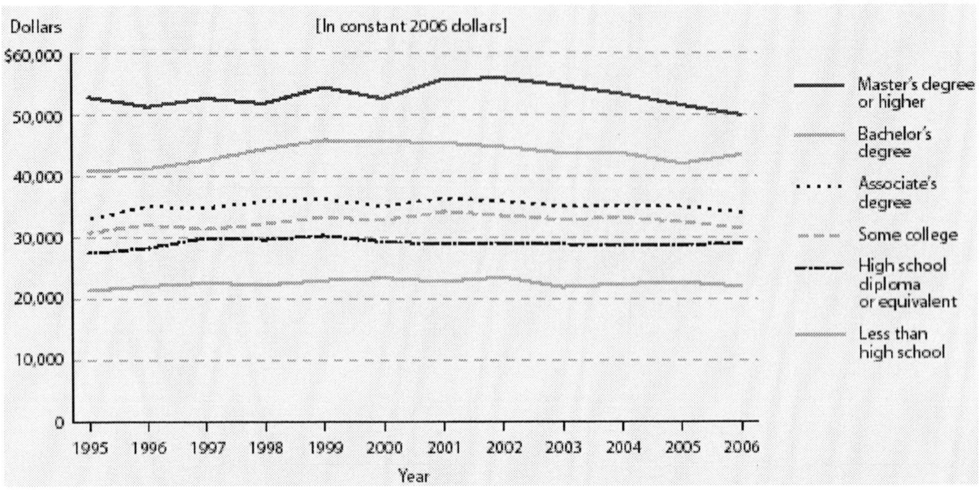

Note: Educational levels represent highest degree obtained. Earnings are presented in 2006 constant dollars by means of the Consumer Price Index (CPI) to eliminate inflationary factors and allow for direct comparison across years. See *supplemental note 11* for further discussion. *Full-year worker* refers to those who were employed 50 or more weeks during the previous year; *full-time worker* refers to those who were usually employed 35 or more hours per week. The Current Population Survey (CPS) questions used to obtain educational attainment were changed in 1992. In 1994, the survey instrument for the CPS was changed and weights were adjusted. See *supplemental note 2* for further discussion on both of these changes.

Source: U.S. Department of Commerce, Census Bureau, Current Population Survey (CPS), March and Annual Social and Economic Supplement, selected years, 1996–2007.

ANNUAL EARNINGS: Median annual earnings of full-time, full-year wage and salary workers ages 25–34, by educational attainment: 1995–2006.

Section 3.
Student Effort and Educational Progress

In: The Condition of Education in America
Editor: Maurice H. Logan
ISBN: 978-1-60692-298-9

Chapter 10

INTRODUCTION

	Indicator–Year
Student Attitudes and Aspirations	
Time Spent on Homework	21–2007
Student Preparedness	22–2007
Postsecondary Expectations of 12th-Graders	23–2006
Student Effort	
Student Absenteeism	24–2006
Elementary/Secondary Persistence and Progress	
Grade Retention	25–2006
Public High School Graduation Rates by State	21–2008
Students With Disabilities Exiting School With a Regular High School Diploma	22–2008
Event Dropout Rates by Family Income, 1972–2001	16–2004
Status Dropout Rates by Race/Ethnicity	23–2008
High School Sophomores Who Left Without Graduating Within 2 Years	27–2006
Transition to College	
Immediate Transition to College	24–2008
International Comparison of Transition to Postsecondary Education	17–2004
Postsecondary Persistence and Progress	
Remediation and Degree Completion	18–2004
Transfers From Community Colleges to 4-Year Institutions	19–2003
Institutional Retention and Student Persistence at 4-Year Institutions	20–2003
Trends in Undergraduate Persistence and Completion	19–2004
Postsecondary Participation and Attainment Among Traditional-Age Students	22–2005
Completions	
Educational Attainment	25–2008
Degrees Earned	26–2008
Degrees Earned by Women	27–2008
Time to Bachelor's Degree Completion	21–2003
Postsecondary Attainment of 1988 8th-Graders	22–2003
Advanced Degree Completion Among Bachelor's Degree Recipients	32–2006
Persistence and Attainment of Students With Pell Grants	23–2003

The indicators in this section of The Condition of Education report on the progress students make through the education system. There are 24 indicators in this section: 7, prepared for this year's volume, appear on the following pages, and all 24, including indicators from previous volumes, appear on the Web (see Website Contents on the facing page for a full list of the indicators). Particular attention is paid to how various subgroups in the population proceed through school and attain different levels of education as well as the factors that are associated with their success along the way.

The first two subsections focus on the educational aspirations and effort of students. The indicators include student measures of time spent on homework, preparedness for academic activities, postsecondary expectations, and patterns of school attendance.

The third subsection traces the progress of students through elementary and secondary education to graduation from high school or some alternate form of completion. Measures include the percentage of students who graduate high school on time (in 4 years) and the percentage who leave high school before completion (drop out). Dropouts are measured by event rates (the percentage of students in an age range who leave school in a given year) and status rates (the percentage of students in an age range who are not enrolled in school and who have not completed high school). Indicators on the following pages and on the website show the status dropout rate by race/ethnicity as well as characteristics of students in the spring of their sophomore year in 2002 who had dropped out 2 years later. In addition, the averaged freshman graduation rate estimates the on-time graduation rate for each state.

The fourth subsection examines the transition to college. An important measure is the percentage of students who make the transition to college within 1 year of completing high school. An indicator on the website compares the rate of first-time enrollment in postsecondary education in the United States to the rates in other countries.

The fifth subsection concerns the percentage of students who enter postsecondary education who earn a credential and how much time they take to do so. This subsection also includes relationships between the qualifications and characteristics of students who enter postsecondary education and their success in earning a credential.

An overall measure of the progress of the population through the education system is attainment, which is the highest level of education completed by a certain age. This is the focus of the final subsection. The Condition of Education annually examines the level of attainment for those ages 25–29. Other indicators examine factors related to the level of attainment and the number of undergraduate and graduate degrees earned over time by sex and race/ethnicity.

The indicators on student effort and educational progress from previous editions of The Condition of Education, which are not included in this volume, are available at http://nces.ed.gov/programs/coe/list/i3.asp.

In: The Condition of Education in America
Editor: Maurice H. Logan
ISBN: 978-1-60692-298-9

Chapter 11

ELEMENTARY/SECONDARY PERSISTENCE AND PROGRESS

PUBLIC HIGH SCHOOL GRADUATION RATES BY STATE

About three-quarters of the freshman class graduated from high school on time with a regular diploma in 2004–05. This indicator examines the percentage of public high school students who graduate on time with a regular diploma. To do so, i t uses the averaged freshman graduation rate—an estimate of the percentage of an incoming freshman class that graduates 4 years later. The averaged freshman enrollment count is the sum of the number of 8th-graders 5 years earlier, the number of 9th-graders 4 years earlier (because this is when current year seniors were freshmen), and the number of 10th-graders 3 years earlier, divided by 3. The intent of this averaging is to account for the high rate of grade retention in the freshman year, which adds 9th-grade repeaters from the previous year to the number of students in the incoming freshman class each year.

Among public high school students in the class of 2004–05, the averaged freshman graduation rate was 74.7 percent (see supplemental table 21-1). Nebraska had the highest graduation rate at 87.8 percent. Sixteen other states had rates above 80 percent: Wisconsin, Iowa, Vermont, North Dakota, Minnesota, New Jersey, Arizona, Utah, Pennsylvania, South Dakota, Montana, Idaho, Connecticut, Missouri, Ohio, and New Hampshire. Nevada had the lowest rate at 55.8 percent. Ten other states and the District of Columbia had graduation rates below 70 percent: Tennessee, Alabama, New Mexico, New York, Florida, Alaska, Louisiana, Mississippi, Georgia, and South Carolina.

The overall averaged freshman graduation rate among public school students increased from 71.7 percent for the class of 2000–01 to 74.7 percent for the class of 2004–05. Between these years, there was an increase in the graduation rate in 44 states and the District of Columbia; 9 states (Arizona, Hawaii, Kentucky, Missouri, North Carolina, Oregon, Tennessee, Vermont, and Washington) and the District of Columbia had an increase of greater than 5 percentage points. The graduation rate decreased in 6 states (Alaska, Massachusetts, Michigan, Nevada, New Jersey, and New Mexico), with Nevada being the only state experiencing a decline of greater than 5 percentage points.

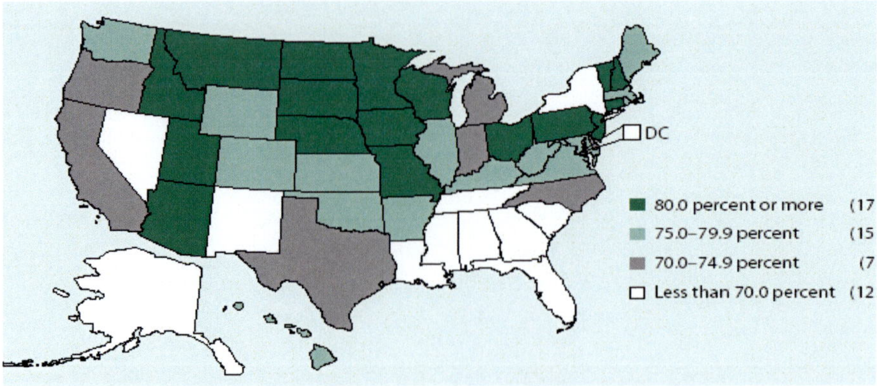

Source: U.S. Department of Education, National Center for Education Statistics, Common Core of Data (CCD), "State Nonfiscal Survey of Public Elementary/Secondary Education," 1986–87 through 2005–06; and Seastrom, M., Hoffman, L., and Chapman, C. (2006). *The Averaged Freshman Graduation Rate for Public High Schools From the Common Core of Data: School Years 2002–03 and 2003–04* (NCES 2006-606rev).

HIGH SCHOOL GRADUATION: Averaged freshman graduation rate for public high school students, by state: School year 2004–05.

STUDENTS WITH DISABILITIES EXITING SCHOOL WITH A REGULAR HIGH SCHOOL DIPLOMA

Between 1996–97 and 2005–06, the percentage of students with disabilities exiting school with a regular high school diploma increased from 43 to 57 percent.

The Individuals with Disabilities Education Act (IDEA) mandates that youth with disabilities are provided a free and appropriate public school education. In 2005–06, the percentage of students with disabilities exiting school with a regular high school diploma was 57 percent, an increase from 43 percent in 1996–97 (see supplemental table 22-1). About 94 percent of these students were between the ages of 17 and 19 years old (see supplemental table 22-2). In addition to the increase in the percentage of regular high school diplomas received over this period, the percentage of students with disabilities exiting with a certificate of attendance[18] increased from 9 to 15 percent, while the percentage who dropped out[19] without a credential decreased from 46 to 26 percent (see supplemental table 22-1).

Among students with disabilities, those with visual impairments and those with hearing impairments were the two groups with the highest percentages exiting with a regular high school diploma. For example, in 2005–06, some 72 percent of students with a visual impairment exited with a regular high school diploma. In contrast, students with mental retardation had the lowest percentage (37 percent), followed by students with an emotional

---

[18] Students who exited an educational program and received a certifi cate of completion, modifi ed diploma, or some similar document. This includes students who received a high school diploma, but did not meet the same standards for graduation as those for students without disabilities.

[19] "Dropped out" is defi ned as the total who were enrolled at some point in the reporting year, were not enrolled at the end of the reporting year, and did not exit for any of the other reasons described. For the purpose of calculating dropout rates, the Office of Special Education Programs (OSEP) counts as dropouts students who moved and were not known to continue.

disturbance (43 percent) and students with multiple disabilities (44 percent) (see supplemental table 22-2). About 62 percent of students with a specific learning disability exited with a regular high school diploma. In 2005–06, students with specific learning disabilities accounted for 60 percent of all exiting students with disabilities.

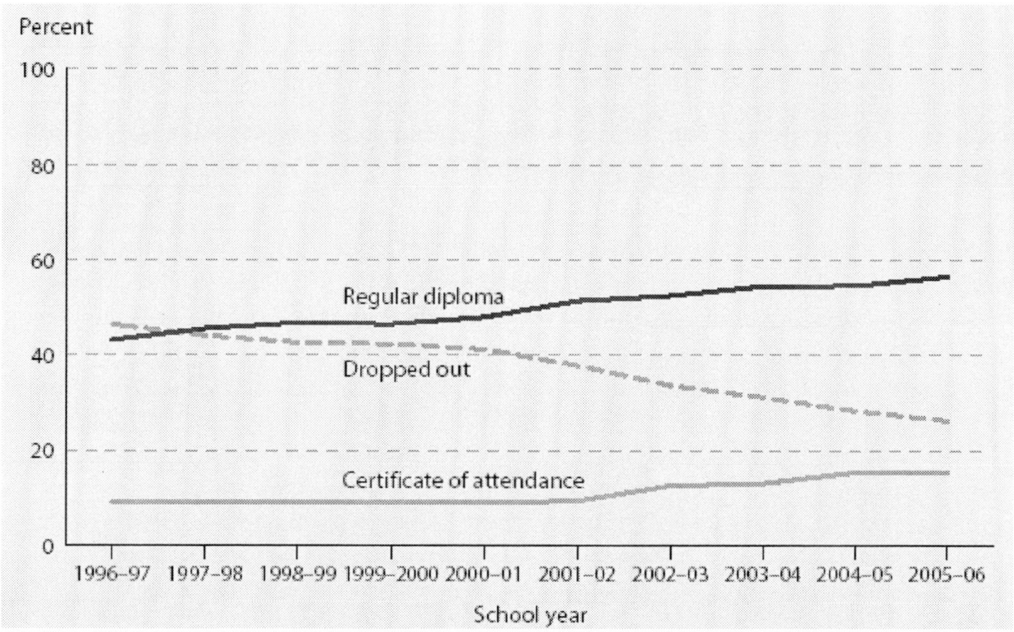

Note: Students who exited school by reaching the maximum age and those who died are not shown, but are included in the total. Special education services through the Individuals with Disabilities Education Act (IDEA) are available for eligible youth identified by a team of qualified professionals as having a disability that adversely affects their academic performance and as in need of special education and related services. The Office of Special Education Programs (OSEP) calculates the graduation rate by dividing the number of students age 14 or older who graduated with a regular high school diploma by the number of students in the same age group who are known to have left school (i.e., graduated with a regular high school diploma, received a certificate of completion, reached a maximum age for services, died, and are not known to be continuing in an education program or dropped out). See *supplemental note 8* for more information about the student disabilities presented here.

Source: U.S. Department of Education, Office of Special Education Programs (OSEP), Data Analysis System (DANS), *Children with Disabilities Exiting Special Education, 2005–06* (OMB #1820-0521). Retrieved November 28, 2007, from https://www. ideadata.org/arc_toc8.asp#partbEX.

STUDENTS WITH DISABILITIES EXITING SCHOOL WITH DIPLOMAS: Percentage of students ages 14–21 with disabilities served under Individuals with Disabilities Education Act (IDEA) (Part B) who exited school, by exit status: School years 1996–97 through 2005–06.

In 2005–06, students with disabilities in 29 states and the District of Columbia exited school with a regular high school diploma at a rate higher than the national rate of 57 percent for students with disabilities (see supplemental table 22-3). The percentage who exited high school with a regular diploma ranged from a high of 91 percent in the District of Columbia to a low of 21 percent in Nevada. In many states, a large percentage of students with disabilities exited with a certificate of attendance. In 14 states, the percentage of students with disabilities exiting with such a certificate was greater than the national average of 15 percent. For example, 54 percent of students with disabilities exiting school in Mississippi received a certificate of attendance.

STATUS DROPOUT RATES BY RACE/ETHNICITY

Status dropout rates for Whites, Blacks, and Hispanics ages 16–24 have each generally declined between 1972 and 2006. Over this time period, status dropout rates for Whites remained lower than rates for Hispanics and Blacks.

The *status dropout rate* represents the percentage of persons in an age group who are not enrolled in school and have not earned a high school diploma or equivalent credential, such as a General Educational Development (GED) certificate. For this indicator, status dropout rates are reported for 16- through 24-year-olds. The status dropout rate for this age group declined from 15 percent in 1972 to 9 percent in 2006 (see supplemental table 23-1). A decline was also seen between 2000 and 2006, the more recent years of this time span (11 to 9 percent).

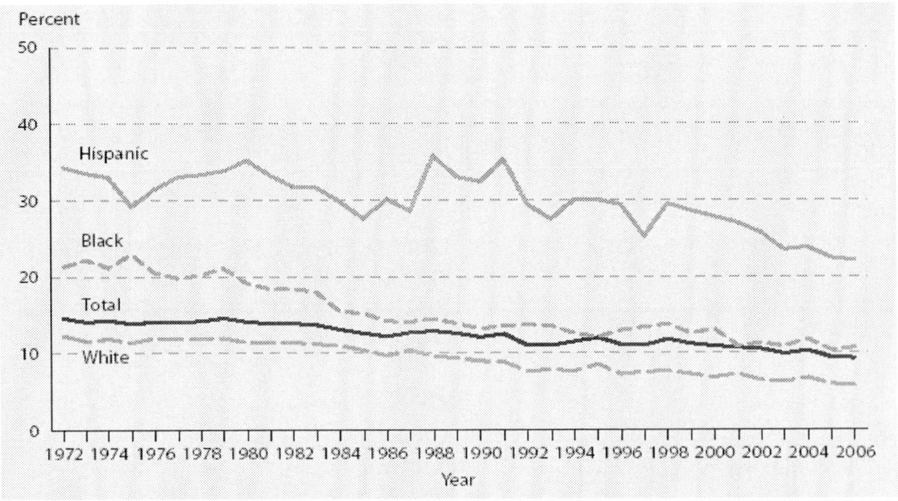

Note: The *status dropout rate* reported in this indicator is one of a number of rates measuring high school dropout and completion behavior in the United States. See *supplemental note 7* for more information about the rate reported here. Total includes other race/ethnicity categories not separately shown. Race categories exclude persons of Hispanic ethnicity.

Source: U.S. Department of Commerce, Census Bureau, Current Population Survey (CPS), October Supplement, 1972–2006.

STATUS DROPOUTS: Status dropout rates of 16- through 24-year-olds, by race/ethnicity: October 1972–2006

Status dropout rates and changes in these rates over time differ by race/ethnicity. In general, the status dropout rates for Whites, Blacks, and Hispanics each declined between 1972 and 2006. However, for each year between 1972 and 2006, the status dropout rate was lowest for Whites and highest for Hispanics. For example, in 2006, the status dropout rate for Whites was 6 percent, compared with 11 percent for Blacks and 22 percent for Hispanics. Although the gaps between the rates of Blacks and Whites and between the rates of Hispanics and Whites have decreased, the patterns have not been consistent. The Black-White gap narrowed during the 1980s, with no measurable change during the 1970s or between 1990 and 2006. In contrast, the Hispanic-White gap narrowed between 1990 and 2006, with no measurable change in the gap during the 1970s and 1980s.

In 2006, Hispanics who were born outside of the United States[20] represented 7 percent of the 16- through 24-year-old population and 28 percent of all status dropouts in this age group (see supplemental table 23-2). Higher dropout rates among these Hispanic immigrants partially account for the persistently high dropout rates for all Hispanic young adults. Among Hispanic 16- through 24-year-olds who were born outside the United States, the status dropout rate was 36 percent in 2006—triple the rates for both first-generation and second-generation or higher Hispanics in this age group (12 percent each). Yet, regardless of immigration status, greater percentages of Hispanics born in the United States were status dropouts than their non-Hispanic counterparts.

[20] The United States refers to the 50 states and the District of Columbia.

In: The Condition of Education in America
Editor: Maurice H. Logan
ISBN: 978-1-60692-298-9

Chapter 12

TRANSITION TO COLLEGE

IMMEDIATE TRANSITION TO COLLEGE

The rate of college enrollment immediately after high school completion increased from 49 percent in 1972 to 67 percent by 1997, but has since fluctuated between 62 and 69 percent.

The immediate college enrollment rate is defined as the percentage of all high school completers[21] ages 16–24 who enroll in college (2- or 4-year) in the fall immediately after high school. In most years between 1972 and 1980, this rate was approximately 50 percent. It subsequently increased to 67 percent by 1997 and then decreased to 62 percent by 2001. Since 2002, the rate has fluctuated between 64 and 69 percent (see supplemental table 24-1).

Differences were evident in the immediate college enrollment rate among racial/ethnic groups between 1972 and 2006. Although the enrollment rates increased overall during this period for both Whites and Blacks, the gap between the two has widened and narrowed at various times, resulting in no overall change in the gap. In 2006, the enrollment rate for Black high school completers was 13 percentage points lower than for their White counterparts (55 vs. 69 percent). For Hispanics, the immediate college enrollment rate has fluctuated over time, but increased overall between 1972 and 2006. Nonetheless, the gap between Hispanics and Whites has widened over this period. In 2006, the immediate college enrollment rate was 58 percent for Hispanics, compared with 69 percent for Whites.

From 1972 through 2006, the immediate enrollment rate of high school completers increased faster for females than for males (see supplemental table 24-2). Much of the growth in the overall rate for females was due to increases in the rate of attending 4-year institutions.

Differences in immediate enrollment rates by family income and parents' education have persisted. Despite an overall narrowing of the gap between students from low-income families and their peers from high-income families, the immediate college enrollment rate was higher for students from high-income families in each year between 1972 and 2006 (see supplemental table 24-1).[22] Likewise, compared with completers whose parents had a

[21] Refers to those who completed 12 years of school for survey years 1972–1991 and to those who earned a high school diploma or equivalent certifi cate such as a General Educational Development (GED) certifi cate for all years since 1992. See supplemental note 2 for more information.

[22] Low income refers to the bottom 20 percent of all family incomes, high income refers to the top 20 percent of all family incomes, and middle income refers to the 60 percent in between. See supplemental note 2 for further information.

bachelor's degree or higher, those whose parents had less education had lower rates of immediate college enrollment in each year between 1992 and 2006 (see supplemental table 24-3).[23]

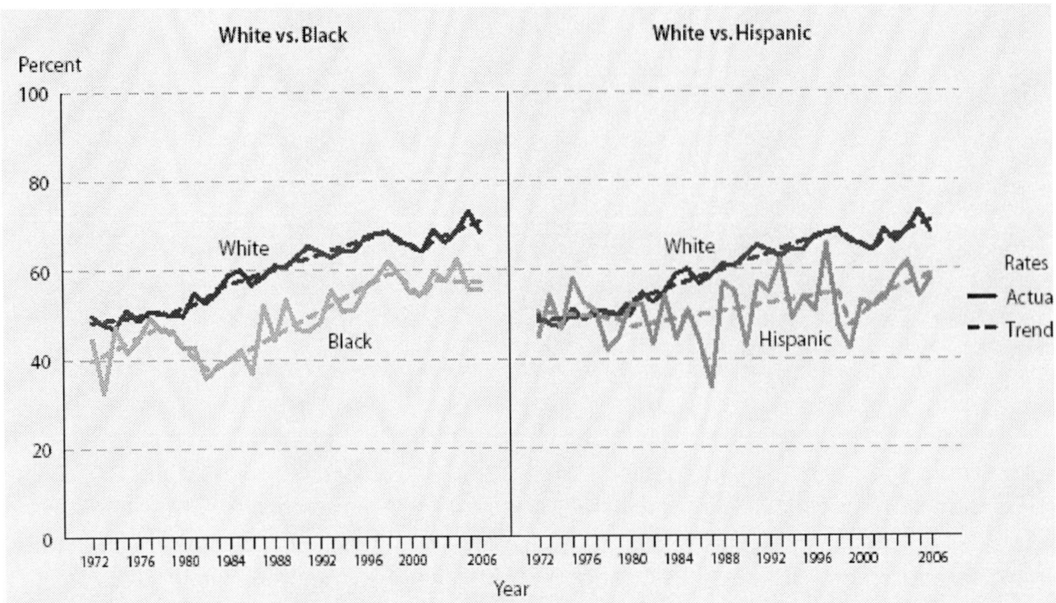

Note: Includes those ages 16–24 completing high school in a given year. Actual rates are annual estimates; trend rates show the linear trend of these annual values over the period shown. See *supplemental note 2* for further information. Race categories exclude persons of Hispanic ethnicity. The erratic nature of the Hispanic rate reflects, in part, the small sample size of Hispanic high school completers. Some estimates have been revised from previous publications.

Source: U.S. Department of Commerce, Census Bureau, Current Population Survey (CPS), October Supplement, 1972–2006.

COLLEGE ENROLLMENT RATES: Actual and trend rates of high school completers who were enrolled in college the October immediately following high school completion, by race/ethnicity: 1972–2006.

---

[23] The earliest year with comparable data available for parents' educational attainment is 1992.

In: The Condition of Education in America
Editor: Maurice H. Logan
ISBN: 978-1-60692-298-9

Chapter 13

COMPLETIONS

EDUCATIONAL ATTAINMENT

In 2007, some 87 percent of 25- to 29-year-olds had received a high school diploma or equivalency certificate. This rate has remained between 85 and 88 percent over the last 30 years.

In 2007, some 87 percent of 25- to 29-year-olds had received a high school diploma or equivalency certificate (see supplemental table 25-1).1 Although this percentage increased 7 percentage points between 1971 and 1976, the high school completion rate has remained between 85 and 88 percent over the last 30 years.

In 1971, a lower percentage of Blacks than Whites completed high school (59 vs. 82 percent). Between 1971 and 1982, the gap between Blacks and Whites decreased 15 percentage points to 8 percentage points, but since 1982 the gap has been between 4 and 10 percentage points. In 2007, the high school completion rate for Blacks was still below that of Whites (88 vs. 93 percent). The high school completion rate for Hispanics increased between 1971 and 2007 (48 vs. 65 percent). Unlike the gap between Blacks and Whites, the gap between Hispanics and Whites fluctuated but was not measurably different in 2007 than in 1971.

The rate at which 25- to 29-year-olds completed at least some college education increased from 34 to 58 percent between 1971 and 2007 (see supplemental table 25-2). However, increases in the rate were not consistent throughout this period. The rate increased during the 1970s, leveled off during the 1980s, and increased in the 1990s. Since the late 1990s, the rate has leveled off again. For each racial/ethnic group, the percentage completing at least some college was higher in 2007 than 1971. However, the rate of increase was lower for Hispanics than for Whites or Blacks. In 2007, about 66 percent of White 25- to 29-year-olds had completed at least some college, compared with 50 percent of their Black peers and 34 percent of their Hispanic peers.

HIGH SCHOOL: Percentage of 25- to 29-year-olds who completed high school, by race/ethnicity: March 1971–2007

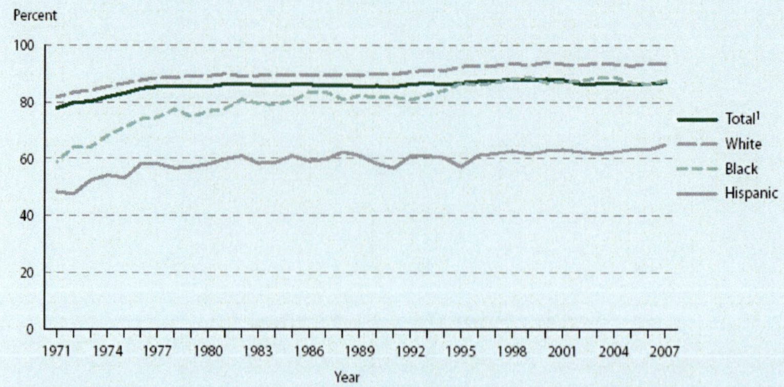

SOME COLLEGE: Percentage of 25- to 29-year-olds who completed at least some college, by race/ethnicity: March 1971–2007

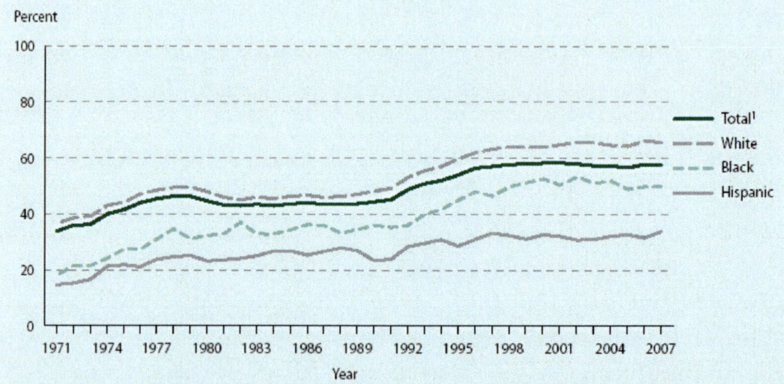

BACHELOR'S DEGREE OR HIGHER: Percentage of 25- to 29-year-olds with a bachelor's degree or higher, by race/ethnicity: March 1971–2007

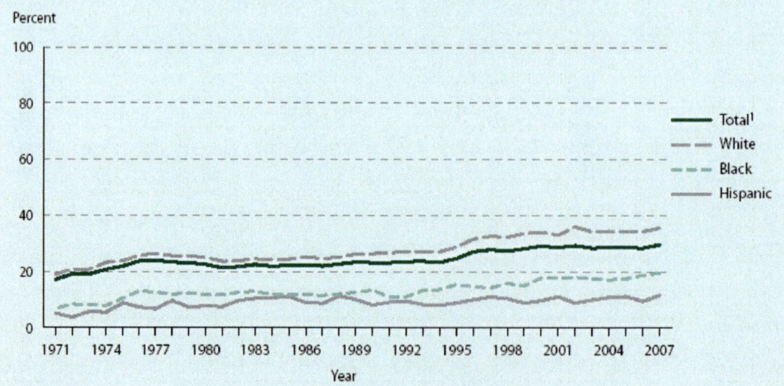

Note: This indicator uses March Current Population Survey (CPS) data to estimate the percentage of civilian, noninstitutionalized people ages 25 through 29 who are out of high school and who have earned a high school credential. Prior to 1992, *high school completers* referred to those who completed 12 years of schooling, and *some college* meant completing 1 or more years of college; beginning in 1992, *high school completers* referred to those who received a high school diploma or equivalency certificate, and *some college* meant completing any college at all. In 1994, the survey instrument for the CPS was changed and weights were adjusted. See *supplemental notes 2* and *7* for further discussion. Some estimates are revised from previous publications. Race categories exclude persons of Hispanic ethnicity.

Source: U.S. Department of Commerce, Census Bureau, Current Population Survey (CPS), March Supplement, 1971–2007.

In 2007, some 30 percent of 25- to 29-yearolds had completed a bachelor's degree or higher. In most years, about half as many 25- to 29-year-olds had completed a bachelor's degree or higher as had completed at least some college. Between 1971 and 1996, the percentage of 25- to 29-year-olds who had completed a bachelor's degree or higher increased from 17 to 27 percent (see supplemental table 25-3). Although this change represents an increase of 10 percentage points, the rate has remained between 27 and 30 percent since 1996. While the percentage of 25- to 29-year-olds with a bachelor's degree or higher increased for all three racial/ethnic groups, the gaps between Whites and their Black and Hispanic peers widened between 1971 and 2007.

Degrees Earned

Between 1995–96 and 2005–06, the number of associate's and bachelor's degrees earned by minority students grew at a faster rate than for White students.

Between 1995–96 and 2005–06, enrollments in postsecondary degree-granting institutions increased by 23 percent, from 14.3 million to 17.5 million students (NCES 2008-022, table 3). This growth in enrollment was accompanied by increases in the number of degrees earned, with the number of associate's degrees increasing by 28 percent, bachelor's degrees by 28 percent, master's degrees by 46 percent, first-professional degrees by 14 percent, and doctoral degrees by 26 percent (see supplemental table 26-1). For example, the annual number of bachelor's degrees earned increased from 1.2 million in 1995–96 to 1.5 million in 2005–06.

Between 1995–96 and 2005–06, the number of associate's degrees earned by minority students grew at a faster rate than for White students and accounted for over 60 percent of the increase in the total number of associate's degrees awarded (see supplemental table 26-2). While the number of bachelor's degrees earned by White students increased by 19 percent (from 905,800 to 1.1 million), the number of bachelor's degrees earned by minority students increased by 64 percent (from 221,300 to 363,300) and accounted for 44 percent of the total increase during this period. Minority students accounted for 37 percent of the increase in the number of master's degrees, 59 percent of the increase in the number of first-professional degrees, and 27 percent of the increase in the number of doctoral degrees awarded. Nonresident aliens (foreign students) accounted for 13 percent of the increase in the number of master's degrees awarded and 40 percent of the increase in doctoral degrees awarded. Despite slower growth, however, White students still earned the majority of each type of degree awarded in each year during this period. For example, Whites earned 72 percent of all bachelor's degrees in 2005–06, compared with 78 percent in 1995–96.

Among minority students, Blacks earned 10 percent each of all bachelor's and master's degrees awarded in 2005–06. From 1995–96 to 2005–06, Blacks accounted for 16 percent of the increase in the number of bachelor's degrees awarded and 18 percent of the increase in the number of master's degrees awarded. Asians earned 12 percent of all first-professional degrees awarded in 2005–06 and accounted for 37 percent of the increase in first-professional degrees awarded.

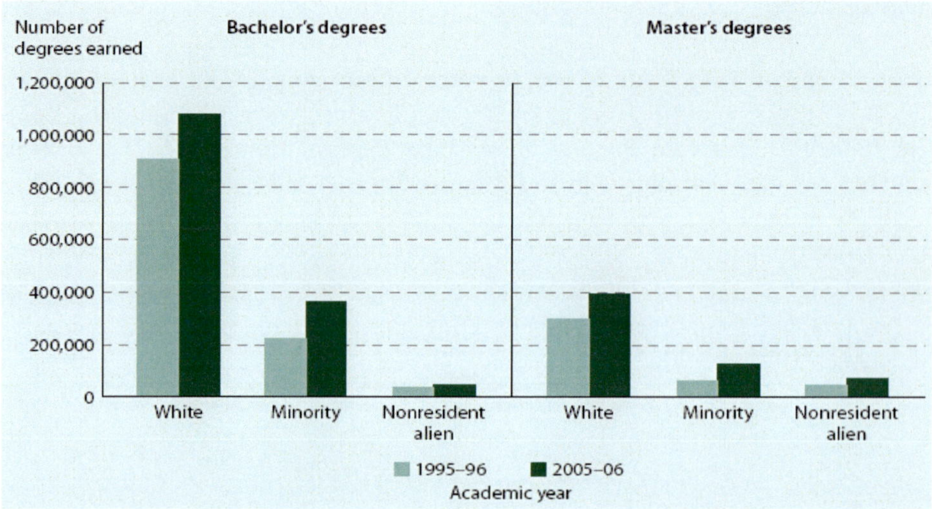

Note: Race categories exclude persons of Hispanic ethnicity. Nonresident aliens are shown separately because information about their race/ethnicity is not available. Detail may not sum to totals because of rounding. The contribution of growth is calculated as the increase in the number of degrees for a particular level divided by the increase in the total number of degrees.

Source: U.S. Department of Education, National Center for Education Statistics, 1995–96 Integrated Postsecondary Education Data System, "Completions Survey" (IPEDS-C:96), and Fall 2006.

DEGREES CONFERRED: Number of bachelor's and master's degrees earned by White, minority, and nonresident alien students: Academic years 1995–96 and 2005–06.

Degrees Earned by Women

Women have earned a greater percentage of bachelor's degrees than men since the early 1980s overall, but men still earn a greater percentage of degrees in some fields, including computer and information sciences and engineering.

From 1995–96 to 2005–06, the number of degrees earned by women grew at a faster rate than for men and accounted for over 65 percent of the increase in the total bachelor's and master's degrees awarded, and for nearly 85 percent of the increase in the total doctoral degrees awarded. At each degree level, degrees earned by women as a percentage of total degrees earned also increased during this time frame (see supplemental table 27-1). Though women have earned a greater number and percentage of bachelor's and master's degrees overall than men have since the early 1980s (NCES 2008-022, table 258), men continue to earn the majority of degrees at the doctoral level.

Women earned 58 percent of all bachelor's and 60 percent of all master's degrees awarded in 2005–06 (up from 55 and 56 percent, respectively, in 1995–96). During this period, the number of degrees earned by women increased by 33 percent at the bachelor's level (from 642,000 to 855,000) and by 57 percent at the master's level (from 227,000 to

356,000). The increase in education degrees earned by women accounted for 42 percent of the overall growth in master's degrees earned by women. Although women earned 50 percent of bachelor's and 43 percent of master's degrees in business in 2005–06, the increase in degrees in this field contributed to over 20 percent of the total growth in degrees earned by women at both levels from 1995–96 to 2005–06. Women earned over 75 percent of bachelor's and master's degrees awarded in health professions, education, and psychology in 2005–06, but less than 30 percent of degrees awarded in computer and information sciences and in engineering at both levels.

Overall, women earned 49 percent of doctoral degrees awarded in 2005–06 (up from 40 percent in 1995–96). During this period, doctoral degrees earned by women increased by 54 percent (from 17,800 to 27,400). Increases in the number of degrees earned in health professions accounted for over 40 percent of the overall growth in doctoral degrees earned by women. In 2005–06, women earned less than 40 percent of doctoral degrees awarded in business, physical sciences, mathematics and statistics, computer and information sciences, and engineering. In contrast, women earned over 70 percent of doctoral degrees in psychology and health professions that year.

Field of study	1990–91	1995–96	2005–06	Change in percentage points between 1995–96 and 2005–06
Total[1]	53.9	55.1	57.5	2.4
Health professions and related clinical sciences	83.9	81.5	86.0	4.5
Education	78.9	75.1	79.1	3.9
Psychology	72.6	73.0	77.5	4.5
English language and literature/letters	66.9	65.9	68.6	2.6
Communication, journalism, and related programs	60.8	58.8	63.4	4.7
Biological and biomedical sciences	50.8	52.6	61.5	8.9
Visual and performing arts	62.6	59.2	61.4	2.3
Social sciences and history	45.1	47.9	50.0	2.0
Business	47.2	48.6	49.8	1.2
Agriculture and natural resources	32.7	36.8	47.7	10.8
Mathematics and statistics	47.3	46.1	45.1	-1.1
Physical sciences and science technologies	31.6	36.0	41.8	5.8
Computer and information sciences and support services	29.4	27.5	20.6	-7.0
Engineering and engineering technologies	14.1	16.2	17.9	1.7

[1] Includes other fields not shown separately.

Source: U.S. Department of Education, National Center for Education Statistics (NCES). *Digest of Education Statistics, 2007* (NCES 2008-022), tables 258, 286, 288, 290–294, 296, 299–301, 303, 305, and 307, data from U.S. Department of Education, NCES, 1979–80 Higher Education General Information Survey (HEGIS), "Degrees and Other Formal Awards Conferred" and 1990–91, 1995–96, and 2005–06 Integrated Postsecondary Education Data System, "Completions Survey" (IPEDS-C:91 and 96), and IPEDS, Fall 2006.

BACHELOR'S DEGREES: Percentage of bachelor's degrees women earned and change in the percentage of degrees women earned, by field of study: Academic years 1990–91, 1995–96, and 2005–06.

SECTION 4. CONTEXTS OF ELEMENTARY AND SECONDARY EDUCATION

In: The Condition of Education in America
Editor: Maurice H. Logan
ISBN: 978-1-60692-298-9

Chapter 14

INTRODUCTION

	Indicator–Year
School Characteristics and Climate	
Size of High Schools	30–2003
Student Perceptions of Their School's Social and Learning Environment	29–2005
Parents' Attitudes Toward Schools	38–2006
Rates of School Crime	36–2007
School Violence and Safety	28–2008
Poverty Concentration in Public Schools by Locale and Race/Ethnicity	29–2008
Concentration of Public School Enrollment by Locale and Race/Ethnicity	30–2008
Teachers and Staff	
Characteristics of School Principals	34–2007
Characteristics of Full-Time School Teachers	33–2007
Beginning Teachers	29–2003
Elementary/Secondary School Teaching Among Recent College Graduates	37–2006
Teacher Turnover	31–2008
Public School Staff	32–2008
Student Support Staff in Public Schools	35–2007
High School Guidance Counseling	27–2004
Learning Opportunities	
Early Development of Children	35–2005
Early Literacy Activities	33–2006
Care Arrangements for Children After School	33–2004
Afterschool Activities	29–2007
Availability of Advanced Courses in High Schools	25–2005
Student/Teacher Ratios in Public Elementary and Secondary Schools	33–2008
Out-of-Field Teaching in Middle and High School Grades	28–2003
Out-of-Field Teaching by Poverty Concentration and Minority Enrollment	24–2004
Special Programs	
Public Alternative Schools for At-Risk Students	27–2003
Inclusion of Students With Disabilities in General Classrooms	31–2007
School Choice	
Charter Schools	32–2007
Parental Choice of Schools	36–2006
Profile and Demographic Characteristics of Public Charter Schools	28–2005
Finance	Indicator–Year
Changes in Sources of Public School Revenue	34–2008
Public Elementary and Secondary Expenditures by Type and Function	35–2008
Variations in Instruction Expenditures per Student	36–2008
Public Elementary and Secondary Expenditures by District Poverty	37–2008
Public Elementary and Secondary Expenditures by District Location	35–2004
Public Effort to Fund Elementary and Secondary Education	39–2005
International Comparisons of Expenditures for Education	38–2008

The indicators in this section of *The Condition of Education* measure features of the context of learning in elementary and secondary schools. This includes the content of learning and expectations for student performance; processes of instruction; mechanisms of choice in education; characteristics of teachers and the teaching profession; the climate for learning and other organizational aspects of schools; and financial resources. There are 35 indicators in this section: 11, prepared for this year's volume, appear on the following pages, and all 35, including indicators from previous years, appear on the Web (see Website Contents on the facing page for a full list of the indicators).

The first subsection considers the climate for learning, which is shaped by different factors in the school environment, including parent, teacher, and student attitudes; the concentration of poverty and racial/ethnic groups in schools; and schools' physical security and freedom from violence. Indicators in this volume present measures of these last three factors, while the Web displays indicators for the full subsection.

The indicators in the second subsection look at teachers and school staff. One indicator in this volume examines the nature of teacher attrition by various individual and professional characteristics. Other indicators on the Web examine the characteristics of principals, beginning teachers, and guidance counselors.

The third subsection focuses on learning opportunities afforded children. One indicator in this volume measures student/teacher ratios in public schools. Additional indicators on the Web highlight the availability of advanced-level academic courses, participation in early literacy activities, and afterschool activities.

Subsection four looks at special programs that serve the particular educational needs of special populations. Indicators appearing on the Web examine the extent to which students with disabilities are included in regular classrooms for instructional purposes and the characteristics of public alternative schools for at-risk students.

School choice provides parents with the opportunity to choose a school for their children beyond the assigned public school. Parents may choose a private school, they may live in a district that offers choice among public schools, or they may select a school by moving into that school's community. Indicators in the school choice subsection on the Web examine parental choice of charter schools and profile the characteristics of public charter schools.

The final subsection details financial support for education. Fundamentally, these financial sources of support are either private, in which individuals decide how much they are willing to pay for education, or public, in which case funding decisions are made by citizens through their governments. In this subsection of *The Condition of Education*, the primary focus is on describing the forms and amounts of financial support to education from public and private sources, how those funds are distributed among different types of schools, and on what they are spent. Among the indicators in this volume of *The Condition of Education* are indicators on variations in expenditures per student and trends in expenditures per student in elementary and secondary education.

The indicators on contexts of elementary and secondary schooling from previous editions of *The Condition of Education*, which are not included in this volume, are available at http://nces.ed.gov/programs/coe/list/i4.asp.

In: The Condition of Education in America
Editor: Maurice H. Logan
ISBN: 978-1-60692-298-9

Chapter 15

SCHOOL CHARACTERISTICS AND CLIMATE

SCHOOL VIOLENCE AND SAFETY

During the 2005–06 school year, 17 percent of public schools experienced at least one serious violent incident at school.

In the School Survey on Crime and Safety, public school principals were asked to provide the number of violent incidents,1 thefts of items valued at $10 or greater,2 and other incidents3 that occurred at their school, as well as the number of these incidents reported to the police. During the 2005–06 school year, 86 percent of public schools indicated that one or more incidents had taken place at school (see supplemental table 28-1). During the same year, 61 percent of schools reported at least one incident to the police.

In the 2005–06 school year, 78 percent of public schools experienced one or more violent incidents, 17 percent experienced one or more serious violent incidents, 46 percent experienced one or more thefts, and 68 percent experienced one or more of other types of incidents. Thirty-eight percent of public schools reported at least one violent incident to the police, 13 percent reported at least one serious violent incident to the police, 28 percent reported at least one theft to the police, and 51 percent reported at least one of the other specified incidents to the police.

The percentage of schools experiencing at least one violent incident was lower in 2005–06 than in 2003–04 (78 vs. 81 percent), but the percentage of schools experiencing violent incidents was lowest in 1999–2000 (71 percent). While the percentage of schools reporting at least one violent incident to the police was not measurably different in 2005–06 than in 1999–2000 (38 vs. 36 percent), a larger percentage of schools reported at least one violent incident to the police in 2003–04 (44 percent) than in 1999–2000 or 2005–06.

The prevalence of violent incidents at public schools varied by school level. A smaller percentage of primary schools (67 percent) than middle schools (94 percent) or high schools (95 percent) experienced a violent incident in 2005–06 (see supplemental table 28-2).

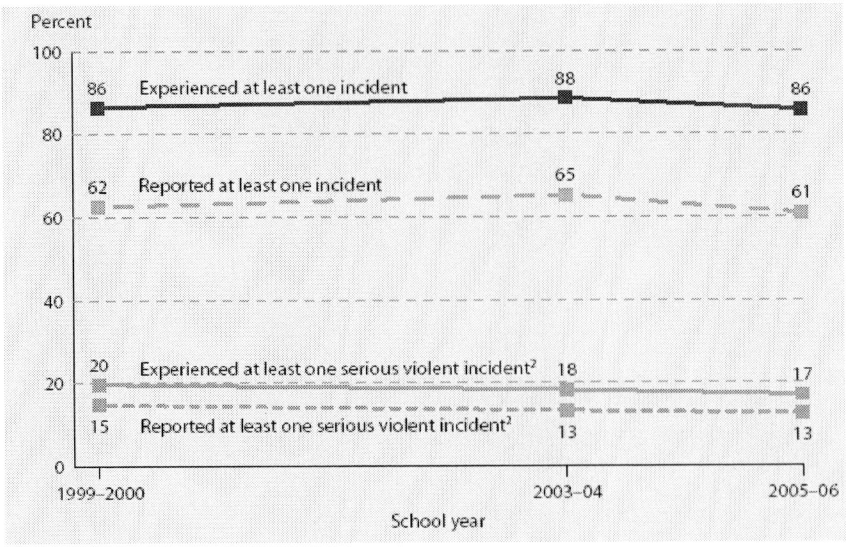

Note: "At school" was defined for respondents to include activities that happen in school buildings, on school grounds, on school buses, and at places that hold school-sponsored events or activities. Respondents were instructed to respond only for those times that were during normal school hours or when school activities or events were in session. Reported crimes are computed by dividing the number of public schools that reported crimes to the police by all public schools, including those that did not report experiencing crime. For more information, please see *supplemental note 3*.

Source: U.S. Department of Education, National Center for Education Statistics, 1999–2000, 2003–04, and 2005–06 School Survey on Crime and Safety (SSOCS), 2000, 2004, and 2006.

SCHOOL VIOLENCE AND SAFETY: Percentage of public schools experiencing at least one incident and reporting at least one incident that occurred at school to the police, by selected incidents: School years 1999–2000, 2003–04, and 2005–06.

Poverty Concentration in Public Schools by Locale and Race/Ethnicity

Larger percentages of Black, Hispanic, and American Indian/Alaska Native students attended high-poverty schools than White or Asian/Pacific Islander students in 2005–06.

The percentage of students eligible for the free or reduced-price lunch program provides a proxy measure for the concentration of low-income students within a school. For the purpose of this indicator, high-poverty schools are defined as public schools with more than 75 percent of students eligible for free or reducedprice lunch.[24] In 2005–06, approximately 15 percent of all elementary and secondary public school students (or 7.1 million students) attended high-poverty schools (see supplemental table 29-1).

Nationally, larger percentages of Black, Hispanic, and American Indian/Alaska Native students attended high-poverty schools than did White or Asian/Pacific Islander students in 2005–06, and higher percentages of Asian/Pacific Islander than White students attended these schools. Some 32 percent of Black, 34 percent of Hispanic, and 24 percent of American

[24] Private school students are excluded because large proportions of private schools do not participate in the free or reduced-price lunch program.

Indian/Alaska Native students were enrolled in high-poverty schools, compared with 4 percent of White and 10 percent of Asian/Pacific Islander students. In contrast, nationally, larger percentages of White (19 percent) and Asian/Pacific Islander (24 percent) students attended low-poverty schools (public schools with 10 percent or less of students eligible for free or reduced-price lunch) than did Black (4 percent), Hispanic (7 percent), and American Indian/ Alaska Native (5 percent) students.

Overall, a similar pattern existed among racial/ethnic groups within different school locales. In each locale (cities, suburban areas, towns, and rural areas), higher percentages of Black, Hispanic, and American Indian/Alaska Native students attended high-poverty schools than did their White and Asian/Pacific Islander peers in 2005–06. Among students attending city schools, for example, 44 percent of Blacks, 46 percent of Hispanics, and 27 percent of American Indians/Alaska Natives attended high-poverty schools, compared with 9 percent of Whites and 17 percent of Asians/Pacific Islanders. In rural areas, higher percentages of Black (25 percent), Hispanic (21 percent), and American Indian/Alaska Native (33 percent) students attended high-poverty schools than did their White and Asian/Pacific Islander (4 percent for both) peers.

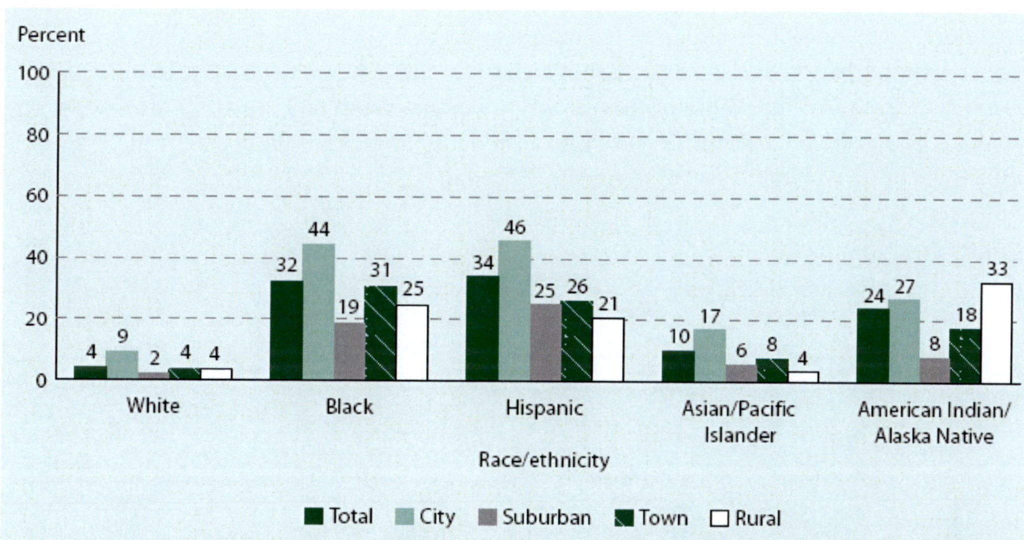

Note: Figure represents percentages of students in public schools with more than 75 percent of students eligible for free or reduced-price lunch. The National School Lunch Program is a federally assisted meal program. To be eligible, a student must be from a household with an income at or below 130 percent of the poverty threshold for free lunch or between 130 percent and 185 percent of the poverty threshold for reduced-price lunch. Approximately 10,745 public schools (or 11 percent) did not report information on the number of students eligible for free or reducedprice school lunch. For details on Census-defined areas and poverty thresholds, see *supplemental note 1*. Race categories exclude persons of Hispanic ethnicity.

Source: U.S. Department of Education, National Center for Education Statistics, Common Core of Data (CCD), "Public Elementary/Secondary School Universe Survey," 2005–06.

POVERTY CONCENTRATION: Percentage of public elementary and secondary school students in high-poverty schools, by race/ethnicity and locale: School year 2005–06.

Concentration of Public School Enrollment by Locale and Race/Ethnicity

In 2005–06, larger percentages of Black and Hispanic public school students attended schools with high minority enrollments than White, American Indian/Alaska Native, and Asian/Pacific Islander public school students.

In 2005–06, public schools with high minority enrollments (defined as schools in which 75 percent or more of the students were Black, Hispanic, Asian/Pacific Islander, or American Indian/Alaska Native) enrolled 23 percent of all public elementary and secondary students (see supplemental table 30-1). However, about half of all Hispanic (56 percent) and Black (50 percent) students attended such schools—larger percentages than Asian/Pacific Islander (31 percent), American Indian/Alaska Native (29 percent), or White (3 percent) students at such schools.

The percentage of students in schools with high minority enrollments varied across school locales in 2005–06, with a larger percentage of public school students in cities (45 percent) attending such schools than in suburban areas (20 percent), towns (10 percent), or rural areas (7 percent). In cities, greater percentages of Hispanic and Black students attended such schools than did Asian/Pacific Islander, American Indian/Alaska Native, and White students. In suburban areas and towns, however, a greater percentage of Hispanic students attended such schools than did students of any other race/ethnicity. In rural areas, a greater percentage of American Indian/Alaska Native students attended schools with high minority enrollments than did students of any other race/ethnicity.

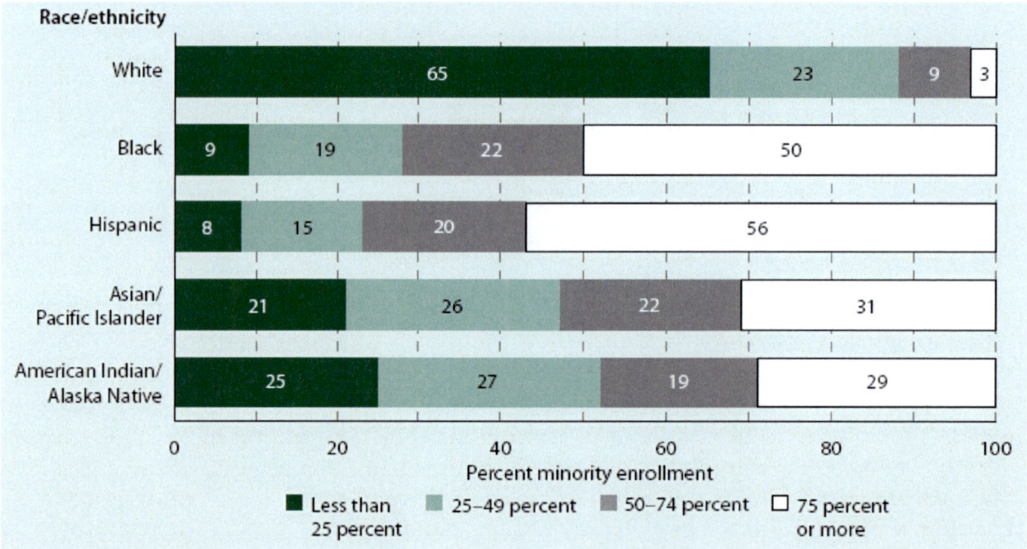

Note: Minority enrollment includes Black, Hispanic, Asian/Pacific Islander, and American Indian/Alaska Native students. Race categories exclude persons of Hispanic ethnicity. Detail may not sum to totals because of rounding.

Source: U.S. Department of Education, National Center for Education Statistics, Common Core of Data (CCD),"Public Elementary/Secondary School Universe Survey," 2005–06.

MINORITY CONCENTRATION: Percentage distribution of public elementary and secondary school students of each racial/ethnic group, by percent minority enrollment in school: School year 2005–06.

Examining the concentration of specific racial/ethnic groups provides a more detailed snapshot of the extent to which students are in racially and ethnically diverse schools. Nationally, public schools in which 75 percent or more of the students were Black enrolled 31 percent of all Black students and less than 1 percent of students of each other race/ethnicity in 2005–06 (see supplemental table 30-2). Public schools in which 75 percent or more of the students were Hispanic enrolled 33 percent of Hispanic public school students, 3 percent of Asian/Pacific Islander public school students, and 2 percent or less of public school students of each other race/ethnicity (see supplemental table 30-3). Public schools in which 75 percent or more of the students were White enrolled 64 percent of White public school students, 24 percent of American Indian/Alaska Native, 20 percent of Asian/Pacific Islander, 9 percent of Black, and 8 percent of Hispanic public school students (see supplemental table 30-4).

In: The Condition of Education in America
Editor: Maurice H. Logan

ISBN: 978-1-60692-298-9

Chapter 16

TEACHERS AND STAFF

TEACHER TURNOVER

Teacher turnover is higher in high-poverty than in low-poverty public schools.

At the end of the 2003–04 school year, 17 percent of the elementary and secondary teacher workforce (or 621,000 teachers) left the public and private schools where they had been teaching (see supplemental tables 31-1 and 31-2). Almost half of this teacher turnover was due to transfers: 8 percent of the teacher workforce (or 289,000 teachers) transferred to a different school. The remainder (9 percent of the teacher workforce or 333,000 teachers) was due to teachers who left teaching: teachers who took a job in a field other than elementary or secondary teaching (4 percent), returned to school for further education (0.3 percent), left for family reasons (e.g., to raise children or take care of other family members) (1 percent), retired (2 percent), and left for miscellaneous "other"[25] reasons (1 percent).

The percentage of teacher turnover at the end of 2003–04 was larger than at the end of 1987–88, 1990–91, and 1993–94 but was not measurably different from that at the end of 1999–2000. This relative increase in turnover from earlier years was not due to changes in the percentages of teachers who transferred, pursued further education, or left for family reasons: the percentages of teachers in these categories at the end of 2003–04 were not measurably different from the earlier school years. Virtually all of this relative increase was due to increases in the percentages of teachers who retired (which was greater at the end of 2003–04 than 1987–88, 1990–91, or 1993–94) and teachers who took another job or left teaching for miscellaneous other reasons (both of which were greater at the end of 2003–04 than 1987–88 or 1990–91).

In public schools, the turnover rate for highpoverty schools was greater than for low-poverty schools at the end of 2003–04 (21 vs. 14 percent) (see supplemental table 31-3). Schools were considered high poverty if 75 percent or more of their students were eligible for free or reduced-price lunch, and low poverty if less than 15 percent of their students were

---

[25] Leavers in this category left teaching for a variety of personal reasons, ranging from "starting their own business" to becoming "a member of a contemplative religious community." However, the most common reason reported by leavers who left for "other" reasons was to take a year-long sabbatical or leave of absence from teaching.

eligible.[26] Much of the difference between the two turnover rates is due to the higher transfer rate among teachers in high- versus low-poverty schools (11 vs. 6 percent). This same difference in transfer rates was observed for teachers in high- and low-poverty schools in 1991–92, 1993–94, and 1999–2000, but no difference was measurable in 1987–88.[27]

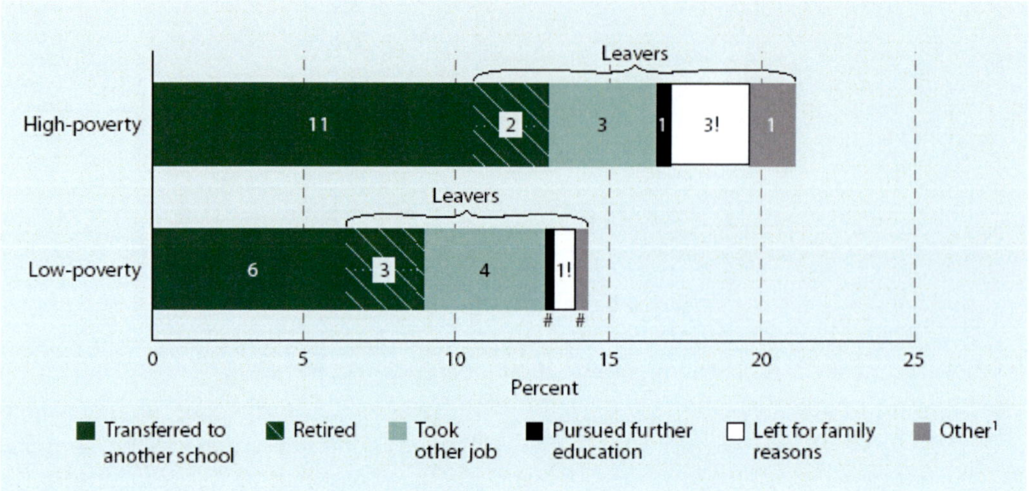

Note: Figure created from unrounded data. Detail may not sum to totals because of rounding.

Source: U.S. Department of Education, National Center for Education Statistics, Schools and Staffing Survey (SASS), "Public School Data File," 2003–04, and Teacher Follow-up Survey (TFS), "Current Teacher Data File" and "Former Teacher Data File," 2004–05.

TEACHER TURNOVER: Percentage of 2003–04 public K–12 teachers who did not teach in the same school the following school year, by poverty level of school and the reason teachers left.

PUBLIC SCHOOL STAFF

In 2003–04, professional instructional staff accounted for 64 percent of public school staff, with teachers making up the majority of all staff.

In 2003–04, public schools employed over 5.5 million staff (see supplemental table 32-1).[28] Of these staff, 2.8 million were employed by elementary schools, 1.4 million by secondary schools, and 950,000 by middle schools. Professional instructional staff[29] accounted for 64 percent of public school staff, with teachers making up 57 percent of all

---

[26] Poverty differences in private schools are not examined because a large proportion of private schools do not participate in the free or reducedprice lunch program. Public schools for which data are missing or that do not participate in the program were excluded.

[27] High- and low-poverty schools can only be identifi ed in 1990–91 based on the percentage of students who receive free or reduced-price lunches and not on the percentage eligible to receive free or reduced-price lunches.

[28] Data are for full- and part-time staff. Not all schools have each type of staff member. Fulltime-equivalent calculations were completed for part-time staff within each staff category.

[29] Professional instructional staff include principals, teachers, instructional coordinators and supervisors, librarians/library media specialists, and school counselors.

staff. Student services professional staff[30] and school aides accounted for 5 and 13 percent of public school staff, respectively.

The average number of students per staff member varied by staff type and by school characteristics (see supplemental table 32-2).[31] In terms of school enrollment size, the average number of students per staff member was consistently higher for larger schools than for smaller schools. This finding held for all staff except school counselors. For example, for social workers and psychologists, there was an average of 156 students per staff member in schools with less than 300 students, compared with an average of 1,106 students per staff member in schools with 1,500 or more students.

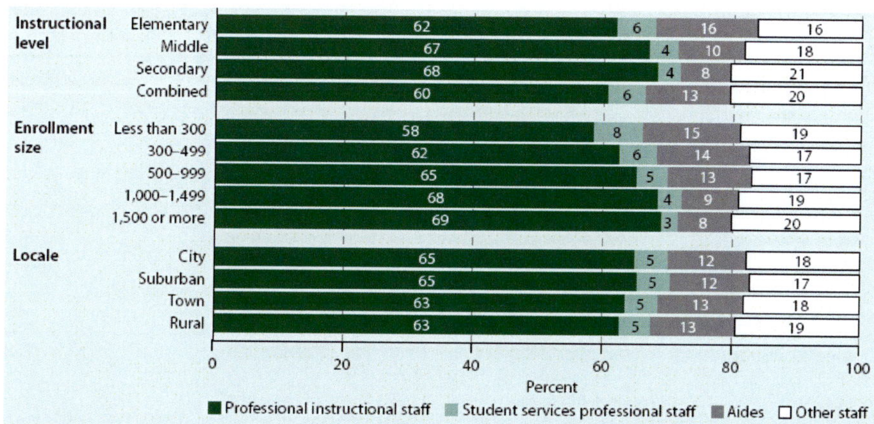

Note: Elementary schools are defined as schools with at least one grade lower than 5 and no grade higher than 8. Middle schools are defined as schools with no grade lower than 5 and no grade higher than 8. Secondary schools are defined as schools with no grade lower than 7 and at least one grade higher than 8. Combined schools have at least one grade lower than 7 and at least one grade higher than 8; schools with only ungraded classes are also included in combined schools. Detail may not sum to totals because of rounding. See *supplemental note 3* for more information on The Schools And Staffing Survey (SASS).

Source: U.S. Department of Education, National Center for Education Statistics, Schools and Staffing Survey (SASS), "Public School Data File," 2003–04.

PUBLIC SCHOOL STAFF: Percentage distribution of staff employed in public schools, by instructional level, enrollment size, and locale: School year 2003–04.

In contrast with patterns for enrollment size, the average number of students per staff member was generally lower for schools with larger percentages of students approved for free or reduced-price lunch than for schools with smaller percentages of students approved for this benefit. This finding held for principals, nurses, social workers and psychologists, speech therapists, other professional staff, special needs aides, and other aides.[32] For example, on average, there were 669 students per speech therapist in schools with 10 percent or fewer students approved for free or reduced-price lunch, compared with 512 students per speech therapist in schools with more than 75 percent of students approved for this benefit.

---

[30] Student services professional staff include nurses, social workers and psychologists, speech therapists, and other professional staff.

[31] Data for each staff category are derived from schools with staff members in those categories.

[32] Other aides include regular Title I aides, library media center instructional and noninstructional aides, and other classroom instructional and noninstructional aides.

Differences in the average number of students per staff member were also found by school locale. Schools in rural areas generally had lower average numbers of students per staff member than did schools in other locales for principals, teachers, librarians/library media specialists, school counselors, nurses, social workers and psychologists, speech therapists, and other aides. For example, for nurses, rural schools had an average of 481 students per staff member, compared with 563 in towns, 688 in suburban areas, and 685 in cities.

In: The Condition of Education in America
Editor: Maurice H. Logan

ISBN: 978-1-60692-298-9

Chapter 17

LEARNING OPPORTUNITIES

STUDENT/TEACHER RATIOS IN PUBLIC ELEMENTARY AND SECONDARY SCHOOLS

Student/teacher ratios tend to be higher in public schools with larger enrollments than in public schools with smaller enrollments.

The ratio of students to teachers, which is sometimes used as a proxy measure for class size, declined between 1990 and 2005 from 17.6 to 16.1 students per teacher for all regular[33] schools (see supplemental table 33-1). This pattern changes, however, when public elementary, secondary, and combined schools are examined separately.

The student/teacher ratio for regular public elementary schools declined from 1990 through 2005 (from 18.2 to 15.8), with most of the decline occurring after 1996. Generally, elementary schools in each enrollment category showed similar patterns except in the largest schools (1,500 students or more), where the student/teacher ratio fluctuated between 19.6 and 21.2 over this period.

In contrast, student/teacher ratios for all regular public secondary schools increased between 1990 and 1996 (from 16.7 to 17.6) and then declined to 16.8 in 2005. Secondary schools in each enrollment category showed similar patterns.

In regular public combined schools (schools that include both elementary and secondary grades), student/teacher ratios were lower in 2005 (15.3) than in 1990 (15.8). This pattern varied by the school enrollment: the student/teacher ratio for the largest enrollment category was higher in 2005 than in 1990, the student/ teacher ratios for the middle three enrollment categories were lower in 2005 than in 1990, and the student/teacher ratio for the smallest enrollment category was of similar magnitude in 2005 and 1990 (11.1 versus 11.0).

In every year from 1990 through 2005, the student/teacher ratio was positively associated with the enrollment for elementary, secondary, and combined regular public schools: the student/teacher ratio for any given enrollment category was always larger than that of any smaller enrollment category. For example, in 2005, regular secondary schools with 1,500 students or more enrolled 6.6 more students per teacher, on average, than regular secondary schools with enrollments under 300.

---

[33] Regular schools include all schools except special education schools, vocational schools, and alternative schools. Charter schools can be of any school type.

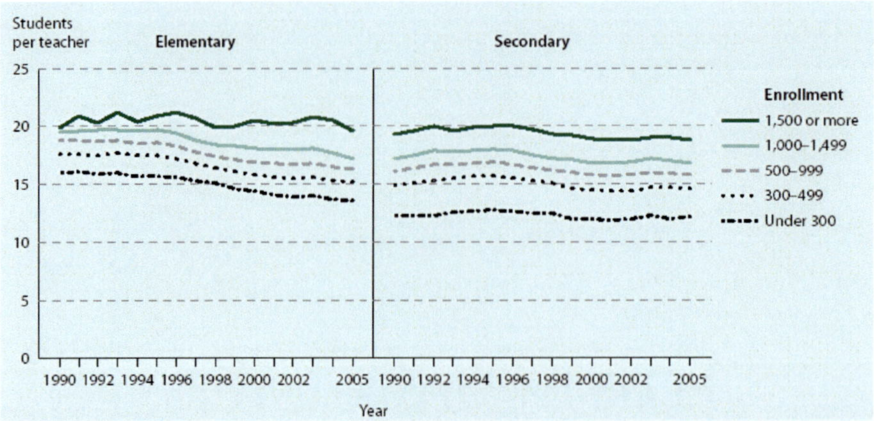

Note: Student/teacher ratios do not provide a direct measure of class size. The ratio is determined by dividing the total number of fulltime- equivalent teachers into the total student enrollment. These teachers include classroom teachers; prekindergarten teachers in some elementary schools; art, music, and physical education teachers; and teachers who do not teach regular classes every period of the day. This analysis excludes schools that did not report both enrollment and teacher data.

Source: U.S. Department of Education, National Center for Education Statistics, Common Core of Data (CCD), "Public Elementary/Secondary School Universe Survey," 1990–91 through 2005–06.

STUDENT/TEACHER RATIO: Student/teacher ratios in regular public elementary and secondary schools, by school level and enrollment: Fall 1990–2005.

In: The Condition of Education in America
Editor: Maurice H. Logan

ISBN: 978-1-60692-298-9

Chapter 18

FINANCE

CHANGES IN SOURCES OF PUBLIC SCHOOL REVENUE

Federal, state, and local revenues all increased from 1989–90 to 2004–05, though at different rates.

From 1989–90 to 2004–05, total elementary and secondary public school revenues increased 55 percent in constant dollars. During this period, the total amount from each revenue source (federal, state, and local) increased, though not at the same rate (see supplemental table 34-1). Federal and state revenues increased at a faster rate than all local revenues (both property tax revenue and other local revenue). Federal revenue increased 134 percent, compared with an increase of 54 percent for state revenue and 45 percent for local revenue. The total amount of revenue from each revenue source increased in each region as well.

The percentage of total revenue for public elementary and secondary education from local sources declined, from 47 percent in 1989–90 to 44 percent in 2004–05, while the percentage of total revenue flowing to public schools from federal sources increased from 6 percent in 1989–90 to 9 percent in 2004–05 (see supplemental table 34-2). The percentage from state sources was the same in 1989–90 as in 2004–05 (47 percent).

In each region, as in the nation, state and local sources were the two largest sources of revenue in 2004–05. There were, however, differences in the percentages contributed by these two revenue sources in the four regions. In the Northeast, a majority of all revenue was from local sources (52 percent) in 2004–05. Another 42 percent was from state sources. In the Midwest, about the same percentage of revenue was from local sources (45 percent) as from state sources (46 percent) in 2004–05. In the South, as in the Midwest, about the same percentage of revenue came from state sources (44 percent) and local sources (45 percent) in 2004–05. In the West, a majority of revenue was from state sources (56 percent) in 2004–05, with 33 percent from local sources.

The percentage of revenue from federal sources increased in each region from 1989–90 to 2004–05. In 2004–05, the percentage of revenue from federal sources ranged from about 7 percent in the Northeast and 8 percent in the Midwest to 11 percent in the South and West.

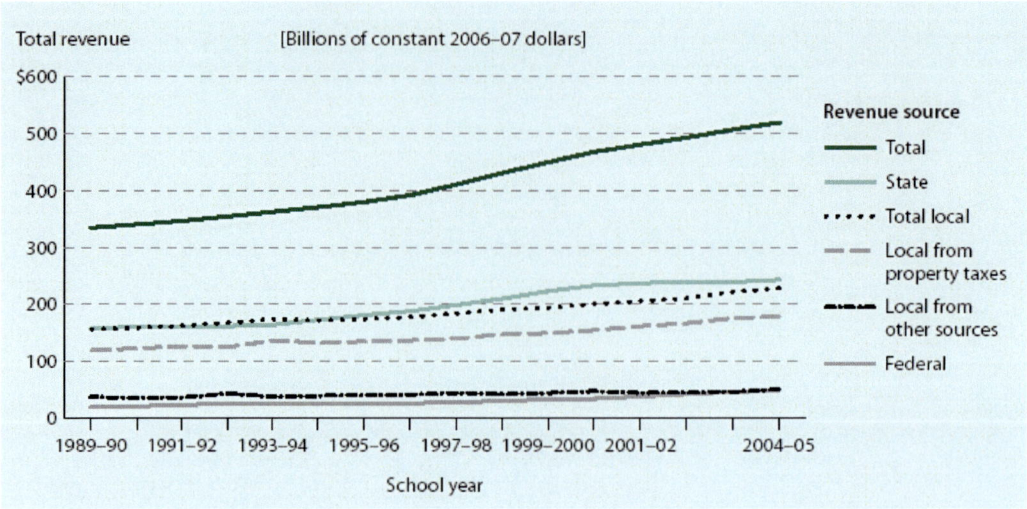

Note: Other local government revenue includes revenue from such sources as local nonproperty taxes, investments, and revenue from student activities, textbook sales, transportation and tuition fees, and food services. Property tax revenue and other local government revenues were imputed for Texas for 1992–93. See *supplemental note 11* for information about revenue for public elementary and secondary schools. Estimates are revised from previous publications.

Source: U.S. Department of Education, National Center of Education Statistics, Common Core of Data (CCD), "National Public Education Financial Survey," 1989–90 to 2004–05.

REVENUES BY SOURCE: Total revenue for public elementary and secondary schools, by revenue source: School years 1989–90 to 2004–05.

Public Elementary and Secondary Expenditures by Type and Function

The percentage of current expenditures spent on salaries declined 4 percentage points from 1989–90 to 2004–05, from 66 to 62 percent. During this period, the percentage spent on employee benefits increased 3 percentage points.

Total expenditures per student rose 29 percent in constant dollars between 1989–90 and 2004–05, from $8,437 to $10,892 (see supplemental table 35-1). This rate of increase in total expenditures was not evenly distributed among the types of expenditures. Spending on interest on school debt increased the most (94 percent), followed by capital outlays (66 percent), other total expenditures[34] (41 percent), and current expenditures (24 percent).

Among the functions of current expenditures, spending on student and staff support increased the most (48 percent), followed by instruction (26 percent) and transportation (20 percent). Spending on three other functions of current expenditures also increased: operation and maintenance (11 percent), food services (11 percent), and administration (10 percent). Of the seven functions of current expenditures, only spending on enterprise operations declined (39 percent) (see supplemental table 35-2).

---

[34] Other expenditures include funds for adult education, community colleges, private school programs funded by local and state education agencies, and community services.

In the 2004–05 school year, 61 percent of the $9,266 spent on current expenditures in public elementary and secondary schools went toward instruction expenditures such as teacher salaries and employee benefits. About 13 percent went toward student and staff support, 10 percent toward operation and maintenance, 8 percent toward administration, and 4 percent each toward transportation and food services.

From 1989–90 to 2004–05, the amount of current expenditures spent on salaries increased 16 percent (see supplemental table 35-1). Despite this increase, the percentage of current expenditures spent on salaries declined 4 percentage points, from 66 to 62 percent. The percentage of current expenditures spent on employee benefits increased almost 3 percentage points during this period, and the percentage spent on purchased services and supplies each increased 1 percentage point. In each year, the percentage spent on tuition and other expenditures was about 2 percent. The greatest increase was for employee benefits, which rose 43 percent, from $1,246 to $1,787 per student.

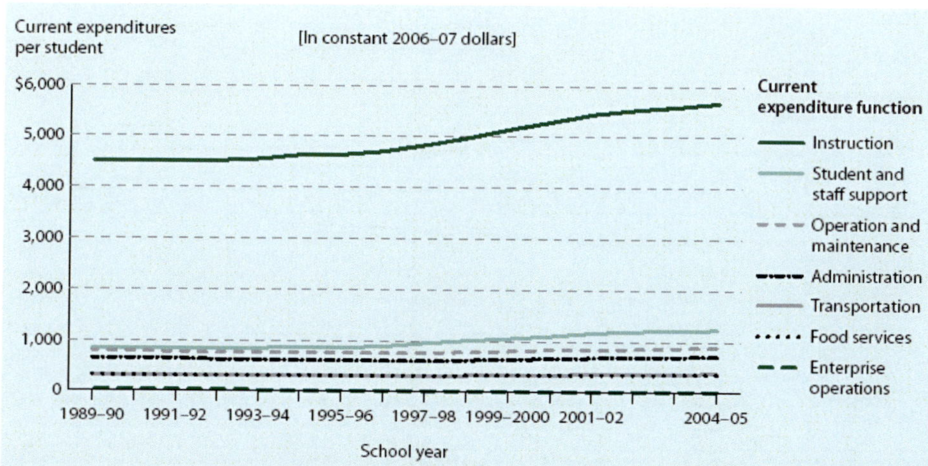

Note: Expenditures have been adjusted for the effects of inflation using the Consumer Price Index (CPI) and are in constant 2006–07 dollars. See *supplemental note 11* for information about this index and about classifications of expenditures for elementary and secondary education. All analyses were performed with unrounded numbers.

Source: U.S. Department of Education, National Center for Education Statistics, Common Core of Data (CCD), "National Public Education Financial Survey," 1989–90 through 2004–05.

EXPENDITURES BY FUNCTION: Current expenditures per student in fall enrollment in public elementary and secondary schools, by expenditure function: School years 1989–90 through 2004–05.

VARIATIONS IN INSTRUCTION EXPENDITURES PER STUDENT

Between 1997–98 and 2004–05, differences between states accounted for a greater percentage of the variation in instruction expenditures per student among unified public school districts than did differences within states.

A number of methods can be used to measure the variation in the amount school districts spend per student on instruction. This indicator uses the Theil coefficient because it provides a national measure of differences in instruction expenditures per student that can be decomposed into separate components to measure school district-level variations both between and within states. In this indicator, a coefficient of zero indicates that there is no variation in the instruction expenditures per student in unified public school districts for kindergarten through grade 12, and the Theil coefficient, which has a maximum possible value of 1.0, increases as the amount of variation present increases.

Across U.S. districts, the total variation, after controlling for geographic cost differences,[35] in instruction expenditures per student increased between the 1997–98 and 2004–05 school years (see supplemental table 36-1). The between- state variation also increased during that time, but the within-state component remained largely unchanged. In the 1997–98 school year, 57 percent of the variation in instruction expenditures per student was due to the between-state differences and 43 percent was due to withinstate differences. As the between-state component of the variation increased from 1997–98 to 2004–05 and the within-state component remained largely unchanged, the percentage of the total variation due to the between-state component increased to 66 percent in 2004–05 and that due to the within-state component decreased to 34 percent.

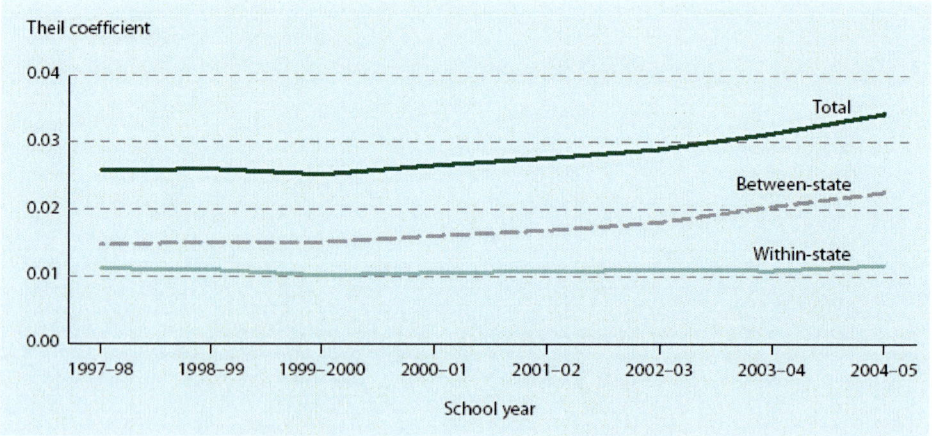

Note: For more information about the *Theil coefficient,* see supplemental table 36-1 and *supplemental note 11*. Public elementary and secondary unified districts are those districts that serve both elementary and secondary grades. In 2004–05, approximately 91 percent of all public elementary and secondary school students were enrolled in unified school districts.

Source: U.S. Department of Education, National Center for Education Statistics (NCES), Common Core of Data (CCD), "NCES Longitudinal School District Fiscal-Nonfiscal (FNF) File, Fiscal Years 1990 to 2002"; "School District Finance Survey (Form F-33)," 2002–03 to 2004–05; and NCES Comparable Wage Index Files, "School District CWI."

VARIATIONS IN EXPENDITURES: Variation in instruction expenditures per student in unified public elementary and secondary school districts controlling for geographic cost differences, by source of variation: School years 1997–98 to 2004–05.

[35] Instruction expenditures in this indicator have been adjusted for geographic cost differences using the Comparable Wage Index (CWI). In indicator 35, expenditures were not presented by geographic area so no such adjustment was required. Rather, in indicator 35, the Consumer Price Index (CPI) was used to adjust for the effects of infl ation. The CWI is available from 1997–98 to 2004–05. See supplemental note 11 for more information.

Changes in the variation in instruction expenditures per student over time may also reflect differences across school districts in the amount of services or goods purchased, such as the number of classroom teachers hired. These changes may, in part, reflect various state litigation, school finance reform efforts, and changes in the composition of student enrollment.

PUBLIC ELEMENTARY AND SECONDARY EXPENDITURES BY DISTRICT POVERTY

Current expenditures per student in 2004–05 were highest in high-poverty school districts and next highest in low-poverty school districts.

Current expenditures per student in public elementary and secondary schools vary by the level of poverty in a district. For example, in 2004–05, current expenditures per student, which include instructional, administrative, and operation and maintenance expenditures, were highest in high-poverty districts ($9,892), next highest in low-poverty districts ($9,263), and lowest in middle-poverty districts ($8,536) (see supplemental table 37-1). Districts were ranked by the percentage of school-age children (5- to 17-year-olds) in poverty and then divided into five groups with approximately equal public school enrollments. The low-poverty district category consists of those districts with the lowest percentages of school-age children in poverty. Conversely, the high-poverty district category consists of those with the highest percentages of school-age children in poverty. All expenditures in this indicator have been adjusted to account for inflation and geographic cost of living differences.[36]

Between 1997–98 and 2004–05, current expenditures per student increased by 20 percent in constant dollars, from $7,602 to $9,094. Current expenditures per student increased the most for the high-poverty districts (26 percent), and the least for the middle-poverty districts (16 percent). Expenditures in the other three categories increased between 18 and 20 percent.

In 2004–05, current expenditures per pupil also differed by the type of community in which the school district was located. When adjusted for geographic cost differences, current expenditures per student were highest in districts located in towns ($9,430) and rural areas ($9,426) and lowest in the suburbs ($8,862) (see supplemental table 37-2). In every district poverty category, rural areas had either the highest or second highest current expenditures per pupil.

There were differences in the types of communities in which low- and high-poverty school districts were located. For example, among students in low-poverty districts, 69 percent were enrolled in the suburbs, while 10 percent were enrolled in cities (see supplemental table 37-3). In contrast, 69 percent of the students in high-poverty districts were enrolled in cities, while the suburbs enrolled 7 percent.

---

[36] The NCES Comparable Wage Index (CWI) was used to adjust for geographic cost differences. As the CWI measures geographic differences in wages, it is more appropriate to use the CWI for expenditure categories with larger percentages of salaries, such as current expenditures and instruction expenditures, than for other expenditures with smaller percentages of salaries such as total expenditures. All expenditures in this indicator are in constant 2006–07 dollars. The Consumer Price Index (CPI) was used to adjust expenditures into constant dollars. See supplemental note 11 for information on the CWI, the CPI, and classifi cations of expenditures.

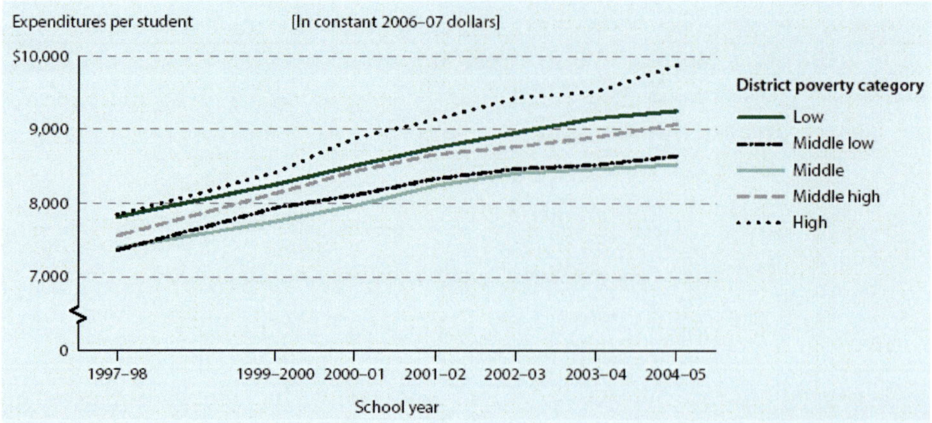

Note: See *supplemental note 1* for further information on poverty and community types. Regular districts include elementary/secondary combined districts and separate elementary or secondary districts. They exclude Department of Defense districts and Bureau of Indian Education districts.

Source: U.S. Department of Commerce, Census Bureau, "Small Area Income and Poverty Estimates," 1997–98 and 1999–2000 to 2004–05; and U.S. Department of Education, National Center for Education Statistics (NCES), Common Core of Data (CCD), "School District Finance Survey (Form F-33)," 1997–98 and 1999–2000 to 2004–05, and NCES Comparable Wage Index Files, "2005 School District CWI."

CURRENT EXPENDITURES PER STUDENT: Public school district geographic cost-adjusted expenditures per student, by district poverty category: Various school years, 1997–98 to 2004–05.

INTERNATIONAL COMPARISONS OF EXPENDITURES FOR EDUCATION

At the postsecondary level in 2004, U.S. expenditures per student were $22,476, which was higher than the OECD average of $11,418.

Two measures used to compare countries' investments in education are *expenditures per student from both public and private sources* and *total education expenditures as a percentage of gross domestic product (GDP)*. The latter measure allows a comparison of countries' expenditures relative to their ability to finance education. Private sources include payments from households for school-based expenses such as tuition, transportation fees, book rentals, or food services, as well as funds raised by institutions.

In 2004, expenditures per student for the United States were $9,368 at the combined elementary and secondary level, which was 42 percent higher than the average of $6,604 for the member countries of the Organization for Economic Cooperation and Development (OECD) reporting data (see supplemental table 38-1). At the postsecondary level, U.S. expenditures per student were $22,476, which was nearly twice as high as the OECD average of $11,418. Expenditures per student varied widely across the OECD countries, ranging from $1,262 in Turkey to $15,157 in Luxembourg at the combined elementary and secondary level, and from $4,412 in Poland to $21,966 in Switzerland and $22,476 in the United States at the postsecondary level.

EXPENDITURES FOR EDUCATION: Annual expenditures per student, by GDP per capita for elementary and secondary education in selected OECD countries: 2004

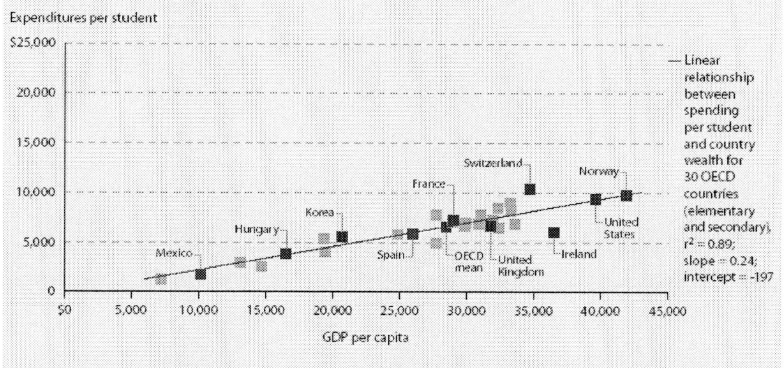

EXPENDITURES FOR EDUCATION: Annual expenditures per student, by GDP per capita for postsecondary education in selected OECD countries: 2004

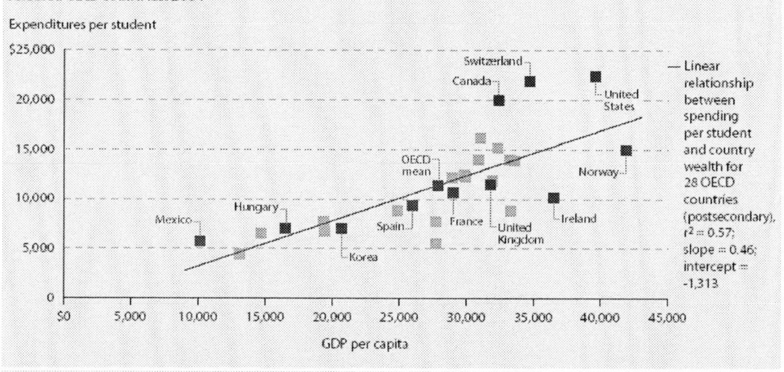

EXPENDITURES FOR EDUCATION: Annual total education expenditures as a percentage of GDP, by GDP per capita in selected OECD countries: 2004

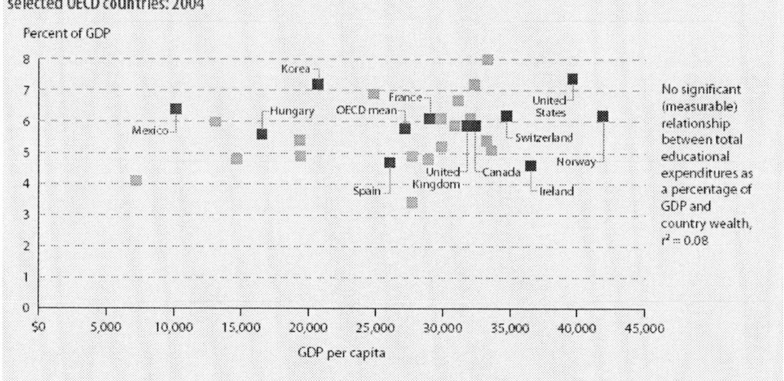

Note: Per student expenditures are based on public and private full-time-equivalent (FTE) enrollment figures and on current expenditures and capital outlays from both public and private sources where data are available. Purchasing power parity (PPP) indices are used to convert other currencies to U.S. dollars (i.e., absolute terms). Within-country consumer price indices are used to adjust the PPP indices to account for inflation because the fiscal year has a different starting date in different countries. Luxembourg data are excluded from the graphs because of anomalies with respect to their GDP per capita data (large revenues from international finance institutions distort the wealth of the population). The OECD average for GDP per capita for each graph is based on the number of countries with data available (30 for first graph; 28 for second graph; 29 for third graph).

Source: Organization for Economic Cooperation and Development (OECD), Center for Educational Research and Innovation. (2007). *Education at a Glance: OECD Indicators, 2007,* tables B1.1b, B2.1, and X2.1.

A country's wealth (defined as GDP per capita) was positively associated with expenditures per student on education. Among the OECD countries reporting data in 2004, the countries that spent the highest percentage of their GDP on total education expenditures[37] were Iceland (8.0 percent), the United States (7.4 percent), Korea (7.2 percent), and Denmark (7.2 percent). Looking at education expenditures by level, the United States spent 4.1 percent of its GDP on elementary and secondary education, higher than the average of 3.8 percent for all OECD countries reporting data. Compared with the United States, 12 countries spent a higher percentage of their GDP on elementary and secondary education, and 16 countries spent a lower proportion on education. Iceland (5.4 percent) spent the highest percentage of GDP. At the postsecondary level, 2.9 percent of the GDP of the United States was spent on education, higher than the average of 1.4 percent for all OECD countries reporting data. The United States also spent a greater percentage of its GDP on postsecondary education than any other OECD countries reporting data.

[37] Total education expenditures include expenditures at the elementary/secondary, postsecondary, and postsecondary nontertiary levels.

Section 5.
Contexts of Postsecondary Education

In: The Condition of Education in America
Editor: Maurice H. Logan
ISBN: 978-1-60692-298-9

Chapter 19

INTRODUCTION

The indicators in this section of *The Condition of Education* examine features of postsecondary education, many of which parallel those presented in the previous section on elementary and secondary education. There are 21 indicators in this section: 5, prepared for this year's volume, appear on the following pages, and all 21, including indicators from previous years, are on the Web (see Website Contents on the facing page for a full list of the indicators).

Postsecondary education is characterized by diversity in both the types of institutions and characteristics of the students. Postsecondary institutions vary in terms of the types of degrees awarded, control (public or private), and whether they are operated on a not-for-profit or for-profit basis. Beyond these basic differences, postsecondary institutions have distinctly different missions and provide a wide range of learning environments. For example, some institutions are research universities with strong graduate programs, while others focus on undergraduate education; some have a religious affiliation, while others do not; and some have selective entrance policies, while others have more open admissions. The student bodies of postsecondary institutions are diverse in other ways as well. For example, many students hold down jobs and regard themselves as employees first and students second; many delay entry into postsecondary education rather than enroll immediately after high school; and a sizable number come from foreign countries. Indicators in *The Condition of Education* measure these and other dimensions of diversity that are fundamental to the character of postsecondary education.

The courses and programs of study that students take are an important feature of postsecondary education. Data on degree completion show trends in the fields of study for undergraduate and graduate degree recipients. In addition, one indicator in this volume compares the distribution of degrees awarded by institution type. Indicators on the Web also present information on distance education courses taught by faculty and on the provision of and participation in remedial education.

Like elementary and secondary schools, postsecondary institutions provide special support and accommodations for special populations of students. One indicator on the Web measures the services and accommodations that are available for students with disabilities in postsecondary education.

Faculty teach students, conduct research, and serve their institutions and communities. One indicator in this volume of *The Condition of Education* highlights trends in faculty salaries and benefits at different postsecondary levels and across types of institutions.

Finally, *The Condition of Education* examines financial support for education. One indicator in this year's volume shows the number and characteristics of college students who are employed. Additional indicators on the Web look at the institutional aid available to students, the total and net access price of attending postsecondary institutions, and the debt burden of college graduates.

The indicators on the contexts of postsecondary education from previous editions of *The Condition of Education*, which are not included in this volume, are available at http://nces.ed.gov/ programs/coe/list/i5.asp.

In: The Condition of Education in America
Editor: Maurice H. Logan
ISBN: 978-1-60692-298-9

Chapter 20

PROGRAMS AND COURSES

UNDERGRADUATE FIELDS OF STUDY

In 2005–06, degrees in the field of business made up 21 percent of the bachelor's degrees awarded. Over 318,000 bachelor's degrees were awarded in business that year.

In each year shown (1990–91, 1995–96, and 2005–06), three broad areas of study—liberal arts and sciences, general studies, and humanities; health professions; and business—made up 65 to 69 percent of associate's degrees awarded (see supplemental table 39-1). In 2005–06, nearly 245,000 degrees were awarded in the first area, and over 114,000 degrees were awarded in each of the other two areas. Other prevalent degrees at this level in 2005–06 included engineering (32,600 degrees) and computer and information sciences (31,200 degrees).

Overall, 158,000 more associate's degrees were awarded in 2005–06 than in 1995–96 (a 28 percent increase). Increases in the number of associate's degrees awarded in the three major areas of study above and in computer and information sciences contributed to 85 percent of this overall growth. The number of degrees awarded in computer and information sciences has increased by 150 percent since 1995–96. Fields including visual and performing arts had a smaller impact on the overall growth but had notable increases during this period (61 percent increase for a total of 21,800 degrees in 2005–06). Also, during this period, the number of associate's degrees awarded in engineering decreased by 23 percent.

In each year shown, between 63 and 66 percent of bachelor's degrees were awarded in seven fields: business; social sciences and history; education; health professions; psychology; visual and performing arts; and engineering (see supplemental table 39-2). In 2005–06, some 318,000 degrees were awarded in business, 161,000 were awarded in social sciences and history, 107,000 were awarded in health professions, and between 81,600 and 92,000 degrees were awarded in each of the other four fields.

Overall, 320,000 more bachelor's degrees were awarded in 2005–06 than in 1995–96 (a 28 percent increase). Increases in the number of bachelor's degrees awarded in business; social sciences and history; visual and performing arts; communication, journalism, and related programs; and computer and information sciences made up 66 percent of this overall growth. Fields including parks, recreation, leisure and fitness studies had a smaller impact on the overall growth in bachelor's degrees awarded but had notable increases during this period (96 percent increase for a total of 25,500 degrees in 2005–06).

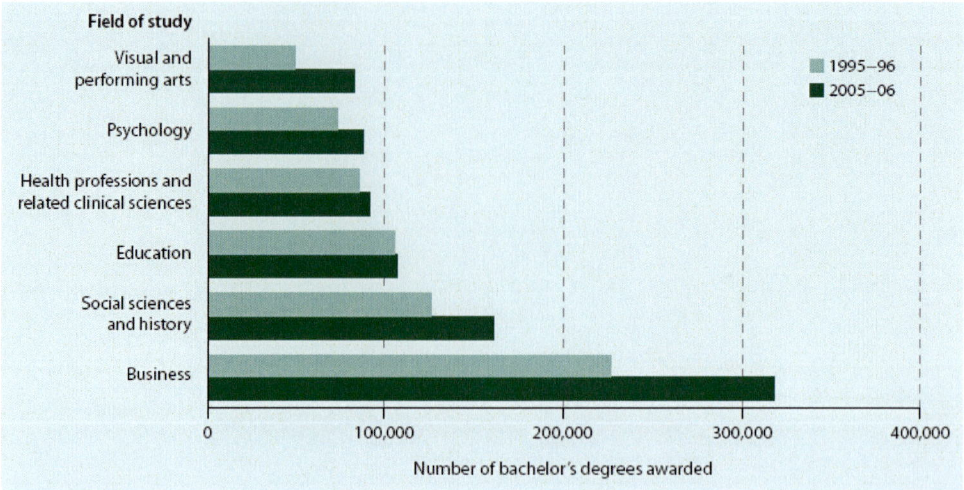

Note: The six most common fields of study at the bachelor's degree level in academic year 2005–06 are featured for academic years 1995–96 and 2005–06; the remaining fields of study are not shown. The contribution of growth is calculated as the increase in the number of degrees for a particular field divided by the increase in the total number of degrees. See *supplemental note 10* for more information on fields of study. The new *Classification of Instructional Programs* was initiated in 2002–03. Estimates for earlier years have been reclassified when necessary to conform to the new taxonomy. See *supplemental note 9* for more information on the Classification of Postsecondary Education Institutions. See *supplemental note 3* for more information on the Integrated Postsecondary Education Data System (IPEDS).

Source: U.S. Department of Education, National Center for Education Statistics (NCES). *Digest of Education Statistics, 2007* (NCES 2008-022), tables 259 and 261, data from U.S. Department of Education, NCES, 1995–96 and 2005–06 Integrated Postsecondary Education Data System, "Completions Survey" (IPEDS-C:96), and Fall 2006.

FIELDS OF STUDY: Number of bachelor's degrees awarded by degree-granting institutions in selected fields of study: Academic years 1995–96 and 2005–06.

GRADUATE FIELDS OF STUDY

In 2005–06, of the 594,000 master's degrees awarded, over 50 percent were in the fields of education (29 percent) and business (25 percent).

In each year shown (1990–91, 1995–96, and 2005–06), six fields—education, business, health professions, engineering, public administration and social services, and psychology—accounted for 72 to 77 percent of the total number of master's degrees awarded (see supplemental table 40-1). In 2005–06, about 175,000 degrees (29 percent) were awarded in education and 146,000 degrees (25 percent) were awarded in business.

Overall, 188,000 more master's degrees were awarded in 2005–06 than in 1995–96 (a 46 percent increase). The increase in the number of education and business degrees earned contributed to over 65 percent of this growth. Although they had less impact on the overall growth, during this time, the number of degrees earned in architecture increased by 44 percent (totaling 5,700 in 2005–06) and the number earned in mathematics and statistics increased by 30 percent (totaling 4,700 in 2005–06).

In each year shown, between 71 and 74 percent of doctoral degrees were awarded in seven fields: education, engineering, health professions, biological and biomedical sciences, psychology, physical sciences, and social sciences and history. In 2005–06, some 7,600 degrees were awarded in education, 7,500 were awarded in engineering, and 7,100 were awarded in health professions (each accounting for 13 to 14 percent of all degrees).

Overall, 11,400 more doctoral degrees were awarded in 2005–06 than in 1995–96 (a 26 percent increase). The increase in doctoral degrees awarded in health professions accounted for 48 percent of this overall growth, and the increase in education and engineering degrees accounted for an additional 21 percent of the overall growth. Although the increase in degrees awarded in computer and information sciences made a smaller contribution to the overall growth (5 percent), the number of degrees in this field increased by 63 percent (from 870 to 1,400) between 1995–96 and 2005–06. During this period, the number of degrees awarded decreased in English language and literature/letters, theology and religious vocations, and agriculture and natural resources.

The number of first-professional degrees awarded increased by 11,000 (a 14 percent increase) between 1995–96 and 2005–06. The increase in the number of degrees awarded in pharmacy (264 percent) accounted for 62 percent of this overall growth.

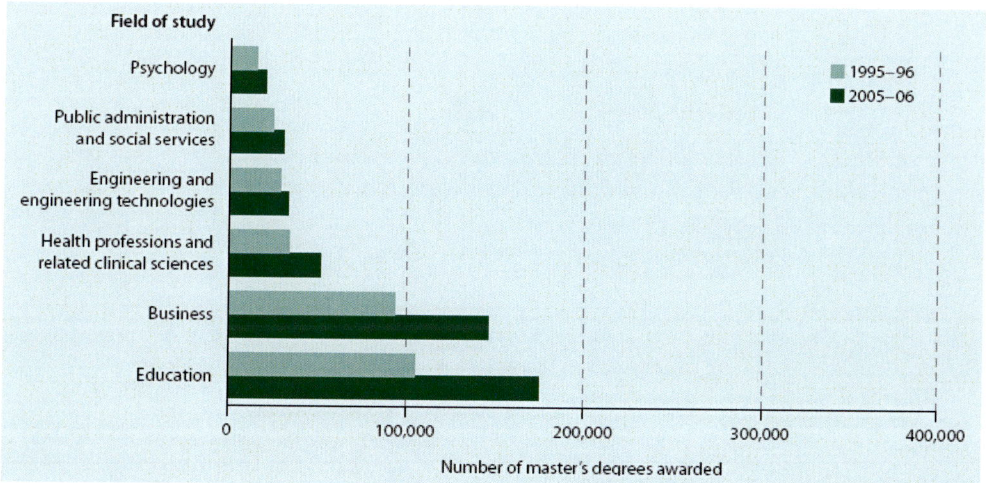

Note: The six most common fields of study at the master's degree level in academic year 2005–06 are featured for academic years 1995–96 and 2005–06; the remaining fields of study are not shown. The contribution of growth is calculated as the increase in the number of degrees for a particular field divided by the increase in the total number of degrees. See supplemental note 10 for more information on fields of study. The new Classification of Instructional Programs was initiated in 2002–03. Estimates for earlier years have been reclassified when necessary to conform to the new taxonomy. See supplemental note 9 for more information on the Classification of Postsecondary Education Institutions. See supplemental note 3 for more information on the Integrated Postsecondary Education Data System (IPEDS).

Source: U.S. Department of Education, National Center for Education Statistics (NCES). *Digest of Education Statistics, 2007* (NCES 2008-022), table 262, data from U.S. Department of Education, NCES, 1995–96 and 2005–06 Integrated Postsecondary Education Data System, "Completions Survey" (IPEDS-C:96), and Fall 2006.

FIELDS OF STUDY: Number of master's degrees awarded by degree-granting institutions in selected fields of study: Academic years 1995–96 and 2005–06.

DEGREES CONFERRED BY PUBLIC AND PRIVATE INSTITUTIONS

The number of associate's, bachelor's, master's, and doctoral degrees conferred by private for-profit institutions increased by a larger percentage between 1995–96 and 2005–06 than the number conferred by private not-for-profit and public institutions.

Although the number of degrees conferred increased between 1995–96 and 2005–06, the percentage increase varied among types of institutions. For associate's, bachelor's, master's, and doctoral degrees, the percentage increases were slower for public and private not-for-profit institutions than for private for-profit institutions. For example, the number of bachelor's degrees conferred by public and private notfor- profit institutions increased by 23 percent between 1995–96 and 2005–06 (from 774,100 to 995,400 at public institutions and from 379,900 to 467,800 at private not-for-profit institutions), compared with 474 percent (10,800 to 62,000) at private for-profit institutions (see supplemental table 41-1). At the master's degree level, the number of degrees conferred by public institutions increased 29 percent (from 227,200 to 293,500), compared with 46 percent at private not-for-profit institutions (175,300 to 255,400) and 1,069 percent at private for-profit institutions (3,900 to 45,100).

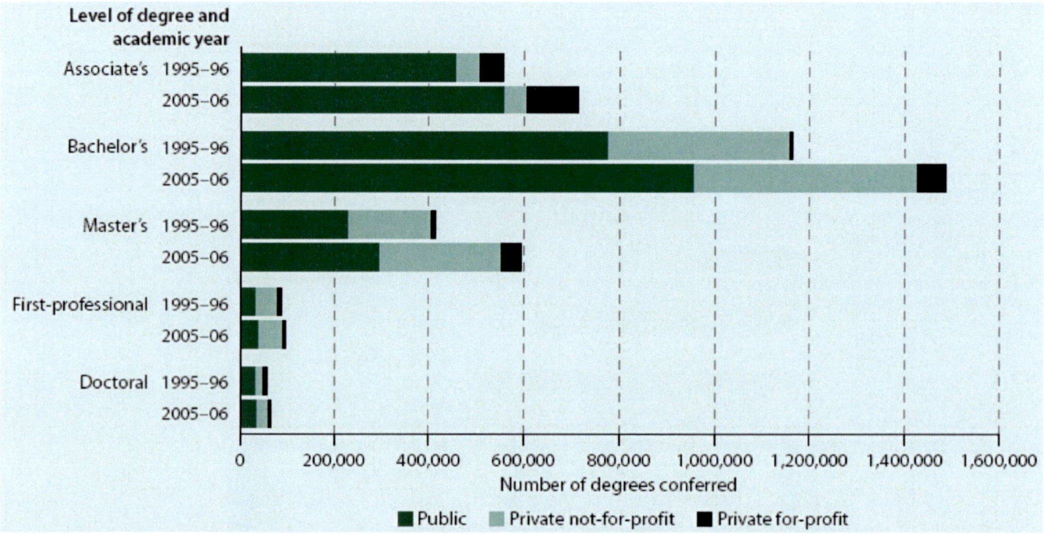

Note: Includes institutions that participated in Title IV federal financial aid programs. See *supplemental note 9* for more information on these programs. See *supplemental note 3* for more information on the Integrated Postsecondary Education Data System (IPEDS). See the glossary for definitions of first-professional degree programs. Detail may not sum to totals because of rounding.

Source: U.S. Department of Education, National Center for Education Statistics, 1995–96 and 2005–06 Integrated Postsecondary Education Data System, "Completions Survey" (IPEDS-C:96), and Fall 2006.

DEGREES CONFERRED BY PUBLIC AND PRIVATE INSTITUTIONS: Number of degrees conferred by degree-granting institutions, by level of degree and control of institution: 1995–96 and 2005–06.

The shift was evident in the share of degrees awarded. Between 1995–96 and 2005–06, the percentage of associate's degrees decreased from 82 to 78 percent for public institutions and from 9 to 7 percent for private not-for-profit institutions. In contrast, the percentage of these degrees conferred by private for-profit institutions increased from 9 to 15 percent. The percentage of bachelor's degrees conferred decreased from 66 to 64 percent for public institutions and from 33 to 31 percent for private not-for-profit institutions, while it increased from 1 to 4 percent for private for-profit institutions. The largest shift at the advanced degree level was in the percentage of master's degrees conferred by private for-profit institutions, which increased from 1 to 8 percent during this period. The percentage of master's degrees conferred by public institutions decreased from 56 to 49 percent, while the percentage conferred by private not-for-profit institutions remained at about 43 percent.

Yet, despite relatively large percentage increases in the number and share of degrees conferred by private for-profit institutions, the number of degrees awarded remained substantially smaller than at public or private not-for-profit institutions, with the exception of associate's degrees.

In: The Condition of Education in America
Editor: Maurice H. Logan
ISBN: 978-1-60692-298-9

Chapter 21

FACULTY AND STAFF

FACULTY SALARY, BENEFITS, AND TOTAL COMPENSATION

Average inflation-adjusted salaries for full-time instructional faculty in colleges and universities were 20 percent higher in 2006–07 than in 1979–80; however, recent increases have been relatively small (1 percent between 1999–2000 and 2006–07).

The average salary for full-time instructional faculty in colleges and universities increased by 20 percent overall between 1979–80 and 2006–07 after adjusting for inflation (see supplemental table 42-1). Average salaries were higher in 2006–07 than in 1979–80 for faculty with academic ranks.[38] The increase was greatest for instructors, whose average salary increased by 38 percent, followed by that for professors, whose average salary increased by 26 percent. The average salary increased at all types of institutions as well, ranging from a low of 8 percent at public 2-year colleges to a high of 37 percent at private doctoral universities. In 2006–07, the average faculty salary was $69,500, with institutional averages ranging from $41,800 at private 2-year colleges to $91,300 at private doctoral universities.

Much of the growth in faculty salaries between 1979–80 and 2006–07 occurred during the earlier years. After increasing by 14 percent during the 1980s and 4 percent during the 1990s, average salaries for faculty increased by 1 percent between 1999–2000 and 2006–07 after adjusting for inflation. Between 1999–2000 and 2006–07, faculty salaries increased by less than 1 percent at public doctoral universities and private master's degree universities, and decreased by 2 percent at public master's degree universities and by 1 percent at public 2-year colleges. Faculty salaries increased by an average of 2 percent at private doctoral universities and private (nonuniversity) 4-year colleges. Although faculty salaries increased by 16 percent at public (nonuniversity) 4-year colleges and by 4 percent at private 2-year colleges, these institutions together employed less than 5 percent of postsecondary faculty.

Fringe benefits for faculty (adjusted for inflation) have increased by a higher percentage than salaries since 1979–80 (69 vs. 20 percent). In contrast to the generally small changes in faculty salaries between 1999–2000 and 2006–07, fringe benefits rose substantially among most types of institutions. Overall, average fringe benefits for faculty increased 17 percent between 1999–2000 and 2006–07, compared with 1 percent for average salaries after

[38] Academic ranks include professor, associate professor, assistant professor, instructor, and lecturer. About 8 percent of faculty in 2006–07 did not have an academic rank.

adjusting for inflation. The percentage of faculty compensation received in the form of benefits rose from 16 percent in 1979–80 to 21 percent in 2006–07.

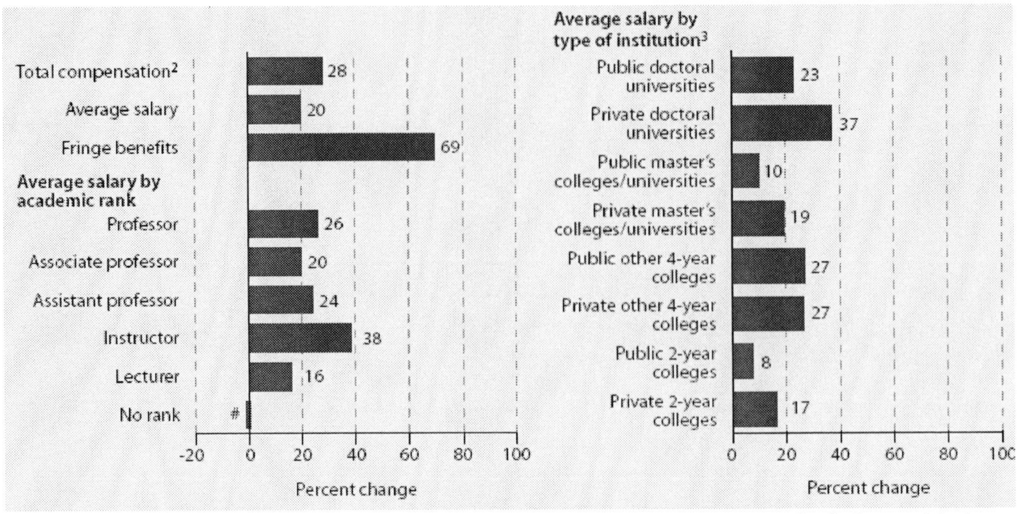

[2] Total compensation is the sum of salary and fringe benefits. Salary does not include outside income. Fringe benefits may include, for example, retirement plans, medical/dental plans, group life insurance, or other benefits.

[3] Institutions in this indicator are classified based on the number of highest degrees awarded. For example, institutions that award 20 or more doctoral degrees per year are classified as doctoral universities. See *supplemental note 9* for more information about Classifications of Postsecondary Education Institutions.

Note: Full-time instructional faculty on lessthan-9-month contracts were excluded. In 2006–07, there were about 3,600 of these faculty, accounting for less than 1 percent of all full-time instructional faculty at degree-granting institutions. Salaries reflect an average of all faculty on 9- through 12-month contracts, rather than a weighted average based on contract length that appears in some other NCES reports. Salaries, benefits, and compensation adjusted by the Consumer Price Index (CPI) to constant 2006–07 dollars. Detail may not sum to totals because of rounding. See *supplemental note 11* for more information about the CPI. See *supplemental note 3* for more information about the Integrated Postsecondary Education Data System (IPEDS).

Source: U.S. Department of Education, National Center for Education Statistics, 1979–80 Higher Education General Information Survey (HEGIS), "Faculty Salaries, Tenure, and Fringe Benefits Survey"; and 2006–07 Integrated Postsecondary Education Data System, Fall 2006 and Winter 2006–07.

FACULTY SALARIES: Percentage change in total compensation, average salary, and fringe benefits, and in average salary, by academic rank and type of institution for full-time instructional faculty at degree-granting institutions (adjusted for inflation): Academic years 1979–80 to 2006–07.

In: The Condition of Education in America
Editor: Maurice H. Logan

ISBN: 978-1-60692-298-9

Chapter 22

FINANCE

EMPLOYMENT OF COLLEGE STUDENTS

In 2006, about 46 percent of full-time and 81 percent of part-time college students ages 16–24 were employed.

The percentage of full-time college students ages 16–24 who were employed increased between 1970 and 2000 from 34 to 52 percent, and in the more recent years, between 2001 and 2006, the percentage fluctuated between 46 and 49 percent. Along with the increase in the percentage of students who worked, the number of hours these students worked per week increased between 1970 and 2006. In 1970, some 10 percent of full-time students worked 20–34 hours per week, and 4 percent worked 35 or more hours per week; in 2006, however, about 22 percent of these students worked 20–34 hours per week, and 8 percent worked 35 or more hours per week (see supplemental table 43-1). In the more recent years, between 2001 and 2006, there were no measurable changes in the percentages of full-time students working 20 or more hours per week.

In contrast to the increase among full-time college students, there was no measurable change between 1970 and 2006 in the percentage of part-time college students ages 16–24 who were employed. In 2006, approximately 81 percent of part-time college students were employed. However, part-time college students worked fewer hours per week in 2006 than they did in 1970, with the percentage of students working 35 or more hours a week decreasing from 60 to 45 percent. In the more recent years, from 2001 to 2006, there were no measurable changes in these employment percentages.

In 2006, the percentage of full-time college students ages 16–24 who were employed differed by sex, race/ethnicity, and school type. A higher percentage of female than male full-time students were employed (49 vs. 44 percent) (see supplemental table 43-2). Also, the employment rates of full-time students were higher among White and Hispanic students (49 and 48 percent, respectively) than among Black and Asian students (37 and 38 percent, respectively). In terms of school type, a higher percentage of full-time students at 2-year colleges than at 4-year institutions were employed (54 vs. 44 percent). Within school types, the percentage of full-time students who were employed varied by school control: a higher percentage of students who attended public colleges than private colleges were employed among students attending 2-year colleges (55 vs. 40 percent) and 4-year institutions (47 vs. 37 percent).

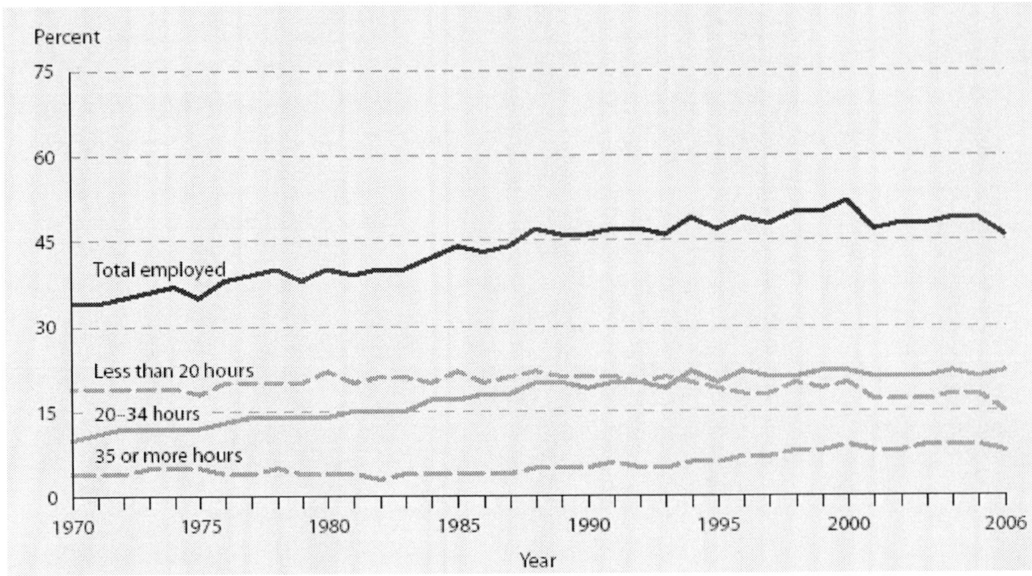

Note: College includes both 2- and 4-year institutions. College students were classified as attending full time if they were taking at least 12 hours of classes (or at least 9 hours of graduate classes) during an average school week and were classified as part time if they were taking fewer hours. Percent employed estimates include those who were employed but not at work during the survey week. *Hours worked per week* refers to the number of hours the respondent worked at all jobs during the survey week. These estimates exclude those who were employed but not at work during the survey week; therefore, detail may not sum to total percentage employed.

Source: U.S. Department of Commerce, Census Bureau, Current Population Survey (CPS), October Supplement, 1970–2006.

EMPLOYMENT OF COLLEGE STUDENTS: Percentage of 16- to 24-year-old full-time college students who were employed, by hours worked per week: October 1970 through October 2006.

Appendix 1

SUPPLEMENTAL TABLES

Enrollment Trends by Age

Table 1-1. Percentage of the population ages 3–34 enrolled in school, by age group: October 1970–2006

							Ages 18–19						
October	Total, ages 3–34	Ages 3–41	Ages 5–6	Ages 7–13	Ages 14–17	Total	In elementary/ secondary	In post-secondary	Total	Ages 20–24 Ages 20–21	Ages 22–24	Ages 25–29	Ages 30–34
1970	56.4	20.5	89.5	99.2	94.1	47.7	10.5	37.3	21.5	31.9	14.9	7.5	4.2
1971	56.2	21.2	91.6	99.1	94.5	49.2	11.5	37.7	21.9	32.2	15.4	8.0	4.9
1972	54.9	24.4	91.9	99.2	93.3	46.3	10.4	35.9	21.6	31.4	14.8	8.6	4.6
1973	53.5	24.2	92.5	99.2	92.9	42.9	10.0	32.9	20.8	30.1	14.5	8.5	4.5
1974	53.6	28.8	94.2	99.3	92.9	43.1	9.9	33.2	21.4	30.2	15.1	9.6	5.7
1975	53.7	31.5	94.7	99.3	93.6	46.9	10.2	36.7	22.4	31.2	16.2	10.1	6.6
1976	53.1	31.3	95.5	99.2	93.7	46.2	10.2	36.0	23.3	32.0	17.1	10.0	6.0
1977	52.5	32.0	95.8	99.4	93.7	46.2	10.4	35.7	22.9	31.8	16.5	10.8	6.9
1978	51.2	34.2	95.3	99.1	93.7	45.4	9.8	35.6	21.8	29.5	16.3	9.4	6.4
1979	50.3	35.1	95.8	99.2	93.6	45.0	10.3	34.6	21.7	30.2	15.8	9.6	6.4
1980	49.7	36.7	95.7	99.3	93.4	46.4	10.5	35.9	22.3	31.0	16.3	9.3	6.4
1981	48.9	36.0	94.0	99.2	94.1	49.0	11.5	37.5	22.5	31.6	16.5	9.0	6.9
1982	48.6	36.4	95.0	99.2	94.4	47.8	11.3	36.5	23.5	34.0	16.8	9.6	6.3
1983	48.4	37.5	95.4	99.2	95.0	50.4	12.8	37.6	22.7	32.5	16.6	9.6	6.4
1984	47.9	36.3	94.5	99.2	94.7	50.1	11.5	38.6	23.7	33.9	17.3	9.1	6.3
1985	48.3	38.9	96.1	99.2	94.9	51.6	11.2	40.4	24.0	35.3	16.9	9.2	6.1
1986	48.2	38.9	95.3	99.2	94.9	54.6	13.1	41.5	23.6	33.0	17.9	8.8	6.0
1987	48.6	38.3	95.1	99.5	95.0	55.6	13.1	42.5	25.5	38.7	17.5	9.0	5.8
1988	48.7	38.2	96.0	99.7	95.1	55.6	13.9	41.8	26.1	39.1	18.2	8.3	5.9
1989	49.0	39.1	95.2	99.3	95.7	56.0	14.4	41.6	27.0	38.5	19.9	9.3	5.7
1990	50.2	44.4	96.5	99.6	95.8	57.2	14.5	42.7	28.6	39.7	21.0	9.7	5.8

October	Total, ages 3–34	Ages 3–4[1]	Ages 5–6	Ages 7–13	Ages 14–17	Total	In elementary/ secondary	In post-secondary	Total	Ages 20–24 Ages 20–21	Ages 22–24	Ages 25–29	Ages 30–34
							Ages 18–19						
1991	50.7	40.5	95.4	99.6	96.0	59.6	15.6	44.0	30.2	42.0	22.2	10.2	6.2
1992	51.4	39.7	95.5	99.4	96.7	61.4	17.1	44.3	31.6	44.0	23.7	9.8	6.1
1993	51.8	40.4	95.4	99.5	96.5	61.6	17.2	44.4	30.8	42.7	23.6	10.2	5.9
1994	53.3	47.3	96.7	99.4	96.6	60.2	16.2	43.9	32.0	44.9	24.0	10.8	6.7
1995	53.7	48.7	96.0	98.9	96.3	59.4	16.3	43.1	31.5	44.9	23.2	11.6	5.9
1996	54.1	48.3	94.0	97.7	95.4	61.5	16.7	44.9	32.5	44.4	24.8	11.9	6.1
1997	55.6	52.6	96.5	99.1	96.6	61.5	16.7	44.7	34.3	45.9	26.4	11.8	5.7
1998	55.8	52.1	95.6	98.9	96.1	62.2	15.7	46.4	33.0	44.8	24.9	11.9	6.6
1999	56.0	54.2	96.0	98.7	95.8	60.6	16.5	44.1	32.8	45.3	24.5	11.1	6.2
2000	55.9	52.1	95.6	98.2	95.7	61.2	16.5	44.7	32.5	44.1	24.6	11.4	6.7
2001	56.4	52.4	95.3	98.3	95.8	61.1	17.1	44.0	34.1	46.1	25.5	11.8	6.9
2002	56.2	56.3	95.5	98.3	96.4	63.3	18.0	45.3	34.4	47.8	25.6	12.1	6.6
2003	56.2	55.1	94.5	98.3	96.2	64.5	17.9	46.6	35.6	48.3	27.8	11.8	6.8
2004	56.2	54.0	95.4	98.4	96.5	64.4	16.6	47.8	35.2	48.9	26.3	13.0	6.6
2005	56.5	53.6	95.4	98.6	96.5	67.6	18.3	49.3	36.1	48.7	27.3	11.9	6.9
2006	56.0	55.7	94.6	98.3	96.4	65.5	19.3	46.2	35.0	47.5	26.7	11.7	7.2

[1] Beginning in 1994, new procedures were used to collect preprimary enrollment data. As a result, pre-1994 data may not be comparable to data from 1994 or later.

Note: Detail may not sum to totals because of rounding. Includes enrollment in any type of graded public, parochial, or other private schools. Includes nursery schools, kindergartens, elementary schools, high schools, colleges, universities, and professional schools. Attendance may be on either a full-time or part-time basis and during the day or night. Excludes enrollments in less-than-2-year postsecondary institutions and enrollments in "special" schools, such as trade schools, business colleges, or correspondence schools. The age breakouts used in this indicator reflect the different schooling stages that are typical for students given their age. For example, students at ages 18–19 are typically transitioning from elementary/secondary education into postsecondary education or the workforce. See *supplemental note 2* for more information on the Current Population Survey (CPS).

Source: U.S. Department of Education, National Center for Education Statistics, *Digest of Education Statistics, 2007* (NCES 2008-022), table 7, data from U.S. Department of Commerce, Census Bureau, Current Population Survey (CPS), October, 1970–2006.

Table 2-1. Percentage distribution of the early education and child care arrangements of the 2001 birth cohort at about 4 years old, by type of arrangement and selected child and family characteristics: School year 2005–06

	Percentage distribution by primary type of care arrangement[2]							
			Home-based care		Center-based care[3]			
Child or family characteristic	Percentage distribution of population[1]	No regular nonparental arrangement	Relative care	Nonrelative care	Total	Head Start	Other than Head Start	Multiple arrangements[4]
Total	100.0	20.0	13.1	7.6	57.5	12.7	44.8	1.9
Sex of child								
Male	51.2	19.3	13.1	7.5	58.0	12.9	45.1	2.1
Female	48.8	20.7	13.1	7.6	56.9	12.4	44.5	.7
Race/ethnicity of child								
White	53.8	17.9	11.0	9.2	60.1	6.8	53.3	1.9
Black	13.8	16.0	13.9	4.3	62.4	25.4	37.1	3.3
Hispanic	25.1	27.2	15.9	6.2	49.4	18.6	30.9	1.2
Asian	2.6	17.5	16.0	3.4	60.7	5.5	55.3	2.3!
Pacific Islander	0.2	22.3!	45.0!	‡	19.9!	5.0!	14.9!	‡
American Indian/Alaska Native	0.5	20.0	14.0	5.3	59.6	31.1	28.5	1.1!
More than one race	4.0	17.8	17.5	8.9	53.9	12.2	41.7	1.8!
Age of child								
Less than 48 months	16.4	27.3	13.9	8.7	48.0	10.6	37.4	2.2
48.0 to 52.9 months	38.1	19.9	13.0	8.3	56.8	12.0	44.8	2.0
53.0 to 57.9 months	36.5	16.5	13.1	6.7	62.2	14.4	47.8	1.5
58.0 or more months	9.0	20.9	12.0	6.3	58.1	12.0	46.1	2.7
Mother's employment status								
Full-time (35 hours or more)	39.4	8.5	18.5	13.4	57.4	11.4	46.1	2.1
Part-time (less than 35 hours)	19.7	13.4	15.9	8.5	59.3	10.1	49.2	2.9
Looking for work	5.8	28.5	12.6	2.1!	54.7	24.3	30.4	2.0!
Not in labor force	34.3	35.6	4.6	1.5	57.3	13.7	43.7	1.0!

	Percentage distribution by primary type of care arrangement[2]							
			Home-based care		Center-based care[3]			
Child or family characteristic	Percentage distribution of population[1]	No regular nonparental arrangement	Relative care	Nonrelative care	Total	Head Start	Other than Head Start	Multiple arrangements[4]
No mother in household	0.8	9.6!	36.0	9.5!	41.1	14.4!	26.7	3.8!
Parents' highest level of education								
Less than high school	10.4	34.0	16.5	4.0	43.4	22.2	21.2	2.1!
High school completion	25.0	22.6	17.1	6.7	51.7	21.4	30.3	2.0
Some college/vocational	31.6	20.6	14.9	7.3	55.5	13.0	42.5	1.7
Bachelor's degree	16.8	16.0	8.4	8.1	65.7	3.3	62.4	1.8
Any graduate/professional school	16.2	9.7	6.2	11.2	70.8	2.0	68.8	2.0
Poverty status5								
Below poverty threshold	24.8	27.6	15.0	4.4	51.0	26.3	24.7	2.0
At or above poverty threshold	75.2	17.4	12.5	8.6	59.6	8.2	51.4	1.9
Socioeconomic status6								
Lowest 20 percent	20.0	30.5	15.0	5.0	47.1	24.7	22.4	2.3
Middle 60 percent	60.0	19.6	15.0	7.4	56.2	12.5	43.7	1.8
Highest 20 percent	20.0	10.3	5.5	10.7	71.6	1.0	70.6	1.9

! Interpret data with caution (estimates are unstable).

‡ Reporting standards not met (too few cases).

1 Distribution of weighted Early Childhood Longitudinal Study, Birth Cohort (ECLS-B) survey population between 44 and 65 months of age with data on primary care arrangements.

2 Primary type of care arrangement is the type of nonparental care in which the child spent the most hours.

3 Care provided in places such as early learning centers, nursery schools, and preschools, including Head Start.

4 Children who spent an equal amount of time in each of two or more arrangements.

5 Poverty status based on Census Bureau guidelines from 2002, which identify a dollar amount determined to meet a household's needs, given its size and composition. In 2002, a family of four was considered to live below the poverty threshold if its income was less than or equal to $18,392.

6 Socioeconomic status (SES) was measured by a composite score on parental education and occupations and on family income.

Note: Estimates weighted by W3R0. Estimates for children at about 4 years old pertain to children assessed between 44 and 65 months. See *supplemental note 3* for more information about the Early Childhood Longitudinal Study, Birth Cohort. Race categories exclude persons of Hispanic ethnicity. Detail may not sum to totals because of rounding and suppression of cells that do not meet standards.

Source: U.S. Department of Education, National Center for Education Statistics, Early Childhood Longitudinal Study, Birth Cohort, Longitudinal 9-Month–Preschool Restricted-Use Data File.Past and Projected Public School Enrollments

Table 3-1. Public school enrollment in prekindergarten through grade 12, with projections, by grade level and region: Various years, fall 1965–201; [Totals in thousands]

				Total and percent enrollment, grades preK–12 by region							
	Total enrollment			Northeast		Midwest		South		West	
Fall of year	Grades preK–12	Grades preK–8	Grades 9–12	Total	Percent	Total	Percent	Total	Percent	Total	Percent
1965	42,068	30,466	11,602	8,833	21.0	11,834	28.1	13,834	32.9	7,568	18.0
1970	45,894	32,558	13,336	9,860	21.5	12,936	28.2	14,759	32.2	8,339	18.2
1975	44,819	30,515	14,304	9,679	21.6	12,295	27.4	14,654	32.7	8,191	18.3
1980	40,877	27,647	13,231	8,215	20.1	10,698	26.2	14,134	34.6	7,831	19.2
1985	39,422	27,034	12,388	7,318	18.6	9,862	25.0	14,117	35.8	8,124	20.6
1986	39,753	27,420	12,333	7,294	18.3	9,871	24.8	14,312	36.0	8,276	20.8
1987	40,008	27,933	12,076	7,252	18.1	9,870	24.7	14,419	36.0	8,468	21.2
1988	40,189	28,501	11,687	7,208	17.9	9,846	24.5	14,491	36.1	8,644	21.5
1989	40,543	29,152	11,390	7,200	17.8	9,849	24.3	14,605	36.0	8,889	21.9
1990	41,217	29,878	11,338	7,282	17.7	9,944	24.1	14,807	35.9	9,184	22.3
1991	42,047	30,506	11,541	7,407	17.6	10,080	24.0	15,081	35.9	9,479	22.5
1992	42,823	31,088	11,735	7,526	17.6	10,198	23.8	15,357	35.9	9,742	22.7
1993	43,465	31,504	11,961	7,654	17.6	10,289	23.7	15,591	35.9	9,931	22.8
1994	44,111	31,898	12,213	7,760	17.6	10,386	23.5	15,851	35.9	10,114	22.9
1995	44,840	32,341	12,500	7,894	17.6	10,512	23.4	16,118	35.9	10,316	23.0
1996	45,611	32,764	12,847	8,006	17.6	10,638	23.3	16,373	35.9	10,594	23.2
1997	46,127	33,073	13,054	8,085	17.5	10,704	23.2	16,563	35.9	10,775	23.4
1998	46,539	33,346	13,193	8,145	17.5	10,722	23.0	16,713	35.9	10,959	23.5
1999	46,857	33,488	13,369	8,196	17.5	10,726	22.9	16,842	35.9	11,093	23.7
2000	47,204	33,688	13,515	8,222	17.4	10,730	22.7	17,007	36.0	11,244	23.8
2001	47,672	33,938	13,734	8,250	17.3	10,745	22.5	17,237	36.2	11,440	24.0
2002	48,183	34,116	14,067	8,297	17.2	10,819	22.5	17,471	36.3	11,596	24.1
2003	48,540	34,202	14,338	8,292	17.1	10,809	22.3	17,673	36.4	11,766	24.2
2004	48,795	34,178	14,617	8,271	17.0	10,775	22.1	17,892	36.7	11,857	24.3
2005	49,113	34,205	14,909	8,240	16.8	10,818	22.0	18,104	36.9	11,951	24.3

				Total and percent enrollment, grades preK–12 by region							
	Total enrollment			Northeast		Midwest		South		West	
Fall of year	Grades preK–12	Grades preK–8	Grades 9–12	Total	Percent	Total	Percent	Total	Percent	Total	Percent
Projected											
2006	49,464	34,422	15,041	8,183	16.5	10,809	21.9	18,384	37.2	12,088	24.4
2007	49,644	34,589	15,055	8,123	16.4	10,769	21.7	18,581	37.4	12,172	24.5
2008	49,825	34,903	14,922	8,057	16.2	10,718	21.5	18,802	37.7	12,248	24.6
2009	50,067	35,240	14,826	8,000	16.0	10,674	21.3	19,055	38.1	12,337	24.6
2010	50,353	35,653	14,700	7,948	15.8	10,646	21.1	19,312	38.4	12,447	24.7
2011	50,722	36,096	14,626	7,910	15.6	10,635	21.0	19,599	38.6	12,579	24.8
2012	51,194	36,527	14,667	7,888	15.4	10,647	20.8	19,930	38.9	12,730	24.9
2013	51,701	36,972	14,729	7,879	15.2	10,671	20.6	20,252	39.2	12,900	25.0
2014	52,284	37,403	14,881	7,885	15.1	10,711	20.5	20,598	39.4	13,091	25.0
2015	52,910	37,711	15,199	7,906	14.9	10,759	20.3	20,941	39.6	13,304	25.1
2016	53,503	38,052	15,451	7,927	14.8	10,799	20.2	21,255	39.7	13,522	25.3
2017	54,087	38,399	15,689	7,953	14.7	10,839	20.0	21,553	39.8	13,742	25.4

Note: Some data have been revised from previously published figures. See *supplemental note 1* for more information on geographic regions. Detail may not sum to totals because of rounding.

Source: U.S. Department of Education, National Center for Education Statistics (NCES). *Digest of Education Statistics, 2007* (NCES 2008-022), table 33; Hussar, W. (forthcoming). *Projections of Education Statistics to 2017* (NCES 2008-078), tables 1 and 4; Snyder, T., and Hoffman, C.M. (1995). *State Comparisons of Education Statistics: 1969–70 to 1993–94* (NCES 95-122), tables 10, 11, and 12, retrieved December 4, 2007, from http://nces.ed.gov/pubsearch/pubsinfo.asp?pubid=95122; and table ESE65, retrieved December 4, 2007, from http://www.nces.ed.gov/surveys/AnnualReports/historicaltables.asp.

Trends in Private School Enrollments

Table 4-1. Total enrollment and percentage distribution of students enrolled in private elementary and secondary schools, by school type and grade level: Various years, fall 1989–fall 2005

		Roman Catholic				Other religious[1]				
Grade level and fall of year	Total enrollment (in thousands)	Total	Parochial	Diocesan	Private	Total	Conservative Christian	Affiliated	Unaffiliated	Nonsectarian[2]
Grades K–12										
1989	4,838	54.5	32.2	15.2	7.1	32.3	10.9	12.8	8.5	13.2
1991	4,890	53.0	30.0	15.9	7.1	32.2	12.0	12.5	7.8	14.8
1993	4,836	51.4	29.2	15.5	6.8	33.7	12.6	12.3	8.8	14.9
1995	5,032	50.1	27.2	16.2	6.7	34.7	14.0	11.7	8.9	15.3
1997	5,076	49.5	26.5	16.3	6.7	34.8	14.5	10.9	9.4	15.7
1999	5,163	48.6	25.3	16.2	7.1	35.7	15.0	10.7	10.0	15.7
2001	5,342	47.1	22.9	17.3	6.9	36.0	15.4	10.5	10.1	16.9
2003	5,123	46.2	21.4	17.7	7.0	35.8	15.1	10.8	9.9	18.0
2005	5,058	44.4	19.4	17.7	7.3	37.3	16.3	11.6	9.4	18.3
Grades K–8[3]										
1989	3,588	55.1	40.1	12.5	2.5	34.1	11.8	13.7	8.6	10.8
1991	3,657	53.4	37.4	13.8	2.2	34.2	12.7	13.2	8.3	12.3
1993	3,641	51.8	36.4	13.2	2.1	35.7	13.3	13.0	9.4	12.5
1995	3,760	50.3	34.0	14.2	2.1	36.9	15.0	12.4	9.5	12.8
1997	3,781	49.9	33.2	14.6	2.1	36.9	15.5	11.4	10.0	13.3
1999	3,849	48.8	31.8	14.6	2.4	37.8	15.9	11.3	10.7	13.4
2001	3,951	47.2	28.8	16.0	2.5	38.2	16.4	11.0	10.9	14.5
2003	3,731	46.3	27.4	16.5	2.4	38.3	16.2	11.3	10.9	15.4
2005	3,636	44.5	25.1	16.8	2.7	39.6	17.3	12.3	10.0	15.9

Grades 9–12[3]										
1989	1,126	57.2	10.2	25.0	22.0	27.0	8.7	10.9	7.4	15.8
1991	1,126	55.5	8.6	23.6	23.3	27.2	10.0	11.0	6.2	17.2
1993	1,102	54.0	7.4	24.2	22.4	28.3	10.6	10.8	7.0	17.7
1995	1,160	53.3	7.8	23.7	21.8	29.4	11.7	10.5	7.2	17.3
1997	1,181	52.4	7.3	23.3	21.8	29.8	12.2	9.9	7.6	17.8
1999	1,225	51.1	6.5	22.3	22.3	30.6	12.9	9.5	8.1	18.3
2001	1,293	49.5	6.4	22.5	20.6	31.0	13.3	9.8	7.8	19.5
2003	1,307	48.5	5.7	22.4	20.4	30.0	12.8	10.0	7.2	21.6
2005	1,346	46.3	5.2	21.1	20.0	32.5	14.3	10.1	8.1	21.3

[1] Other religious schools have a religious orientation or purpose, but are not Roman Catholic. Conservative Christian schools are those with membership in at least one of four associations: Accelerated Christian Education, American Association of Christian Schools, Association of Christian Schools International, or Oral Roberts University Education Fellowship. Affiliated schools are those with membership in 1 of 12 associations—Association of Christian Teachers and Schools, Christian Schools International, Council of Islamic Schools in North America, Evangelical Lutheran Education Association, Friends Council on Education, General Conference of the Seventh-Day Adventist Church, Islamic School League of America, National Association of Episcopal Schools, National Christian School Association, National Society for Hebrew Day Schools, Solomon Schechter Day Schools, or Southern Baptist Association of Christian Schools—or indicating membership in "other religious school associations." Unaffiliated schools are those that have a religious orientation or purpose, but are not classified as Conservative Christian or affiliated.

[2] Nonsectarian schools do not have a religious orientation or purpose.

[3] Grades K–8 and 9–12 do not include ungraded students; therefore, these two categories do not sum to grades K–12.

Note: Detail may not sum to totals because of rounding.

Source: U.S. Department of Education, National Center for Education Statistics, Private School Universe Survey (PSS), various years, 1989–90 through 2005–06.

Table 4-2. Private elementary and secondary school enrollment and as a percentage of total enrollment in public and private schools, by region and grade level: Various years, fall 1989–fall 2005

[Totals in thousands]										
	Total enrollment		Northeast		Midwest		South		West	
Grade level and fall of year	Total	Percent of total enrollment	Total	Percent of total Northeast enrollment	Total	Percent of total Midwest enrollment	Total	Percent of total South enrollment	Total	Percent of total West enrollment
Grades K–12										
1989	4,838	10.7	1,346	15.8	1,368	12.3	1,280	8.1	844	8.7
1991	4,890	10.5	1,324	15.3	1,353	12.0	1,304	8.1	909	8.8
1993	4,836	10.1	1,276	14.4	1,309	11.4	1,386	8.3	865	8.1
1995	5,032	10.2	1,289	14.1	1,349	11.5	1,445	8.4	949	8.5
1997	5,076	10.0	1,287	13.8	1,346	11.3	1,510	8.5	933	8.0
1999	5,163	10.1	1,295	13.8	1,345	11.3	1,576	8.7	947	7.9
2001	5,342	10.2	1,337	14.1	1,355	11.4	1,641	8.9	1,008	8.2
2003	5,123	9.7	1,273	13.5	1,271	10.7	1,612	8.6	967	7.7
2005	5,058	9.4	1,203	13.0	1,233	10.3	1,626	8.3	995	7.7
Grades K–81										
1989	3,588	11.0	947	15.9	1,052	13.2	949	8.3	639	9.0
1991	3,657	10.8	935	15.2	1,059	12.9	974	8.2	689	9.1
1993	3,641	10.5	907	14.3	1,021	12.4	1,048	8.6	664	8.5
1995	3,760	10.6	911	14.0	1,042	12.5	1,086	8.7	721	8.9
1997	3,781	10.5	911	13.8	1,036	12.3	1,126	8.8	708	8.5
1999	3,849	10.5	917	13.8	1,035	12.3	1,177	9.1	720	8.5
2001	3,951	10.7	935	14.0	1,039	12.4	1,223	9.2	754	8.6
2003	3,731	10.1	857	13.2	962	11.6	1,191	8.9	720	8.2
2005	3,636	9.7	803	12.7	931	11.2	1,181	8.4	721	8.0
Grades 9–121										

1989	1,126	9.0	362	14.6	288	9.2	291	6.8	185	7.1
1991	1,126	8.9	346	14.1	276	8.9	302	7.0	203	7.3
1993	1,102	8.4	328	13.1	273	8.5	315	7.1	186	6.4
1995	1,160	8.5	334	13.0	286	8.5	330	7.1	209	6.8
1997	1,181	8.3	330	12.5	292	8.5	353	7.2	206	6.3
1999	1,225	8.4	338	12.6	297	8.6	375	7.5	214	6.3
2001	1,293	8.6	364	13.0	302	8.6	389	7.5	239	6.8
2003	1,307	8.4	381	13.0	293	8.1	395	7.3	237	6.4
2005	1,346	8.3	366	12.6	292	8.0	424	7.5	265	6.7

[1] Grades K–8 and 9–12 do not include ungraded students; therefore, these two categories do not sum to grades K–12.

Note: Detail may not sum to totals because of rounding. Calculations were revised and estimates may differ from previously published data. *Supplemental note 1* identifies the states in each region.

Source: U.S. Department of Education, National Center for Education Statistics, Private School Universe Survey (PSS), various years, 1989–90 through 2005–06.

Table 4-3. Number and percentage distribution of students in private schools, by race/ethnicity and selected school characteristics: Fall 2005

				Minority enrollment[1]				
School characteristic	Number (in thousands)	Total students	White	Total minority	Black	Hispanic	Asian/ Pacific Islander	American Indian/Alaska Native
Total	5,058	100.0	75.4	24.6	9.5	9.2	5.1	0.7
NCES private school typology								
Roman Catholic	2,246	44.4	74.1	25.9	7.9	12.6	4.7	0.7
Parochial	982	19.4	74.1	25.9	7.7	13.0	4.6	0.7
Diocesan	896	17.7	75.0	25.0	7.8	12.1	4.5	0.6
Private	368	7.3	72.0	28.0	8.8	12.6	5.5	1.0
Other religious2	1,885	37.3	77.8	22.2	10.8	6.3	4.5	0.5
Conservative Christian	824	16.3	75.3	24.7	12.2	7.7	4.2	0.7
Affiliated	585	11.6	81.0	19.0	8.7	5.3	4.6	0.4
Unaffiliated	476	9.4	78.3	21.7	11.1	5.3	5.0	0.3
Nonsectarian3	927	18.3	73.7	26.3	10.8	7.0	7.4	1.0
Regular	604	12.0	76.7	23.3	8.9	6.0	7.5	0.9
Special emphasis	218	4.3	71.6	28.4	9.9	7.6	9.4	1.6
Special education	104	2.1	61.3	38.7	23.8	11.8	2.2	0.9
School level								
Elementary	2,551	50.4	73.7	26.3	9.7	10.7	5.2	0.7
Secondary	859	17.0	75.4	24.6	8.3	10.5	5.2	0.7
Combined	1,647	32.6	78.2	21.8	9.8	6.4	4.9	0.7
Program emphasis								
Regular	4,570	90.4	76.0	24.0	9.1	9.3	4.9	0.7
Montessori	90	1.8	70.1	29.9	9.1	7.6	11.9	1.3
Special program emphasis	206	4.1	77.5	22.5	7.9	7.1	6.4	1.0
Special education	116	2.3	62.0	38.0	23.5	11.5	2.2	0.8
Alternative	66	1.3	61.8	38.2	17.1	11.5	8.3	1.4
Early childhood	7	0.1	72.1	27.9	13.4	7.0	6.3	1.2

Enrollment								
Less than 50	236	4.7	71.5	28.5	15.1	8.5	3.8	1.1
50–149	763	15.1	71.3	28.7	14.2	9.0	4.5	1.0
150–299	1,322	26.1	70.6	29.4	11.7	11.6	5.5	0.6
300–499	1,090	21.5	78.2	21.8	7.8	8.5	4.9	0.6
500–749	805	15.9	80.0	20.0	5.8	8.3	5.2	0.7
750 or more	842	16.7	80.0	20.0	6.1	7.7	5.7	0.5
Region								
Northeast	1,203	23.8	75.5	24.5	11.6	8.2	4.3	0.4
Midwest	1,233	24.4	84.0	16.0	8.0	4.8	2.4	0.7
South	1,626	32.2	76.2	23.8	11.3	8.8	3.2	0.4
West	995	19.7	63.5	36.5	6.0	16.6	12.5	1.4
Locale								
City	2,142	42.4	68.5	31.5	12.8	11.9	6.3	0.5
Suburban	1,949	38.5	77.4	22.6	8.5	8.7	4.8	0.6
Town	365	7.2	88.2	11.8	3.2	5.3	2.6	0.8
Rural	601	11.9	86.2	13.8	5.1	3.8	3.3	1.6

[1] Race categories exclude persons of Hispanic ethnicity.

[2] Other religious schools have a religious orientation or purpose, but are not Roman Catholic. Conservative Christian schools are those with membership in at least one of four associations: Accelerated Christian Education, American Association of Christian Schools, Association of Christian Schools International, or Oral Roberts University Education Fellowship. Affiliated schools are those with membership in 1 of 12 associations—Association of Christian Teachers and Schools, Christian Schools International, Council of Islamic Schools in North America, Evangelical Lutheran Education Association, Friends Council on Education, General Conference of the Seventh-Day Adventist Church, Islamic School League of America, National Association of Episcopal Schools, National Christian School Association, National Society for Hebrew Day Schools, Solomon Schechter Day Schools, or Southern Baptist Association of Christian Schools—or indicating membership in "other religious school associations." Unaffiliated schools are those that have a religious orientation or purpose, but are not classified as Conservative Christian or affiliated.

[3] Nonsectarian schools do not have a religious orientation or purpose.

Note: Detail may not sum to totals because of rounding. *Supplemental note 1* identifies the states in each region.

Source: U.S. Department of Education, National Center for Education Statistics, Private School Universe Survey (PSS), 2005–06.

Racial/Ethnic Distribution of Public School Students

Table 5-1. Percentage distribution of the race/ethnicity of public school students enrolled in kindergarten through 12th grade: October 1972–2006

		Minority enrollment							
October of year	White	Total	Black	Hispanic	Pacific	Asian Islander	American Indian/ Alaska Native	More than one race	Other
1972	77.8	22.2	14.8	6.0	—	—	—	—	1.4
1973	78.1	21.9	14.7	5.7	—	—	—	—	1.4
1974	76.8	23.2	15.4	6.3	—	—	—	—	1.5
1975	76.2	23.8	15.4	6.7	—	—	—	—	1.7
1976	76.2	23.8	15.5	6.5	—	—	—	—	1.7
1977	76.1	23.9	15.8	6.2	—	—	—	—	1.9
1978	75.5	24.5	16.0	6.5	—	—	—	—	2.1
1979	—	—	—	—	—	—	—	—	—
1980	—	—	—	—	—	—	—	—	—
1981	72.4	27.6	16.0	8.7	—	—	—	—	2.9
1982	71.9	28.1	16.0	8.9	—	—	—	—	3.2
1983	71.3	28.7	16.1	9.2	—	—	—	—	3.4
1984	71.7	28.3	16.1	8.5	—	—	—	—	3.6
1985	69.6	30.4	16.8	10.1	—	—	—	—	3.5
1986	69.1	30.9	16.6	10.8	—	—	—	—	3.6
1987	68.5	31.5	16.6	10.8	—	—	—	—	4.0
1988	68.3	31.7	16.5	11.0	—	—	—	—	4.2
1989	68.0	32.0	16.6	11.4	3.01	(1)	0.9	—	0.1
1990	67.6	32.4	16.5	11.7	3.01	(1)	0.9	—	0.3
1991	67.1	32.9	16.8	11.8	3.21	(1)	0.8	—	0.2
1992	66.8	33.2	16.9	12.0	3.31	(1)	0.8	—	0.2
1993	67.0	33.0	16.6	12.1	3.31	(1)	0.8	—	0.2

		Minority enrollment							
October of year	White	Total	Black	Hispanic	Pacific	Asian Islander	American Indian/ Alaska Native	More than one race	Other
1994	65.8	34.2	16.7	13.7	2.51	(1)	0.8	—	0.5
1995	65.5	34.5	16.9	14.1	2.31	(1)	0.6	—	0.6
1996	63.7	36.3	16.6	14.5	4.11	(1)	1.2	—	—
1997	63.0	37.0	16.9	14.9	3.91	(1)	1.2	—	—
1998	62.4	37.6	17.2	15.4	4.01	(1)	1.1	—	—
1999	61.9	38.1	16.5	16.2	4.51	(1)	1.0	—	—
2000	61.3	38.7	16.6	16.6	4.21	(1)	1.3	—	—
2001	61.3	38.7	16.5	16.6	4.31	(1)	1.3	—	—
2002	60.7	39.3	16.5	17.6	4.01	(1)	1.2	—	—
2003	58.3	41.7	16.1	18.6	3.7	0.3	0.6	2.4	—
2004	57.4	42.6	16.0	19.3	3.9	0.2	0.8	2.4	—
2005	57.6	42.4	15.6	19.7	3.7	0.2	0.7	2.5	—
2006	56.9	43.1	15.6	20.2	3.8	0.2	0.7	2.7	—

— Not available.

[1] From 1989 through 2002, Asian and Pacific Islander students were not reported separately; therefore, Pacific Islander students are included with Asian students during this period.

Note: Estimates include all public school students enrolled in kindergarten through 12th grade. Race categories exclude persons of Hispanic ethnicity. Over time, the Current Population Survey (CPS) has had different response options for race/ethnicity. In 1994, the survey methodology for the CPS was changed and weights were adjusted. In 1996, the Census revised procedures for editing and allocating the race variable to offset an underestimation of Asians/Pacific Islanders. One should use caution when making comparisons between data for 1995 and earlier and data for 1996 and later. See *supplemental note 2* for more information on the CPS. Detail may not sum to totals because of rounding.

Source: U.S. Department of Commerce, Census Bureau, Current Population Survey (CPS), October Supplement, 1972–2006.

Table 5-2. Percentage distribution of the race/ethnicity of public school students enrolled in kindergarten through 12th grade, by region: Selected years, October 1972–2006

		Minority enrollment							
Region and October of Year	White	Total	Black	Hispanic	Asian	Pacific Islander	American Indian/Alaska Native	More than one race	Other
Northeast									
1972	81.4	18.6	12.4	5.5	—	—	—	—	0.7
1981	76.5	23.5	13.3	8.2	—	—	—	—	2.0
1986	73.8	26.2	13.3	10.7	—	—	—	—	2.2
1993	72.2	27.8	15.2	8.8	3.41	(1)	0.1!	—	0.3!
2000	68.1	31.9	15.5	11.4	4.51	(1)	0.4	—	—
2001	67.6	32.4	15.2	12.2	4.41	(1)	0.6	—	—
2002	67.9	32.1	15.1	13.1	3.71	(1)	0.3	—	—
2003	64.8	35.2	16.0	13.7	3.7	‡	0.2!	1.5	—
2004	63.7	36.3	15.5	13.9	5.1	‡	0.2!	1.5	—
2005	63.5	36.5	15.1	14.5	5.2	‡	‡	1.5	—
2006	63.8	36.2	14.7	15.3	4.4	‡	0.2!	1.5	—
Midwest									
1972	87.5	12.5	10.6	1.5	—	—	—	—	0.3
1981	84.4	15.6	12.1	1.9	—	—	—	—	1.6
1986	81.8	18.2	13.0	3.4	—	—	—	—	1.8
1993	80.8	19.2	13.4	3.6	1.31	(1)	0.6	—	0.4
2000	76.3	23.7	15.3	5.5	2.01	(1)	0.8	—	—
2001	77.2	22.8	14.8	4.8	2.01	(1)	1.2	—	—
2002	75.5	24.5	14.5	6.4	2.61	(1)	1.0	—	—
2003	74.4	25.6	14.2	6.4	2.2	0.2!	0.4	2.2	—
2004	74.4	25.6	13.5	6.6	2.3	‡	0.5	2.5	—
2005	74.1	25.9	13.8	7.1	1.9	‡	0.6	2.5	—
2006	73.4	26.6	13.2	7.7	2.6	‡	0.5	2.4	—
South									
1972	69.7	30.3	24.8	5.0	—	—	—	—	0.5
1981	64.1	35.9	25.9	8.5	—	—	—	—	1.4
1986	62.2	37.8	26.6	9.0	—	—	—	—	2.2
1993	60.1	39.9	26.4	10.7	2.01	(1)	0.6	—	0.2!

		Minority enrollment							
Region and October of Year	White	Total	Black	Hispanic	Asian	Pacific Islander	American Indian/Alaska Native	More than one race	Other
2000	55.1	44.9	25.6	16.0	2.11	(1)	1.1	—	—
2001	55.6	44.4	25.6	15.6	2.51	(1)	0.8	—	—
2002	54.2	45.8	26.2	16.6	1.91	(1)	1.0	—	—
2003	53.6	46.4	24.8	16.9	2.1	‡	0.6	2.0	—
2004	53.7	46.3	24.5	16.6	2.4	0.1!	0.6	2.2	—
2005	52.9	47.1	23.9	18.3	1.8	‡	0.6	2.4	—
2006	51.5	48.5	24.5	18.8	1.9	‡	0.7	2.6	—
West									
1972	72.8	27.2	6.4	15.3	—	—	—	—	5.5
1981	66.5	33.5	6.8	18.5	—	—	—	—	8.1
1986	62.5	37.5	6.1	22.0	—	—	—	—	9.4
1993	58.7	41.3	6.1	25.9	7.41	(1)	1.7	—	0.2!
2000	51.1	48.9	5.9	31.6	8.81	(1)	2.6	—	—
2001	49.9	50.1	6.1	32.5	8.81	(1)	2.7	—	—
2002	51.0	49.0	5.8	32.6	8.21	(1)	2.4	—	—
2003	45.9	54.1	5.2	35.5	7.5	1.0	1.2	3.6	—
2004	42.9	57.1	6.0	38.7	6.9	0.6	1.6	3.3	—
2005	45.6	54.4	5.2	36.6	7.2	0.6	1.3	3.6	—
2006	45.2	54.8	5.1	36.9	7.1	0.8	1.0	3.9	—

— Not available.

! Interpret data with caution (estimates are unstable).

‡ Reporting standards not met (too few cases).

[1] From 1989 through 2002, Asian and Pacific Islander students were not reported separately; therefore, Pacific Islander students are included with Asian students during this period.

Note: Figures include all public school students enrolled in kindergarten through 12th grade. Race categories exclude persons of Hispanic ethnicity. Over time, the Current Population Survey (CPS) has had different response options for race/ethnicity. In 1994, the survey methodology for the CPS was changed and weights were adjusted. In 1996, the Census revised procedures for editing and allocating the race variable to offset an underestimation of Asians/Pacific Islanders. One should use caution when making comparisons between data for 1995 and earlier and data for 1996 and later. See *supplemental note 2* for more information on the CPS. Detail may not sum to totals because of rounding.

Source: U.S. Department of Commerce, Census Bureau, Current Population Survey (CPS), October Supplement, selected years, 1972–2006.

Family Characteristics of 5- to 17-Year-Olds

Table 6-1. Percentage distribution of 5- to 17-year-olds, by race/ethnicity and selected family characteristics: Selected years, 1979–2006

Family characteristic	1979	1989	1992	1995	1999	2002	2004	2006
Total U.S. population								
Parents' education								
Less than high school	—	14.9	14.0	12.8	12.6	10.8	10.7	11.0
High school diploma	—	34.2	33.0	28.9	27.5	26.2	25.3	24.7
Some college	—	25.0	27.3	30.1	29.9	29.9	30.3	29.2
Bachelor's degree or higher	19.0	25.8	25.7	28.2	30.0	33.1	33.7	35.2
Family type1								
Two-parent household	74.8	71.8	70.1	68.5	67.2	68.1	66.9	66.8
Mother-only household	17.8	21.8	23.1	23.0	23.5	22.9	23.3	23.2
Father-only household	2.2	3.0	3.2	3.5	4.3	4.4	4.6	4.7
Poverty status2								
Poor	14.7	18.5	20.6	20.8	18.8	15.6	16.9	16.9
Near-poor	19.3	20.9	22.0	21.8	20.7	20.5	20.5	20.8
Nonpoor	66.0	60.7	57.4	57.4	60.5	63.9	62.6	62.3
Citizenship								
U.S.-born	—	—	—	95.6	96.0	95.3	95.3	95.0
Naturalized U.S. citizen	—	—	—	0.3	0.5	0.7	0.7	0.8
Non-U.S. citizen	—	—	—	4.1	3.4	4.0	3.9	4.2
Immigration status								
Born outside the 50 states and the								
District of Columbia	—	—	—	5.5	5.1	5.6	5.5	5.9
First generation3	—	—	—	12.7	14.6	15.5	16.3	18.0
Second generation or more4	—	—	—	81.7	80.3	78.9	78.2	76.0
Total White population								
Parents' education								
Less than high school	—	7.6	6.9	5.5	5.2	4.5	3.8	4.0
High school diploma	—	34.8	32.6	28.5	26.2	24.2	23.1	22.0
Some college	—	26.9	29.9	31.4	31.8	31.3	31.8	30.3
Bachelor's degree or higher	22.3	30.7	30.6	34.5	36.8	39.9	41.3	43.7

Family characteristic	1979	1989	1992	1995	1999	2002	2004	2006
Family type[1]								
Two-parent household	80.7	79.9	78.3	77.2	75.3	75.8	75.1	74.8
Mother-only household	13.2	15.1	16.4	16.3	17.0	16.6	16.5	16.4
Father-only household	2.2	3.0	3.2	3.4	4.5	4.5	4.7	5.0
Poverty status[2] Poor	8.9	10.3	12.4	12.1	10.8	9.5	9.7	9.9
Near-poor	16.6	19.1	19.6	19.3	16.4	16.1	16.1	15.4
Nonpoor	74.5	70.5	68.0	68.6	72.7	74.4	74.2	74.7
Citizenship U.S.-born	—	—	—	98.8	99.0	98.6	98.4	98.4
Naturalized U.S. citizen	—	—	—	#	0.2	0.3	0.3	0.4
Non-U.S. citizen	—	—	—	1.2	0.8	1.1	1.3	1.2
Immigration status Born outside the 50 states and the								
District of Columbia	—	—	—	2.0	1.7	2.1	2.2	2.1
First generation[3]	—	—	—	5.6	5.8	6.3	6.0	6.0
Second generation or more4	—	—	—	92.4	92.5	91.6	91.9	91.9
Total Black population								
Parents' education								
Less than high school	—	23.6	22.5	19.3	16.7	14.0	13.6	13.3
High school diploma	—	39.4	40.6	35.3	36.1	35.3	34.9	33.0
Some college	—	24.6	24.3	32.5	31.7	32.8	33.0	32.5
Bachelor's degree or higher	4.9	12.3	12.7	12.9	15.5	18.0	18.5	21.2
Family type1								
Two-parent household	43.8	38.8	37.5	34.2	35.5	37.7	36.1	35.1
Mother-only household	43.7	48.3	50.5	49.7	49.7	47.8	48.3	50.2
Father-only household	2.4	3.3	2.9	3.8	3.8	5.3	5.0	4.2
Poverty status[2]								
Poor	40.6	41.9	43.8	41.9	36.0	29.0	33.4	33.3
Near-poor	28.4	22.7	24.1	25.5	27.9	26.8	27.3	26.8
Nonpoor	31.1	35.4	32.1	32.5	36.0	44.2	39.4	39.9
Citizenship								
U.S.-born	—	—	—	98.3	98.1	97.1	97.5	97.1
Naturalized U.S. citizen	—	—	—	0.2	0.3	0.3	0.3	0.4
Non-U.S. citizen	—	—	—	1.5	1.6	2.7	2.1	2.5
Immigration status								

Table 6-1. (Continued).

Family characteristic	1979	1989	1992	1995	1999	2002	2004	2006
Born outside the 50 states and the								
District of Columbia	—	—	—	2.7	2.5	3.5	3.1	3.3
First generation3	—	—	—	5.1	6.4	7.8	8.9	9.
Second generation or more4	—	—	—	92.1	91.1	88.8	88.1	1
Total Hispanic population								
Parents' education								
Less than high school	—	47.8	48.2	43.5	40.8	38.0	36.7	32.4
High school diploma	—	27.3	27.2	25.4	26.3	27.7	27.1	28.8
Some college	—	16.0	15.8	22.3	21.1	21.7	23.3	23.8
Bachelor's degree or higher	7.2	8.8	8.8	8.9	11.9	12.6	13.0	14.9
Family type1								
Two-parent household	71.6	64.9	63.5	63.0	63.4	64.4	63.6	65.3
Mother-only household	17.2	28.9	28.2	26.9	26.2	25.6	26.1	24.5
Father-only household	2.1	2.8	3.3	4.3	3.8	3.9	4.2	4.0
Poverty status[2] Poor	26.9	34.5	38.3	39.8	33.6	28.8	29.1	26.5
Near-poor	31.9	29.4	33.0	30.7	31.8	32.5	31.5	32.8
Nonpoor	41.2	36.2	28.7	29.5	34.6	38.7	39.3	40.7
Citizenship								
U.S.-born	—	—	—	81.4	86.3	83.5	85.4	85.9
Naturalized U.S. citizen	—	—	—	1.1	1.0	1.6	0.9	1.2
Non-U.S. citizen	—	—	—	17.5	12.6	14.9	13.8	12.9
Immigration status Born outside the 50 states and the								
District of Columbia	—	—	—	21.2	16.6	18.5	16.4	16.4
First generation[3]	—	—	—	50.2	49.2	53.0	52.3	52.5
Second generation or more4	—	—	—	28.6	34.2	28.5	31.3	31.1

— Not available.

Rounds to zero.

[1] Detail does not sum to total because a small percentage of respondents were not in the survey universe or had no parents present in the home.

[2] *Poor* is defined to include families below the poverty threshold, *near-poor* is defined to include families at 100–199 percent of the poverty threshold, and *nonpoor* is defined to include families at 200 percent or more than the poverty threshold. See *supplemental note 1* for more information.

[3] *First generation* describes an individual born in the 50 states or the District of Columbia with at least one parent born outside the 50 states or the District of Columbia.

[4] *Second generation or more* describes an individual born in the 50 states or the District of Columbia whose parents were both born inside the 50 states or the District of Columbia.

Note: Prior to 1992, *high school completers* referred to those who completed 12 years of schooling, and *some college* meant completing 1 or more years of college; beginning in 1992, *high school completers* referred to those who received a high school diploma or equivalency certificate, and *some college* meant completing any college at all. Included in the totals but not shown separately are estimates for those from other racial/ethnic categories.

In 1994, the survey instrument for the Current Population Survey (CPS) was changed and weights were adjusted. See *supplemental note 2* for further discussion. Some estimates are revised from previous publications. Detail may not sum to totals because of rounding. Race categories exclude persons of Hispanic ethnicity.

Source: U.S. Department of Commerce, Census Bureau, Current Population Survey (CPS), March Supplement, selected years, 1979–2006.

Language Minority School-Age Children

Table 7-1. Number and percentage of children ages 5–17 who spoke a language other than English at home and who spoke English with difficulty: Selected years, 1979–2006

		Spoke a language other than English at home				
				Spoke English with difficulty[1]		
Year	Total population (in millions)	Number (in millions)	Percent of total population	Number (in millions)	Percent of total population	Percent of those who spoke a language other than English at home
1979	44.7	3.8	8.5	1.3	2.8	34.2
1989	42.3	5.2	12.3	1.8	4.3	34.6
1992	47.7	6.3	13.2	2.2	4.6	34.9
1995	47.5	6.7	14.1	2.4	5.2	35.8
1999	52.7	8.8	16.7	2.6	5.0	29.5
2000	52.5	9.5	18.1	2.9	5.5	30.5
2001	53.0	9.8	18.5	2.8	5.4	28.6
2002	53.0	9.8	18.5	2.8	5.3	28.6
2003	53.0	9.9	18.7	2.9	5.5	29.4
2004	52.9	9.9	18.8	2.8	5.3	27.9
2005	52.8	10.6	20.0	2.8	5.4	26.8
2006	53.4	10.8	20.3	2.8	5.2	25.4
		Percentage change compared with 1979				
2006	19.5	185.4	138.9	112.2	84.4	-25.7
		Percentage change compared with 2000				
2006	1.8	14.2	12.2	-4.9	-6.1	-16.7

[1] Data on language spoken at home and difficulty speaking English were obtained from household respondents. Respondents were asked if each child in the household spoke a language other than English at home. If they answered "yes," they were asked how well each child could speak English. Categories used for reporting were "very well," "well," "not well," and "not at all." All those who reported speaking English less than "very well" were considered to have difficulty speaking English. Since the American Community Survey (ACS) does not ask whether household children speak English at home, these data cannot be used to determine whether English or another language is the primary language spoken at home.

Note: Spanish-language versions of both the Current Population Survey (CPS) and the American Community Survey (ACS) were available to respondents. Due to differences between the CPS and the ACS, use caution when comparing data before 2000 (CPS) with data from 2000 onward (ACS). See *supplemental notes 2* and *3* for more information.

Source: U.S. Department of Commerce, Census Bureau, Current Population Survey (CPS), 1979 and 1989 November Supplement and 1992, 1995, and 1999 October Supplement, and American Community Survey (ACS), 2000–06.

Table 7-2. Number and percentage of children ages 5–17 who spoke a language other than English at home and who spoke English with difficulty, by selected characteristics: 2006; [Numbers in thousands]

	Spoke a language other than English at home								
				Spoke English with difficulty1					
				Total		Ages 5–9		Ages 10–17	
Characteristic	Total population	Number	Percent of total population	Number	Percent of total population	Number	Percent of total population	Number	Percent of total population
Total	53,406	10,845	20.3	2,758	5.2	1,372	6.9	1,386	4.1
Language spoken at home									
Spanish	7,787	7,787	100.0	2,071	26.6	1,054	35.4	1,018	21.1
Other Indo-European3	1,434	1,434	100.0	277	19.3	121	23.6	156	16.9
Asian/Pacific Islander4	1,200	1,200	100.0	333	27.8	161	36.2	172	22.9
Other	424	424	100.0	77	18.1	36	21.3	40	15.9
Race/ethnicity5									
White	31,154	1,762	5.7	378	1.2	134	1.2	245	1.2
Black	7,870	429	5.5	99	1.3	34	1.2	65	1.3
Hispanic	10,250	7,038	68.7	1,882	18.4	1,011	24.6	870	14.2
Mexican	6,986	4,998	71.5	1,463	20.9	821	28.5	641	15.6
Puerto Rican	936	465	49.7	78	8.3	32	8.9	46	7.9
Cuban	218	149	68.4	24	11.0	11	13.7	13	9.4
Dominican	274	243	88.6	49	17.9	17	18.0	32	17.9
Central American	614	510	83.2	137	22.3	69	29.1	68	18.0
South American	398	314	78.9	58	14.6	25	16.9	33	13.2
Other Hispanic	823	358	43.5	73	8.9	36	11.2	38	7.5
Asian	2,042	1,321	64.7	350	17.1	172	21.7	178	14.2
Pacific Islander	84	25	30.0	5	6.1	2	7.5 3	3	5.2
American Indian/Alaska Native	436	85	19.6	12	2.8	5	3.4	7	2.5
More than one race	1,383	116	8.4	18	1.3	7	1.2	11	1.4

Table 7-2. Continued

	Spoke a language other than English at home								
				Spoke English with difficulty1					
				Total		Ages 5–9		Ages 10–17	
Characteristic	Total population	Number	Percent of total population	Number	Percent of total population	Number	Percent of total population	Number	Percent of total population
Citizenship									
U.S.-born	50,701	8,571	16.9	1,831	3.6	1,044	5.5	787	2.5
Naturalized U.S. citizen	544	331	60.9	66	12.1	18	13.3	48	11.7
Non-U.S. citizen	2,161	1,942	89.9	861	39.9	310	50.5	551	35.6
Poverty status6									
Poor	9,083	2,742	30.2	881	9.7	464	12.7	417	7.7
Near-poor	11,002	3,276	29.8	885	8.0	468	10.9	417	6.2
Nonpoor	32,348	4,661	14.4	937	2.9	411	3.6	526	2.5
Region									
Northeast	9,321	1,869	20.1	409	4.4	180	5.3	229	3.8
Midwest	11,859	1,338	11.3	363	3.1	179	4.1	184	2.5
South	19,401	3,339	17.2	886	4.6	445	6.1	440	3.6
West	12,825	4,299	33.5	1,101	8.6	568	11.9	533	6.6

[1] Data on language spoken at home and difficulty speaking English were obtained from household respondents. Respondents were asked if each child in the household spoke a language other than English at home. If they answered "yes," they were asked how well each child could speak English. Categories used for reporting were "very well," "well," "not well," and "not at all." All those who reported speaking English less than "very well" were considered to have difficulty speaking English. Since the American Community Survey (ACS) does not ask whether household children speak English at home, these data cannot be used to determine whether English or another language is the primary language spoken at home.

[2] Percentage of the total subgroup population for that particular subgroup. For example, 3.4 percent of all American Indians/Alaska Natives ages 5–9 spoke a language other than English at home and spoke English with difficulty.

[3] An Indo-European language other than Spanish (e.g., French, German, Portuguese, etc.).

[4] Any native language spoken by Asians or Pacific Islanders, which linguists classify variously as Sino-Tibetan, Austroasiatic, or Austronesian languages.

[5] Race categories exclude persons of Hispanic ethnicity.

[6] *Poor* is defined to include families below the poverty threshold, *near-poor* is defined to include families at 100–199 percent of the poverty threshold, and *nonpoor* is defined to include families at 200 percent or more than the poverty threshold. See *supplemental note 1* for more information. Detail may not sum to totals because of missing values for poverty.

Note: Detail may not sum to totals because of rounding. A Spanish-language version of the American Community Survey (ACS) was available to respondents. For the states in each region, see *supplemental note 1*.

Source: U.S. Department of Commerce, Census Bureau, American Community Survey (ACS), 2006.

Children and Youth With Disabilities in Public Schools

Table 8-1. Number and percentage of children and youth ages 3–21 served under the Individuals with Disabilities Education Act (IDEA): 1976–77 through 2006–07

School year	Total served under IDEA (in thousands)	Percentage of total public school enrollment served under IDEA1	Percentage of youth ages 3–21 served under IDEA
1976–77	3,692	8.3	5.0
1977–78	3,755	8.6	5.1
1978–79	3,894	9.2	5.4
1979–80	4,010	9.6	5.6
1980–81	4,146	10.1	5.8
1981–82	4,203	10.5	6.0
1982–83	4,260	10.8	6.1
1983–84	4,304	11.0	6.3
1984–85	4,320	11.0	6.3
1985–86	4,322	11.0	6.4
1986–87	4,379	11.0	6.5
1987–88	4,414	11.0	6.6
1988–89	4,493	11.2	6.7
1989–90	4,599	11.3	6.8
1990–91	4,717	11.4	6.9
1991–92	4,881	11.6	7.1
1992–93	5,042	11.8	7.3
1993–94	5,223	12.0	7.5
1994–95	5,378	12.2	7.6
1995–96	5,572	12.4	7.7
1996–97	5,737	12.6	7.8
1997–98	5,908	12.8	7.9
1998–99	6,056	13.0	8.0
1999–2000	6,195	13.2	8.1

Table 8-1. (Continued).

School year	Total served under IDEA (in thousands)	Percentage of total public school enrollment served under IDEA1	Percentage of youth ages 3–21 served under IDEA
2000–01	6,296	13.3	8.2
2001–02	6,407	13.4	8.3
2002–03	6,523	13.5	8.4
2003–04	6,634	13.7	8.6
2004–05	6,719	13.8	8.7
2005–06	6,713	13.8	8.6
2006–07	6,686	13.5	8.6

[1] Number of children and youth served as a percentage of all children and youth ages 3–21 enrolled in early education centers and elementary and secondary schools.

Note: Special education services through the Individuals with Disabilities Education Act (IDEA) are available for eligible youth identified by a team of qualified professionals as having a disability that adversely affects academic performance and as in need of special education and related services. The total includes youth receiving special education services through IDEA in early education centers and elementary and secondary schools in the 50 states and the District of Columbia and in Bureau of Indian Affairs (BIA) schools through 1993–94. Beginning in 1994–95, estimates exclude BIA schools. See *supplemental note 8* for more information about the student disabilities represented here.

Source: U.S. Department of Education, Office of Special Education and Rehabilitative Services (OSERS), Office of Special Education Programs (OSEP), Data Analysis System (DANS), 1976–2006. Retrieved November 29, 2007, from https://www.ideadata.org/arc_toc8.asp#partbCC and https://www.ideadata.org/docs/PartBTrendData/B1.xls.

Table 8-2. Percentage of children and youth ages 3–21 served under the Individuals with Disabilities Education Act (IDEA), by disability: Selected years, 1976–77 through 2006–07

	1976	1980	1990	1994	1995	1996	1997	1998	1999	2000	2001	2002	2003	2004	2005	2006
Age and disability	–77	–81	–91	–95	–96	–97	–98	–99	–2000	–01	–02	–03	–04	–05	–06	–07
All disabilities	8.3	10.1	11.4	12.2	12.4	12.6	12.8	13.0	13.2	13.3	13.4	13.5	13.7	13.8	13.8	13.5
Specific learning disabilities1	1.8	3.6	5.2	5.6	5.8	5.8	5.9	6.0	6.0	6.1	6.0	5.9	5.8	5.7	5.6	5.4
Speech or language impairments	2.9	2.9	2.4	2.3	2.3	2.3	2.3	2.3	2.3	3.0	2.9	2.9	3.0	3.0	3.0	3.0
Mental retardation	2.2	2.0	1.3	1.3	1.3	1.3	1.3	1.3	1.3	1.3	1.3	1.2	1.2	1.2	1.1	1.1
Emotional disturbance	0.6	0.8	0.9	1.0	1.0	1.0	1.0	1.0	1.0	1.0	1.0	1.0	1.0	1.0	1.0	0.9
Hearing impairments	0.2	0.2	0.1	0.1	0.1	0.1	0.1	0.2	0.2	0.2	0.2	0.2	0.2	0.2	0.2	0.2
Orthopedic impairments	0.2	0.1	0.1	0.1	0.1	0.1	0.1	0.1	0.2	0.2	0.2	0.2	0.2	0.2	0.1	0.1
Other health impairments	0.3	0.2	0.1	0.2	0.3	0.4	0.4	0.5	0.5	0.6	0.7	0.8	1.0	1.1	1.2	1.2
Visual impairments	0.1	0.1	0.1	0.1	0.1	0.1	0.1	0.1	0.1	0.1	0.1	0.1	0.1	0.1	0.1	0.1
Multiple disabilities	—	0.2	0.2	0.2	0.2	0.2	0.2	0.2	0.2	0.3	0.3	0.3	0.3	0.3	0.3	0.3
Deaf-blindness	—	#	#	#	#	#	#	#	#	#	#	#	#	#	#	#
Autism	—	—	—	#	0.1	0.1	0.1	0.1	0.1	0.2	0.2	0.3	0.3	0.4	0.5	0.5
Traumatic brain injury	—	—	—	#	#	#	#	#	#	#	#	#	#	#	0.1	0.1
Developmental delay	—	—	—	—	—	—	#	#	#	0.4	0.5	0.6	0.6	0.7	0.7	0.7
Preschool-age with disability2	†	†	0.9	1.2	1.2	1.2	1.2	1.2	1.2	†	†	†	†	†	†	†

— Not available.

† Not applicable.

Rounds to zero.

[1] A disorder in one or more of the basic psychological processes involved in understanding or in using language, spoken or written, that may manifest itself in an imperfect ability to listen, think, speak, read, write, spell, or to do mathematical calculations, including conditions such as perceptual disabilities, brain injury, minimal brain dysfunction, dyslexia, and developmental aphasia.

[2] Beginning in 1976, data were collected for preschool-aged children by disability type; those data are combined above with data for youth ages 6–21. However, the 1986 Amendments to the Education of the Handicapped Act (now known as IDEA) mandated that data not be collected by disability for students ages

3–5. Accordingly, those data are reported as a separate row for years 1990–91 through 1999–2000. Beginning in 2000–01, states were again required to report preschool children by disability.

Note: Detail may not sum to totals because of rounding. Special education services through the Individuals with Disabilities Education Act (IDEA) are available for eligible youth identified by a team of qualified professionals as having a disability that adversely affects academic performance and as in need of special education and related services. The total includes youth receiving special education services through IDEA in early education centers and elementary and secondary schools in the 50 states and the District of Columbia and in Bureau of Indian Affairs (BIA) schools through 1993–94. Beginning in 1994–95, estimates exclude BIA schools. See *supplemental note 8* for more information about the student disabilities represented here.

Source: U.S. Department of Education, Office of Special Education and Rehabilitative Services (OSERS), Office of Special Education Programs (OSEP), Data Analysis System (DANS), 1976–2006. Retrieved November 29, 2007, from https://www.ideadata.org/arc_toc8.asp#partbCC and https://www.ideadata.org/docs/PartBTrendData/B1.xls.

PAST AND PROJECTED UNDERGRADUATE ENROLLMENTS

Table 9-1. Total undergraduate enrollment in degree-granting 2- and 4-year postsecondary institutions with projections, by sex, attendance status, and level and control of institution: Fall 1970–2017

				[In thousands]					
Sex				Attendance status		Level of institution		Control of institution	
Fall of year	Total	Male	Female	Full-time	Part-time	4-year	2-year	Public	Private
1970	7,376	4,254	3,122	5,280	2,096	5,057	2,319	5,628	1,748
1971	7,743	4,418	3,325	5,512	2,231	5,164	2,579	6,007	1,736
1972	7,941	4,429	3,512	5,488	2,453	5,185	2,756	6,223	1,718
1973	8,261	4,538	3,723	5,580	2,681	5,249	3,012	6,522	1,739
1974	8,798	4,765	4,033	5,726	3,072	5,394	3,404	7,031	1,767
1975	9,679	5,257	4,422	6,169	3,510	5,709	3,970	7,826	1,853
1976	9,429	4,902	4,527	6,030	3,399	5,546	3,883	7,617	1,812
1977	9,717	4,897	4,820	6,094	3,623	5,674	4,043	7,843	1,874
1978	9,691	4,766	4,925	5,967	3,724	5,663	4,028	7,786	1,905
1979	9,998	4,821	5,178	6,080	3,919	5,781	4,217	8,046	1,951
1980	10,475	5,000	5,475	6,362	4,113	5,948	4,526	8,441	2,033
1981	10,755	5,109	5,646	6,449	4,306	6,039	4,716	8,648	2,106
1982	10,825	5,170	5,655	6,484	4,341	6,053	4,772	8,713	2,112
1983	10,846	5,158	5,688	6,514	4,332	6,123	4,723	8,697	2,149
1984	10,618	5,007	5,611	6,348	4,270	6,087	4,531	8,493	2,125
1985	10,597	4,962	5,635	6,320	4,277	6,066	4,531	8,477	2,120
1986	10,798	5,018	5,780	6,352	4,446	6,118	4,680	8,661	2,137
1987	11,046	5,068	5,978	6,463	4,584	6,270	4,776	8,919	2,128
1988	11,317	5,138	6,179	6,642	4,674	6,441	4,875	9,103	2,213
1989	11,743	5,311	6,432	6,841	4,902	6,592	5,151	9,488	2,255
1990	11,959	5,380	6,579	6,976	4,983	6,719	5,240	9,710	2,250
1991	12,439	5,571	6,868	7,221	5,218	6,787	5,652	10,148	2,291
1992	12,537	5,582	6,954	7,243	5,293	6,814	5,722	10,216	2,320

Table 9-1. (Continued).

				[In thousands]					
Sex				Attendance status		Level of institution		Control of institution	
Fall of year	Total	Male	Female	Full-time	Part-time	4-year	2-year	Public	Private
1993	12,324	5,484	6,840	7,179	5,144	6,758	5,566	10,012	2,312
1994	12,538	5,583	6,955	7,244	5,293	7,008	5,530	10,216	2,321
1995	12,232	5,401	6,831	7,145	5,086	6,739	5,493	9,904	2,328
1996	12,327	5,421	6,906	7,299	5,028	6,764	5,563	9,935	2,392
1997	12,451	5,469	6,982	7,419	5,032	6,845	5,606	10,007	2,443
1998	12,437	5,446	6,991	7,539	4,898	6,948	5,489	9,950	2,487
1999	12,681	5,559	7,122	7,735	4,946	7,089	5,593	10,110	2,571
2000	13,155	5,778	7,377	7,923	5,232	7,207	5,948	10,539	2,616
2001	13,716	6,004	7,711	8,328	5,388	7,465	6,251	10,986	2,730
2002	14,257	6,192	8,065	8,734	5,523	7,728	6,529	11,433	2,824
2003	14,480	6,227	8,253	9,045	5,435	7,987	6,493	11,523	2,957
2004	14,781	6,340	8,441	9,284	5,496	8,235	6,546	11,651	3,130
2005	14,964	6,409	8,555	9,446	5,518	8,476	6,488	11,698	3,266
2006	15,184	6,514	8,671	9,571	5,613	8,666	6,519	11,847	3,337
Projected[1]									
2007	15,366	6,615	8,752	9,690	5,677	8,670	6,696	12,022	3,344
2008	15,571	6,719	8,852	9,836	5,735	8,793	6,778	12,201	3,369
2009	15,770	6,816	8,954	9,975	5,795	8,914	6,856	12,378	3,391
2010	15,939	6,895	9,044	10,090	5,849	9,024	6,915	12,507	3,432
2011	16,106	6,971	9,136	10,195	5,911	9,127	6,979	12,636	3,470
2012	16,273	7,039	9,234	10,295	5,978	9,225	7,049	12,766	3,507
2013	16,457	7,105	9,352	10,408	6,050	9,328	7,129	12,911	3,546
2014	16,628	7,161	9,467	10,510	6,118	9,419	7,208	13,046	3,582
2015	16,755	7,195	9,560	10,584	6,171	9,485	7,270	13,148	3,608
2016	16,881	7,232	9,649	10,657	6,224	9,549	7,332	13,248	3,633
2017	17,022	7,281	9,741	10,737	6,285	9,617	7,405	13,362	3,660

[1] Projections based on data through 2006 and middle alternative assumptions concerning the economy. See NCES 2008–078 for more information on projections.

Note: Detail may not sum to totals because of rounding. Some data have been revised from previously published figures. See *supplemental note 3* for more information on the Integrated Postsecondary Education Data System (IPEDS). See *supplemental note 9* for more information about the classification of postsecondary education institutions.

Source: U.S. Department of Education, National Center for Education Statistics (NCES). *Digest of Education Statistics, 2007* (NCES 2008-022), tables 180 and 196, and Hussar, W. (forthcoming). *Projections of Education Statistics to 2017* (NCES 2008-078), tables 16, 18, and 19, data from U.S. Department of Education, NCES, Higher Education General Information Survey (HEGIS), "Fall Enrollment in Colleges and Universities" surveys, 1970–1985, and 1986–2006 Integrated Postsecondary Education Data System, "Fall Enrollment Survey" (IPEDS-EF:86–99), and Spring 2001 through Spring 2007.

MOBILITY OF COLLEGE STUDENTS

Table 10-1. Residence and migration of all freshmen who had graduated from high school in the previous 12 months attending public or private not-forprofit 4-year degree-granting institutions, by state: Fall 1996

State	Total freshmen enrollment in institutions located in the state	State residents enrolled in institutions		Percentage of all enrolled freshmen who are in-state	Percentage of state's freshmen who are attending in-state	Migration of students		
		In any state[1]	In their home state			Out of state	Into state[2]	Net
United States	1,003,639	984,633	728,323	72.6	74.0	256,310	275,316	19,006
Alabama	16,149	13,124	10,945	67.8	83.4	2,179	5,204	3,025
Alaska	1,207	2,309	1,016	84.2	44.0	1,293	191	-1,102
Arizona	10,733	8,672	6,606	61.5	76.2	2,066	4,127	2,061
Arkansas	10,732	9,736	8,507	79.3	87.4	1,229	2,225	996
California	69,413	74,783	60,699	87.4	81.2	14,084	8,714	-5,370
Colorado	14,875	14,301	10,205	68.6	71.4	4,096	4,670	574
Connecticut	13,002	16,732	6,623	50.9	39.6	10,109	6,379	-3,730
Delaware	5,145	3,545	2,239	43.5	63.2	1,306	2,906	1,600
District of Columbia	7,633	2,154	932	12.2	43.3	1,222	6,701	5,479
Florida	28,414	28,228	20,065	70.6	71.1	8,163	8,349	186
Georgia	26,020	25,588	19,836	76.2	77.5	5,752	6,184	432
Hawaii	3,027	3,894	1,968	65.0	50.5	1,926	1,059	-867
Idaho	4,177	4,971	3,403	81.5	68.5	1,568	774	-794
Illinois	37,127	45,323	30,283	81.6	66.8	15,040	6,844	-8,196
Indiana	34,905	29,255	25,391	72.7	86.8	3,864	9,514	5,650
Iowa	16,141	13,293	10,489	65.0	78.9	2,804	5,652	2,848
Kansas	11,791	10,962	9,018	76.5	82.3	1,944	2,773	829
Kentucky	15,938	14,992	12,522	78.6	83.5	2,470	3,416	946
Louisiana	22,650	21,076	18,296	80.8	86.8	2,780	4,354	1,574
Maine	5,489	6,432	3,288	59.9	51.1	3,144	2,201	-943

State	Total freshmen enrollment in institutions located in the state	State residents enrolled in institutions		Percentage of all enrolled freshmen who are in-state	Percentage of state's freshmen who are attending in-state	Migration of students		
		In any state[1]	In their home state			Out of state	Into state[2]	Net
Maryland	14,573	18,487	8,805	60.4	47.6	9,682	5,768	-3,914
Massachusetts	39,697	31,524	19,542	49.2	62.0	11,982	20,155	8,173
Michigan	40,751	40,271	34,935	85.7	86.7	5,336	5,816	480
Minnesota	19,385	21,082	13,629	70.3	64.6	7,453	5,756	-1,697
Mississippi	8,452	6,944	5,632	66.6	81.1	1,312	2,820	1,508
Missouri	22,290	20,922	16,377	73.5	78.3	4,545	5,913	1,368
Montana	4,734	4,620	3,370	71.2	72.9	1,250	1,364	114
Nebraska	9,847	9,347	7,524	76.4	80.5	1,823	2,323	500
Nevada	2,800	3,229	1,975	70.5	61.2	1,254	825	-429
New Hampshire	7,120	5,653	2,527	35.5	44.7	3,126	4,593	1,467
New Jersey	19,259	37,975	16,286	84.6	42.9	21,689	2,973	-18,716
New Mexico	4,342	5,389	3,351	77.2	62.2	2,038	991	-1,047
New York	77,724	82,490	58,827	75.7	71.3	23,663	18,897	-4,766
North Carolina	32,526	25,040	22,309	68.6	89.1	2,731	10,217	7,486
North Dakota	4,865	3,773	2,784	57.2	73.8	989	2,081	1,092
Ohio	48,839	47,934	39,193	80.2	81.8	8,741	9,646	905
Oklahoma	10,571	10,487	8,551	80.9	81.5	1,936	2,020	84
Oregon	9,621	9,348	6,261	65.1	67.0	3,087	3,360	273
Pennsylvania	62,568	57,181	44,220	70.7	77.3	12,961	18,348	5,387
Rhode Island	8,291	4,455	2,160	26.1	48.5	2,295	6,131	3,836
South Carolina	16,152	13,678	11,185	69.2	81.8	2,493	4,967	2,474
South Dakota	4,198	4,166	2,961	70.5	71.1	1,205	1,237	32
Tennessee	20,853	18,196	14,175	68.0	77.9	4,021	6,678	2,657
Texas	56,837	59,833	50,845	89.5	85.0	8,988	5,992	-2,996
Utah	13,095	8,434	7,847	59.9	93.0	587	5,248	4,661
Vermont	4,871	3,097	1,461	30.0	47.2	1,636	3,410	1,774
Virginia	30,722	26,709	19,834	64.6	74.3	6,875	10,888	4,013

Table 10-1. (Continued).

State	Total freshmen enrollment in institutions located in the state	State residents enrolled in institutions		Percentage of all enrolled freshmen who are in-state	Percentage of state's freshmen who are attending in-state	Migration of students		
		In any state[1]	In their home state			Out of state	Into state[2]	Net
Washington	14,191	14,923	10,808	76.2	72.4	4,115	3,383	-732
West Virginia	11,188	9,291	7,951	71.1	85.6	1,340	3,237	1,897
Wisconsin	24,516	25,071	19,695	80.3	78.6	5,376	4,821	-555
Wyoming	1,148	1,479	741	64.5	50.1	738	407	-331
U.S. Service Academies[3]	3,045	†	231[4]	†	†	-231	2,814	3,045
State unknown[5]	†	4,235	†	†	†	4,235	†	-4,235

† Not applicable.

[1] Students residing in a particular state when admitted to an institution anywhere, either in their home state or another state.

[2] Includes students coming to U.S. colleges from foreign countries and other jurisdictions.

[3] Include U. S. Air Force Academy, U. S. Coast Guard Academy, U. S. Merchant Marine Academy, U. S. Military Academy, and the U. S. Naval Academy.

[4] Students whose residence is in the same state as the service school.

[5] Institution unable to determine student's home state.

Note: Includes first-time postsecondary students who were enrolled at public and private not-for-profit 4-year degree-granting institutions that participated in Title IV federal financial aid programs. See *supplemental note 9* for more information.

Source: U.S. Department of Education, National Center for Education Statistics, Fall 2006 Integrated Postsecondary Education Data System (IPEDS), "Fall Enrollment Survey" (IPEDS-EF:96).

Table 10-2. Residence and migration of all freshmen who had graduated from high school in the previous 12 months attending public or private not-forprofit 4-year degree-granting institutions, by state: Fall 2006

State	Total freshmen enrollment in institutions located in the state	State residents enrolled in institutions		Percentage of all enrolled freshmen who are in-state	Percentage of state's freshmen who are attending in-state	Migration of students		
		In any state[1]	In their home state			Out of state	Into state[2]	Net
United States	1,326,915	1,304,229	973,232	73.3	74.6	330,997	353,683	22,686
Alabama	21,739	17,114	14,846	68.3	86.7	2,268	6,893	4,625
Alaska	2,178	3,315	1,946	89.3	58.7	1,369	232	-1,137
Arizona	17,521	14,426	11,477	65.5	79.6	2,949	6,044	3,095
Arkansas	14,073	11,975	10,493	74.6	87.6	1,482	3,580	2,098
California	107,247	114,495	95,558	89.1	83.5	18,937	11,689	-7,248
Colorado	22,361	22,443	16,564	74.1	73.8	5,879	5,797	-82
Connecticut	17,760	22,926	9,453	53.2	41.2	13,473	8,307	-5,166
Delaware	5,100	3,725	1,925	37.7	51.7	1,800	3,175	1,375
District of Columbia	8,776	2,218	632	7.2	28.5	1,586	8,144	6,558
Florida	60,223	57,789	48,194	80.0	83.4	9,595	12,029	2,434
Georgia	37,652	38,369	29,670	78.8	77.3	8,699	7,982	-717
Hawaii	3,201	4,662	2,092	65.4	44.9	2,570	1,109	-1,461
Idaho	7,156	5,999	4,416	61.7	73.6	1,583	2,740	1,157
Illinois	48,271	59,801	38,551	79.9	64.5	21,250	9,720	-11,530
Indiana	42,857	34,619	30,080	70.2	86.9	4,539	12,777	8,238
Iowa	17,922	13,669	10,910	60.9	79.8	2,759	7,012	4,253
Kansas	13,691	13,148	10,405	76.0	79.1	2,743	3,286	543
Kentucky	20,936	18,264	15,790	75.4	86.5	2,474	5,146	2,672
Louisiana	22,520	21,470	19,186	85.2	89.4	2,284	3,334	1,050
Maine	7,371	7,782	4,506	61.1	57.9	3,276	2,865	-411
Maryland	19,171	26,691	12,379	64.6	46.4	14,312	6,792	-7,520
Massachusetts	47,947	40,663	23,915	49.9	58.8	16,748	24,032	7,284

Table 10-2. (Continued).

State	Total freshmen enrollment in institutions located in the state	State residents enrolled in institutions		Percentage of all enrolled freshmen who are in-state	Percentage of state's freshmen who are attending in-state	Migration of students		
		In any state[1]	In their home state			Out of state	Into state[2]	Net
Michigan	48,470	48,582	42,006	86.7	86.5	6,576	6,464	-112
Minnesota	25,155	28,808	18,102	72.0	62.8	10,706	7,053	-3,653
Mississippi	8,808	7,157	5,866	66.6	82.0	1,291	2,942	1,651
Missouri	26,915	24,742	19,139	71.1	77.4	5,603	7,776	2,173
Montana	5,276	4,766	3,555	67.4	74.6	1,211	1,721	510
Nebraska	10,637	10,177	8,058	75.8	79.2	2,119	2,579	460
Nevada	6,494	7,331	5,517	85.0	75.3	1,814	977	-837
New Hampshire	8,808	7,934	3,316	37.6	41.8	4,618	5,492	874
New Jersey	23,684	50,055	20,086	84.8	40.1	29,969	3,598	-26,371
New Mexico	6,729	7,767	5,634	83.7	72.5	2,133	1,095	-1,038
New York	101,299	100,889	73,581	72.6	72.9	27,308	27,718	410
North Carolina	44,324	36,377	31,929	72.0	87.8	4,448	12,395	7,947
North Dakota	5,496	3,851	2,814	51.2	73.1	1,037	2,682	1,645
Ohio	61,401	61,567	50,031	81.5	81.3	11,536	11,370	-166
Oklahoma	17,339	15,075	13,094	75.5	86.9	1,981	4,245	2,264
Oregon	12,709	11,916	8,294	65.3	69.6	3,622	4,415	793
Pennsylvania	81,766	68,470	53,754	65.7	78.5	14,716	28,012	13,296
Rhode Island	11,510	5,487	2,973	25.8	54.2	2,514	8,537	6,023
South Carolina	20,413	16,323	14,018	68.7	85.9	2,305	6,395	4,090
South Dakota	5,470	4,894	3,652	66.8	74.6	1,242	1,818	576
Tennessee	26,822	24,529	19,696	73.4	80.3	4,833	7,126	2,293
Texas	79,356	87,570	72,842	91.8	83.2	14,728	6,514	-8,214
Utah	13,928	9,890	8,890	63.8	89.9	1,000	5,038	4,038
Vermont	5,905	3,955	1,654	28.0	41.8	2,301	4,251	1,950

State	Total freshmen enrollment in institutions located in the state	State residents enrolled in institutions		Percentage of all enrolled freshmen who are in-state	Percentage of state's freshmen who are attending in-state	Migration of students		
		In any state[1]	In their home state			Out of state	Into state[2]	Net
Virginia	36,672	35,035	25,628	69.9	73.1	9,407	11,044	1,637
Washington	19,009	21,137	14,669	77.2	69.4	6,468	4,340	-2,128
West Virginia	11,078	7,735	6,773	61.1	87.6	962	4,305	3,343
Wisconsin	31,979	30,644	23,618	73.9	77.1	7,026	8,361	1,335
Wyoming	1,495	1,637	898	60.1	54.9	739	597	-142
U.S. Service Academies[3]	2,295	†	157[4]	†	†	-157	2,138	2,295
State unknown[5]	†	4,366	†	†	†	4,366	†	-4,366

† Not applicable.

[1] Students residing in a particular state when admitted to an institution anywhere, either in their home state or another state.

[2] Includes students coming to U.S. colleges from foreign countries and other jurisdictions.

[3] Include U. S. Air Force Academy, U. S. Coast Guard Academy, U. S. Merchant Marine Academy, U. S. Military Academy, and the U. S. Naval Academy.

[4] Students whose residence is in the same state as the service school.

[5] Institution unable to determine student's home state.

Note: Includes first-time postsecondary students who were enrolled at public and private not-for-profit 4-year degree-granting institutions that participated in Title IV federal financial aid programs. See *supplemental note 9* for more information.

Source: U.S. Department of Education, National Center for Education Statistics, Fall 2006 Integrated Postsecondary Education Data System (IPEDS), Spring 2007.

Trends in Graduate and First-Professional Enrollments

Table 11-1. Total graduate and first-professional enrollment in degree-granting institutions, with projections, by sex and attendance status: 1976–2017

		[In thousands]									
Total		Graduate					First-professional				
Fall of year	enrollment	Total	Male	Female	Full-time	Part-time	Total	Male	Female	Full-time	Part-time
1976	1,577	1,333	714	619	463	870	244	190	54	220	24
1977	1,570	1,319	700	617	473	845	251	191	60	226	25
1978	1,569	1,312	682	630	468	844	257	192	65	233	24
1979	1,572	1,309	669	640	476	833	263	193	70	239	24
1980	1,620	1,343	675	670	485	860	278	199	78	251	26
1981	1,617	1,343	674	669	484	859	275	193	82	248	26
1982	1,601	1,322	670	653	485	838	278	191	87	252	26
1983	1,619	1,340	677	663	497	843	279	188	90	250	29
1984	1,624	1,345	672	673	501	844	279	185	94	250	29
1985	1,650	1,376	677	700	509	867	274	180	94	247	28
1986	1,706	1,435	693	742	522	913	270	174	97	246	25
1987	1,720	1,452	693	759	527	925	268	170	98	242	27
1988	1,739	1,472	697	774	553	919	267	167	100	241	26
1989	1,796	1,522	710	811	572	949	274	169	106	248	27
1990	1,860	1,586	737	849	599	987	273	167	107	246	28
1991	1,920	1,639	761	878	642	997	281	170	111	252	29
1992	1,950	1,669	772	896	666	1,003	281	169	112	252	29
1993	1,981	1,688	771	917	688	1,000	292	173	120	260	33
1994	2,016	1,721	776	946	706	1,016	295	174	121	263	31
1995	2,030	1,732	768	965	717	1,015	298	174	124	266	31
1996	2,041	1,742	759	983	737	1,005	298	173	126	267	31
1997	2,052	1,753	758	996	752	1,001	298	170	129	267	31
1998	2,070	1,768	754	1,013	754	1,014	302	169	134	271	31
1999	2,110	1,807	766	1,041	781	1,026	303	165	138	271	33

		[In thousands]									
Total		Graduate					First-professional				
Fall of year	enrollment	Total	Male	Female	Full-time	Part-time	Total	Male	Female	Full-time	Part-time
2000	2,157	1,850	780	1,071	813	1,037	307	164	143	274	33
2001	2,212	1,904	796	1,108	843	1,061	309	161	148	277	32
2002	2,355	2,036	847	1,189	926	1,109	319	163	156	286	33
2003	2,431	2,102	867	1,235	985	1,117	329	166	163	296	33
2004	2,491	2,157	879	1,278	1,024	1,133	335	168	166	302	33
2005	2,524	2,186	877	1,309	1,047	1,139	337	170	167	303	34
2006	2,575	2,231	887	1,344	1,077	1,154	343	174	170	309	34
Projected1											
2007	2,610	2,259	909	1,350	1,098	1,161	351	181	170	316	34
2008	2,629	2,275	919	1,356	1,108	1,167	354	183	171	319	35
2009	2,647	2,290	927	1,362	1,116	1,173	357	186	171	322	35
2010	2,673	2,312	939	1,373	1,129	1,182	361	188	173	326	35
2011	2,715	2,348	955	1,392	1,150	1,197	368	192	176	332	36
2012	2,775	2,398	977	1,421	1,181	1,216	377	196	181	341	36
2013	2,842	2,455	1,000	1,455	1,215	1,239	387	201	186	350	37
2014	2,905	2,508	1,021	1,487	1,246	1,262	397	205	191	359	38
2015	2,960	2,556	1,039	1,516	1,272	1,283	405	209	196	366	38
2016	3,011	2,599	1,056	1,543	1,296	1,304	412	212	200	373	39
2017	3,058	2,640	1,073	1,567	1,315	1,325	418	215	203	378	40

[1] Projections based on reported data through 2006 and middle alternative assumptions concerning the economy. See NCES 2008-078 for more information on projections.

Note: Detail may not sum to totals because of rounding. See *supplemental note 3* for more information on the Integrated Postsecondary Education Data System (IPEDS). See the glossary for a definition of first-professional degree. Some estimates have been revised from previous publications.

Source: U.S. Department of Education, National Center for Education Statistics (NCES). *Digest of Education Statistics, 2007* (NCES 2008-022), tables 197 and 198, and Hussar, W. (forthcoming). *Projections of Education Statistics to 2017* (NCES 2008-078), tables 20 and 21, data from U.S. Department of Education, NCES, Higher Education General Information Survey (HEGIS), "Fall Enrollment in Colleges and Universities" surveys, 1976–1985, and Integrated Postsecondary Education Data System (IPEDS), "Fall Enrollment Survey" (IPEDS-EF:87–99), and Spring 2001 through Spring 2007.

Table 11-2. Total graduate and first-professional enrollment and percentage distribution of students in degree-granting institutions, by race/ethnicity: Selected years, 1976–2006

Level of student and race/ethnicity	1976	1980	1990	1995	2000	2006
			Enrollment (in thousands)			
Graduate Total	1,323	1,341	1,586	1,732	1,850	2,231
White	1,116	1,105	1,228	1,282	1,259	1,445
Total minority	134	144	190	271	359	519
Black	78	75	84	119	158	247
Hispanic	26	32	47	68	95	136
Asian/Pacific Islander	25	32	53	76	96	122
American Indian/Alaska Native	5	5	6	8	10	14
Nonresident alien	72	92	167	179	232	266
First-professional Total	244	277	273	298	307	343
White	220	248	221	223	220	242
Total minority	21	26	47	67	78	93
Black	11	13	16	21	24	27
Hispanic	5	7	11	14	15	18
Asian/Pacific Islander	4	6	19	30	37	46
American Indian/Alaska Native	1	1	1	2	2	3
Nonresident alien	3	3	5	7	8	8
			Percentage distribution			
Graduate Total	100.0	100.0	100.0	100.0	100.0	100.0
White	84.4	82.4	77.4	74.0	68.0	64.8
Total minority	10.2	10.7	12.0	15.6	19.4	23.3
Black	5.9	5.6	5.3	6.8	8.5	11.1
Hispanic	2.0	2.4	3.0	3.9	5.2	6.1
Asian/Pacific Islander	1.9	2.4	3.4	4.4	5.2	5.5
American Indian/Alaska Native	0.4	0.4	0.4	0.5	0.6	0.6
Nonresident alien	5.5	6.9	10.5	10.4	12.6	11.9
First-professional Total	100.0	100.0	100.0	100.0	100.0	100.0
White	90.1	89.5	81.0	75.0	71.8	70.4

Level of student and race/ethnicity	1976	1980	1990	1995	2000	2006
Total minority	8.6	9.5	17.0	22.5	25.5	27.2
Black	4.6	4.6	5.8	7.2	7.7	7.8
Hispanic	1.9	2.4	3.9	4.6	5.0	5.4
Asian/Pacific Islander	1.7	2.2	6.8	9.9	12.0	13.3
American Indian/Alaska Native	0.5	0.3	0.4	0.7	0.8	0.7
Nonresident alien	1.3	1.0	2.0	2.5	2.7	2.5

Note: Because of underreporting and nonreporting of racial/ethnic data, some figures are slightly lower than corresponding data in other published tables. See *supplemental note 3* for more information on the Integrated Postsecondary Education Data System (IPEDS). See the glossary for definitions of minority and first-professional degree. Race categories exclude persons of Hispanic ethnicity.

Source: U.S. Department of Education, National Center for Education Statistics (NCES). *Digest of Education Statistics, 2008* (forthcoming), table 216 and NCES. (2003). *Digest of Education Statistics, 2002* (NCES 2003-060), table 207, data from U.S. Department of Education, NCES, Higher Education General Information Survey (HEGIS), “Fall Enrollment in Colleges and Universities” surveys, 1976 and 1980, and Integrated Postsecondary Education Data System (IPEDS), “Fall Enrollment Survey” (IPEDS-EF:90 and IPEDS-EF:95), and Spring 2001 and Spring 2007.

Reading Performance of Students in Grades 4, 8, and 12

Table 12-1. Average reading scale scores and percentage of students at each achievement level, by grade: Selected years, 1992–2007

Grade, scale score, and achievement level	19921	19941	19981	1998	2002	2003	2005	2007
Grade 4								
Average scale score	217	214	217	215	219	218	219	221
Percentage at each achievement level								
Below Basic	38	40	38	40	36	37	36	33
At or above Basic	62	60	62	60	64	63	64	67
At or above Proficient	29	30	31	29	31	31	31	33
At Advanced	6	7	7	7	7	8	8	8
Grade 8								
Average scale score	260	260	264	263	264	263	262	263
Percentage at each achievement level								
Below Basic	31	30	26	27	25	26	27	26
At or above Basic	69	70	74	73	75	74	73	74
At or above Proficient	29	30	33	32	33	32	31	31
At Advanced	3	3	3	3	3	3	3	3
Grade 122								
Average scale score	292	287	291	290	287	—	286	—
Percentage at each achievement level								
Below Basic	20	25	23	24	26	—	27	—
At or above Basic	80	75	77	76	74	—	73	—
At or above Proficient	40	36	40	40	36	—	35	—
At Advanced	4	40	6	6	5	—	5	—

— Not available.

[1] Testing accommodations (e.g., extended time, small group testing) for children with disabilities and limited-English-proficient students were not permitted.

[2] The 2003 and 2007 National Assessment of Educational Progress (NAEP) Reading Assessments were not administered to 12th-grade students.

Note: The NAEP reading scale ranges from 0 to 500. Beginning in 2002, the NAEP national sample for grades 4 and 8 was obtained by aggregating the samples from each state and the District of Columbia, rather than by obtaining an independently selected national sample. As a consequence, the size of the national sample for grades 4 and 8 increased, and smaller differences between years or between types of students were found to be statistically significant than would have been detected in previous assessments.See *supplemental note 4* for more information on NAEP.

Source: U.S. Department of Education, National Center for Education Statistics, National Assessment of Educational Progress (NAEP), selected years, 1992–2007 Reading Assessments, NAEP Data Explorer.

Table 12-2. Average reading scale scores, by grade and selected student and school characteristics: 1992, 2005, and 2007

Grade 4			Grade 8			Grade 121		
Student or school characteristic	19922	2005	2007	19922	2005	2007	19922	2005
Total	217	219	221	260	262	263	292	286
Sex								
Male	213	216	218	254	257	258	287	279
Female	221	222	224	267	267	268	297	292
Race/ethnicity3								
White	224	229	231	267	271	272	297	293
Black	192	200	203	237	243	245	273	267
Hispanic	197	203	205	241	246	247	279	272
Asian/Pacific Islander	216	229	232	268	271	271	290	287
American Indian/Alaska Native	‡	204	203	‡	249	247	‡	279
Parents' education								
Did not finish high school	—	—	—	243	244	245	275	268
Graduated from high school	—	—	—	251	252	253	283	274
Some education after high school	—	—	—	265	265	266	294	287
Graduated from college	—	—	—	271	272	273	301	297
Locale								
Metro-centric codes								
Central city	—	213	—	—	257	—	—	284
Urban fringe/large town	—	223	—	—	266	—	—	288
Rural/small town	—	219	—	—	263	—	—	285
Urban-centric codes								
City	—	—	215	—	—	257	—	—
Suburban	—	—	226	—	—	267	—	—
Town	—	—	219	—	—	262	—	—
Rural	—	—	222	—	—	264	—	—
Students in school eligible for free or reduced-price lunch 10 percent or less	—	238	240	—	279	280	—	297

Table 12-2. Continued

Grade 4			Grade 8			Grade 121		
Student or school characteristic	19922	2005	2007	19922	2005	2007	19922	2005
11–25 percent	—	230	231	—	270	272	—	290
26–50 percent	—	221	223	—	262	263	—	282
51–75 percent	—	211	212	—	252	253	—	273
More than 75 percent	—	197	200	—	240	241	—	266

— Not available.

‡ Reporting standards not met (too few cases).

[1] The 2003 and 2007 National Assessment of Educational Progress (NAEP) Reading Assessments were not administered to 12th-grade students.

[2] Testing accommodations (e.g., extended time, small group testing) for children with disabilities and limited-English-proficient students were not permitted.

[3] Race categories exclude persons of Hispanic ethnicity.

Note: The NAEP reading scale ranges from 0 to 500. Beginning in 2002, the NAEP national sample for grades 4 and 8 was obtained by aggregating the samples from each state and the District of Columbia, rather than by obtaining an independently selected national sample. As a consequence, the size of the national sample for grades 4 and 8 increased, and smaller differences between years or between types of students were found to be statistically significant than would have been detected in previous assessments. See *supplemental note 4* for more information on NAEP.

Source: U.S. Department of Education, National Center for Education Statistics, National Assessment of Educational Progress (NAEP), 1992, 2005, and 2007 Reading Assessments, NAEP Data Explorer.

Table 12-3. Average reading scale scores and achievement-level results for public school 4th- and 8th-graders, by state: 1992, 1998, and 2007

	Grade 4						Grade 8					
			Percentage of students						Percentage of students			
	Average score		At or above Basic		At or above Proficient		Average score		At or above Basic		At or above Proficient	
State	19921	2007	19921	2007	19921	2007	19982	2007	19982	2007	19982	2007
United States	215	220*	60	66*	27	32*	261	261	71	73	30	29
Alabama	207	216*	51	62*	20	29*	255	252	67	62*	22	21
Alaska	—	214	—	62	—	29	—	259	—	71	—	27
Arizona	209	210	54	56	21	24	260	255*	72	65*	27	24
Arkansas	211	217*	56	64*	23	29*	256	258	68	70	23	25
California	202	209*	48	53*	19	23	252	251	63	62	21	21
Colorado	217	224*	64	70*	25	36*	264	266	77	79	30	35*
Connecticut	222	227*	69	73	34	41*	270	267	81	77	40	37
Delaware	213	225*	57	73*	24	34*	254	265*	64	77*	23	31*
District of Columbia	188	197*	30	39*	10	14*	236	241*	44	48	11	12
Florida	208	224*	53	70*	21	34*	255	260*	67	71*	23	28*
Georgia	212	219*	57	66*	25	28	257	259	68	70	25	26
Hawaii	203	213*	48	59*	17	26*	249	251	59	62*	19	20
Idaho	219	223*	67	70*	28	35*	—	265	—	78	—	32
Illinois	—	219	—	65	—	32	—	263	—	75	—	30
Indiana	221	222	68	68	30	33	—	264	—	76	—	31
Iowa	225	225	73	74	36	36	—	267	—	80	—	36
Kansas	—	225	—	72	—	36	268	267	81	81	36	35
Kentucky	213	222*	58	68*	23	33*	262	262	74	73	30	28
Louisiana	204	207	46	52*	15	20*	252	253	63	64	17	19
Maine	227	226	75	73	36	36	271	270	83	83	41	37
Maryland	211	225*	57	69*	24	36*	261	265	70	76*	31	33
Massachusetts	226	236*	74	81*	36	49*	269	273*	79	84*	38	43*

Table 12-3. Continued

	Grade 4						Grade 8					
			Percentage of students						Percentage of students			
	Average score		At or above Basic		At or above Proficient		Average score		At or above Basic		At or above Proficient	
State	1992[1]	2007	1992[1]	2007	1992[1]	2007	1998[2]	2007	1998[2]	2007	1998[2]	2007
Michigan	216	220*	62	66	26	32*	—	260	—	72	—	28
Minnesota	221	225*	68	73*	31	37*	265	268	78	80	36	37
Mississippi	199	208*	41	51*	14	19*	251	250	62	60	19	17
Missouri	220	221	67	67	30	32	262	263	75	75	28	31
Montana	—	227	—	75	—	39	271	271	83	85	40	39
Nebraska	221	223	68	71	31	35	—	267	—	79	—	35
Nevada	—	211	—	57	—	24	258	252*	70	63*	23	22
New Hampshire	228	229	76	76	38	41	—	270	—	82	—	37
New Jersey	223	231*	69	77*	35	43*	—	270	—	81	—	39
New Mexico	211	212	55	58	23	24	258	251*	71	62*	23	17*
New York	215	224*	61	69*	27	36*	265	264	76	75	32	32
North Carolina	212	218*	56	64*	25	29*	262	259*	74	71	30	28
North Dakota	226	226	74	75	35	35	—	268	—	84	—	32
Ohio	217	226*	63	73*	27	36*	—	268	—	79	—	36
Oklahoma	220	217*	67	65	29	27	265	260*	80	72*	30	26
Oregon	—	215	—	62	—	28	266	266	78	77	35	34
Pennsylvania	221	226*	68	73*	32	40*	—	268	—	79	—	36
Rhode Island	217	219	63	65	28	31	264	258*	76	69*	32	27*
South Carolina	210	214*	53	59*	22	26*	255	257	66	69	22	25
South Dakota	—	223	—	71	—	34	—	270	—	83	—	37
Tennessee	212	216	57	61	23	27	258	259	71	71	27	26
Texas	213	220*	57	66*	24	30*	261	261	74	73	27	28
Utah	220	221	67	69	30	34	263	262	77	75	31	30
Vermont	—	228	—	74	—	41	—	273	—	84	—	42

	Grade 4						Grade 8					
			Percentage of students						Percentage of students			
	Average score		At or above Basic		At or above Proficient		Average score		At or above Basic		At or above Proficient	
State	1992[1]	2007	1992[1]	2007	1992[1]	2007	1998[2]	2007	1998[2]	2007	1998[2]	2007
Virginia	221	227*	67	74*	31	38*	266	267	78	79	33	34
Washington	—	224	—	70	—	36	264	265	76	77	32	34
West Virginia	216	215	61	63	25	28	262	255*	75	68*	28	23*
Wisconsin	224	223	71	70	33	36	265	264	78	76	34	33
Wyoming	223	225	71	73	33	36*	263	266*	76	80	31	33

— Not available (state did not participate in assessment).

* Change in score is statistically significant from 1992 or 1998 ($p < .05$).

[1] 1992 was the first year for state-level data in grade 4. Testing accommodations (e.g., extended time, small group testing) for children with disabilities and limited-English-proficient students were not permitted.

[2] 1998 was the first year for state-level data in grade 8. Testing accommodations (e.g., extended time, small group testing) for children with disabilities and limited-English-proficient students were permitted.

Note: The National Assessment of Educational Progress (NAEP) reading scale ranges from 0 to 500. State samples were not collected for grade 12; therefore, state results for grade 12 are not available. At the state level, NAEP includes only students in public schools, while other reported national results in this indicator include both public and private school students. Variations or changes in exclusion rates for students with disabilities and limited- English-proficient students in the NAEP samples may affect comparative performance results. The 2007 NAEP national sample for grades 4 and 8 was obtained by aggregating the samples from each state and the District of Columbia, rather than by obtaining an independently selected national sample. As a consequence, the size of the national samples for grades 4 and 8 increased, and smaller differences between years or between types of students were found to be statistically significant than would have been detected in previous assessments. See *supplemental note 4* for more information on NAEP.

Source: U.S. Department of Education, National Center for Education Statistics, National Assessment of Educational Progress (NAEP), 1992, 1998, and 2007 Reading Assessments, NAEP Data Explorer.

Mathematics Performance of Students in Grades 4 and 8

Table 13-1. Average mathematics scale scores and percentage of students at each achievement level, by grade: Selected years, 1990–2007

Grade, scale score, and achievement level	1990[1]	1992[1]	1996[1]	1996	2000	2003	2005	2007
Grade 4								
Average scale score	213	220	224	224	226	235	238	240
Percentage at each achievement level Below Basic	50	41	36	37	35	23	20	18
At or above Basic	50	59	64	63	65	77	80	82
At or above Proficient	13	18	21	21	24	32	36	39
At Advanced	1	2	2	2	3	4	5	6
Grade 8								
Average scale score	263	268	272	270	273	278	279	281
Percentage at each achievement level Below Basic	48	42	38	39	37	32	31	29
At or above Basic	52	58	62	61	63	68	69	71
At or above Proficient	15	21	24	23	26	29	30	32
At Advanced	2	3	4	4	5	5	6	7
Grade 12								
Average scale score	(2)	(2)	(2)	(2)	(2)	(2)	150	—
Percentage at each achievement level Below Basic	(2)	(2)	(2)	(2)	(2)	(2)	39	—
At or above Basic	(2)	(2)	(2)	(2)	(2)	(2)	61	—
At or above Proficient	(2)	(2)	(2)	(2)	(2)	(2)	23	—
At Advanced	(2)	(2)	(2)	(2)	(2)	(2)	2	—

— Not available.

[1] Testing accommodations (e.g., extended time, small group testing) for children with disabilities and limited-English-proficient students were not permitted.

[2] The 2005 Grade 12 Mathematics Assessment was based on a new framework. The assessment includes more questions on algebra, data analysis, and probability to reflect changes in high school mathematics standards and coursework. Results could not be placed on the old National Assessment of Educational Progress (NAEP) scale and could not be directly compared with previous years; therefore, information on previous assessments are not shown. For more information on NAEP Grade 12 Mathematics Assessments, see http://www.nces.ed.gov/nationsreportcard/mathematics/.

Note: The NAEP mathematics scale ranges from 0 to 500 for grades 4 and 8 and ranges from 0 to 300 for grade 12. Beginning in 2003, the NAEP national sample for grades 4 and 8 was obtained by aggregating the samples from each state and the District of Columbia, rather than by obtaining an independently selected national sample. As a consequence, the size of the national samples for grades 4 and 8 increased, and smaller differences between years or between types of students were found to be statistically significant than would have been detected in previous assessments. The 2007 NAEP Mathematics Assessment was not administered to 12th-grade students. See *supplemental note 4* for more information on NAEP.

Source: U.S. Department of Education, National Center for Education Statistics, National Assessment of Educational Progress (NAEP), selected years, 1990–2007 Mathematics Assessments, NAEP Data Explorer.

Table 13-2. Average mathematics scale scores, by grade and selected student and school characteristics: Selected years, 1990–2007

	Grade 4				Grade 8				Grade 12
Student or school characteristic	19901	2000	2005	2007	1990[1]	2000	2005	2007	2005
Total	213	226	238	240	263	273	279	281	150
Sex									
Male	214	227	239	241	263	274	280	282	151
Female	213	224	237	239	262	272	278	280	149
Race/ethnicity2									
White	220	234	246	248	270	284	289	291	157
Black	188	203	220	222	237	244	255	260	127
Hispanic	200	208	226	227	246	253	262	265	133
Asian/Pacific Islander	225	‡	251	253	275	288	295	297	163
American Indian/Alaska Native	‡	208	226	228	‡	259	264	264	134
Parents' education									
Did not finish high school	—	—	—	—	242	253	259	263	130
Graduated from high school	—	—	—	—	255	261	267	270	138
Some education after high school	—	—	—	—	267	277	280	283	148
Graduated from college	—	—	—	—	274	286	290	292	161
Locale									
Metro-centric codes									
Central city	—	220	233	—	—	266	273	—	147
Urban fringe/large town	—	230	241	—	—	277	283	—	154
Rural/small town	—	226	238	—	—	275	279	—	148
Urban-centric codes									
City	—	—	—	235	—	—	—	275	—
Suburban	—	—	—	244	—	—	—	286	—
Town	—	—	—	238	—	—	—	280	—
Rural	—	—	—	240	—	—	—	282	—
Students in school eligible for free or									
reduced-price lunch									
10 percent or less	—	—	254	256	—	—	298	300	162

Table 13-2. (Continued).

	Grade 4				Grade 8				Grade 12
Student or school characteristic	19901	2000	2005	2007	1990[1]	2000	2005	2007	2005
11–25 percent	—	—	247	248	—	—	289	292	155
26–50 percent	—	—	240	242	—	—	280	282	147
51–75 percent	—	—	232	234	—	—	268	271	136
More than 75 percent	—	—	220	222	—	—	254	259	122

— Not available.

‡ Reporting standards not met (too few cases).

[1] Testing accommodations (e.g., extended time, small group testing) for children with disabilities and limited-English-proficient students were not permitted.

[2] Race categories exclude persons of Hispanic ethnicity.

Note: The National Assessment of Educational Progress (NAEP) mathematics scale ranges from 0 to 500 for grades 4 and 8 and ranges from 0 to 300 for grade 12. Beginning in 2003, the NAEP national sample for grades 4 and 8 was obtained by aggregating the samples from each state and the District of Columbia, rather than by obtaining an independently selected national sample. As a consequence, the size of the national samples for grades 4 and 8 increased, and smaller differences between years or between types of students were found to be statistically significant than would have been detected in previous assessments. The 2007 NAEP Mathematics Assessment was not administered to 12th-grade students. See *supplemental note 4* for more information on NAEP.

Source: U.S. Department of Education, National Center for Education Statistics, National Assessment of Educational Progress (NAEP), selected years, 1990–2007 Mathematics Assessments, NAEP Data Explorer.

Table 13-3. Average mathematics scale scores and achievement-level results for public school 4th- and 8th-graders, by state: 1990, 1992, and 2007

	Grade 4						Grade 8					
			Percentage of students						Percentage of students			
	Average score		At or above *Basic*		At or above Proficient		Average score		At or above Basic		At or above Proficient	
State	19921	2007	19921	2007	19921	2007	19901	2007	19901	2007	19901	2007
United States	219	239*	57	81*	17	39*	262	280*	51	70*	15	31*
Alabama	208	229*	43	70*	10	26*	253	266*	40	55*	9	18*
Alaska	—	237	—	79	—	38	—	283	—	73	—	32
Arizona	215	232*	53	74*	13	31*	260	276*	48	66*	13	26*
Arkansas	210	238*	47	81*	10	37*	256	274*	44	65*	9	24*
California	208	230*	46	70*	12	30*	256	270*	45	59*	12	24*
Colorado	221	240*	61	82*	17	41*	267	286*	57	75*	17	37*
Connecticut	227	243*	67	84*	24	45*	270	282*	60	73*	22	35*
Delaware	218	242*	55	87*	17	40*	261	283*	48	74*	14	31*
District of Columbia	193	214*	23	49*	5	14*	231	248*	17	34*	3	8*
Florida	214	242*	52	86*	13	40*	255	277*	43	68*	12	27*
Georgia	216	235*	53	79*	15	32*	259	275*	47	64*	14	25*
Hawaii	214	234*	52	77*	15	33*	251	269*	40	59*	12	21*
Idaho	222	241*	63	85*	16	40*	271	284*	63	75*	18	34*
Illinois	—	237	—	79	—	36	261	280*	50	70*	15	31*
Indiana	221	245*	60	89*	16	46*	267	285*	56	76*	17	35*
Iowa	230	243*	72	87*	26	43*	278	285*	70	77*	25	35*
Kansas	—	248	—	89	—	51	—	290	—	81	—	40
Kentucky	215	235*	51	79*	13	31*	257	279*	43	69*	10	27*
Louisiana	204	230*	39	73*	8	24*	246	272*	32	64*	5	19*
Maine	232	242*	75	85*	27	42*	—	286	—	78	—	34
Maryland	217	240*	55	80*	18	40*	261	286*	50	74*	17	37*
Massachusetts	227	252*	68	93*	23	58*	—	298	—	85	—	51

Table 13-3. (Continued).

	Grade 4						Grade 8					
			Percentage of students						Percentage of students			
	Average score		At or above *Basic*		At or above Proficient		Average score		At or above Basic		At or above Proficient	
Michigan	220	238*	61	80*	18	37*	264	277*	53	66*	16	29*
Minnesota	228	247*	71	87*	26	51*	275	292*	67	81*	23	43*
Mississippi	202	228*	36	70*	6	21*	—	265	—	54	—	14
Missouri	222	239*	62	82*	19	38*	—	281	—	72	—	30
Montana	—	244	—	88	—	44	280	287*	74	79*	27	38*
Nebraska	225	238*	67	80*	22	38*	276	284*	68	74*	24	35*
Nevada	—	232	—	74	—	30	—	271	—	60	—	23
New Hampshire	230	249*	72	91*	25	52*	273	288*	65	78*	20	38*
New Jersey	227	249*	68	90*	25	52*	270	289*	58	77*	21	40*
New Mexico	213	228*	50	70*	11	24*	256	268*	43	57*	10	17*
New York	218	243*	57	85*	17	43*	261	280*	50	70*	15	30*
North Carolina	213	242*	50	85*	13	41*	250	284*	38	73*	9	34*
North Dakota	229	245*	72	91*	22	46*	281	292*	75	86*	27	41*
Ohio	219	245*	57	87*	16	46*	264	285*	53	76*	15	35*
Oklahoma	220	237*	60	82*	14	33*	263	275*	52	66*	13	21*
Oregon	—	236	—	79	—	35	271	284*	62	73*	21	35*
Pennsylvania	224	244*	65	85*	22	47*	266	286*	56	77*	17	38*
Rhode Island	215	236*	54	80*	13	34*	260	275*	49	65*	15	28*
South Carolina	212	237*	48	80*	13	36*	—	282	—	71	—	32
South Dakota	—	241	—	86	—	41	—	288	—	81	—	39
Tennessee	211	233*	47	76*	10	29*	—	274	—	64	—	23
Texas	218	242*	56	87*	15	40*	258	286*	45	78*	13	35*
Utah	224	239*	66	83*	19	39*	—	281	—	72	—	32
Vermont	—	246	—	89	—	49	—	291	—	81	—	41
Virginia	221	244*	59	87*	19	42*	264	288*	52	77*	17	37*

	Grade 4						Grade 8					
			Percentage of students						Percentage of students			
	Average score		At or above *Basic*		At or above Proficient		Average score		At or above Basic		At or above Proficient	
Washington	—	243	—	84	—	44	—	285	—	75	—	36
West Virginia	215	236*	52	81*	12	33*	256	270*	42	61*	9	19*
Wisconsin	229	244*	71	85*	24	47*	274	286*	66	76*	23	37*
Wyoming	225	244*	69	88*	19	44*	272	287*	64	80*	19	36*

— Not available (state did not participate in assessment).

* Change in score is statistically significant from 1990 or 1992 ($p < .05$).

[1] Testing accommodations (e.g., extended time, small group testing) for children with disabilities and limited-English-proficient students were not permitted.

Note: State samples were not collected for grade 12; therefore, state results for grade 12 are not available. At the state level, the National Assessment of Educational Progress (NAEP) includes only students in public schools, while other reported national results in this indicator include both public and private school students. Variations or changes in exclusion rates for students with disabilities and limited-English-proficient students in the NAEP samples may affect comparative performance results. The 2007 NAEP national sample for grades 4 and 8 was obtained by aggregating the samples from each state and the District of Columbia, rather than by obtaining an independently selected national sample. As a consequence, the size of the national samples for grades 4 and 8 increased, and smaller differences between years or between types of students were found to be statistically significant than would have been detected in previous assessments. See *supplemental note 4* for more information on testing accommodations and on NAEP.

Source: U.S. Department of Education, National Center for Education Statistics, National Assessment of Educational Progress (NAEP), 1990, 1992, and 2007 Mathematics Assessments, NAEP Data Explorer.

Writing Performance of Students in Grades 8 and 12

Table 14-1. Average writing scale scores and percentage of students at each achievement level, by grade: 1998, 2002, and 2007

Grade, scale score, and achievement level	1998	2002	2007
Grade 8			
Average scale score	150	153	156
Percentage at each achievement level			
Below Basic	16	15	12
At or above Basic	84	85	88
At or above Proficient	27	31	33
At Advanced	1	2	2
Grade 12			
Average scale score	150	148	153
Percentage at each achievement level			
Below Basic	22	26	18
At or above Basic	78	74	82
At or above Proficient	22	24	24
At Advanced	1	2	1

Note: National Assessment of Educational Progress (NAEP) writing scores range from 0 to 300. The achievement levels define what students should know and be able to do: *Basic* indicates partial mastery of fundamental skills; *Proficient* indicates demonstrated competency over challenging subject matter; and *Advanced* indicates superior performance.

Source: U.S. Department of Education, National Center for Education Statistics, National Assessment of Educational Progress (NAEP), 1998, 2002, and 2007 Writing Assessments, NAEP Data Explorer.

Table 14-2. Average writing scale scores, by grade and selected student and school characteristics: 1998, 2002, and 2007

School or student characteristic	1998	2002	2007	1998	2002	2007
Total	150	153	156	150	148	153
Sex						
Male	140	143	146	140	136	144
Female	160	164	166	159	160	162
Race/ethnicity1 White	157	161	164	155	154	159
Black	131	135	141	134	130	137
Hispanic	131	137	142	136	136	139
Asian/Pacific Islander	154	161	167	150	151	160
American Indian/Alaska Native	130	137	143	129	‡	140
Parents' education						
Did not finish high school	—	136	139	—	129	134
Graduated from high school	—	144	147	—	139	141
Some education after high school	—	156	158	—	149	152
Graduated from college Locale2	—	165	166	—	158	163
City	—	—	151	—	—	152
Suburban	—	—	161	—	—	156
Town	—	—	153	—	—	150
Rural	—	—	155	—	—	151
Free or reduced-price lunch Eligible	132	136	141	133	132	138
Not eligible	157	162	164	152	152	157
Information not available	157	161	170	155	156	165

— Not available.

‡ Reporting standards not met.

[1] Race categories exclude persons of Hispanic ethnicity.

[2] Adoption of the new urban-centric locale classification codes does not permit comparison across assessment years.

Note: National Assessment of Educational Progress (NAEP) writing scores range from 0 to 300. The achievement levels define what students should know and be able to do: *Basic* indicates partial mastery of fundamental skills; *Proficient* indicates demonstrated competency over challenging subject matter; and *Advanced* indicates superior performance.

Source: U.S. Department of Education, National Center for Education Statistics, National Assessment of Educational Progress (NAEP), 1998, 2002, and 2007 Writing Assessments, NAEP Data Explorer.

Table 15-1. Percentage of 12th-grade students at each economics achievement level, by student and school characteristics: 2006

Student or school characteristic	Below *Basic*	At or above *Basic*[1]	At or above *Proficient*[1]	At *Advanced*[1]
Total				
Sex				
Male	21	79	45	4
Female	21	79	38	2
Race/ethnicity[2] White	13	87	51	4
Black	43	57	16	#
Hispanic	36	64	21	#
Asian/Pacific Islander	20	80	44	4!
American Indian/Alaska Native	28	72	26	2
Highest level of parental education				
Did not finish high school	41	59	17	#
Graduated from high school	31	69	27	1!
Some education after high school	18	82	39	1
Graduated from college	13	87	54	5
Region West	‡	‡	‡	‡
Midwest	17	83	45	3
South	23	77	37	2
Northeast	19	81	46	4
Locale City Suburban	25 19	75 81	39 45	4 4
Town	21	79	38	2
Rural	20	80	40	2
Students in school eligible for free or reduced-price lunch 10 percent or less	10	90	58	6
11–25 percent	17	83	46	3
26–50 percent	23	77	37	2
51–75 percent	35	65	23	1!
More than 75 percent	42	58	18	1

Rounds to zero.
! Interpret data with caution (estimates are unstable).
‡ Reporting standards not met (too few cases).
[1] Included in the at or above *Proficient* achievement level is the at *Advanced* achievement level; included in the at or above *Basic* achievement level is the at or above *Proficient* achievement level.
[2] Race categories exclude persons of Hispanic ethnicity.
Note: See *supplemental note 4* for more information on the National Assessment of Educational Progress (NAEP) and NAEP achievement levels.
Source: Mead, N., and Sandene, B. (2007). *The Nation's Report Card: Economics 2006* (NCES 2007-475), data from U.S. Department of Education, National Center for Education Statistics, NAEP Data Explorer.

Table 15-2. Average economics scale scores of 12th-grade students, by content area and student and school characteristics: 2006

Student or school characteristic	Overall	Market economy	National economy	International economy
Total	150	150	150	150
Sex				
Male	152	152	152	152
Female	148	148	148	148
Race/ethnicity[1]				
White	158	158	158	158
Black	127	128	127	129
Hispanic	133	133	132	133
Asian/Pacific Islander	153	153	153	152
American Indian/Alaska Native	137	138	138	134
Highest level of parental education				
Did not finish high school	129	128	129	133
Graduated from high school	138	138	137	138
Some education after high school	150	151	150	149
Graduated from college	160	160	161	160
Region				
West	‡	‡	‡	‡
Midwest	153	153	154	153
South	147	147	147	147
Northeast	153	153	153	154
Locale				
City	148	148	148	148
Suburban	153	153	153	152
Town	148	147	148	149
Rural	149	149	149	149
Students in school eligible for free or reduced-price lunch 10 percent or less	164	164	164	163
11–25 percent	153	153	154	153
26–50 percent	147	147	146	147
51–75 percent	134	134	134	134
More than 75 percent	130	130	129	132

‡ Reporting standards not met (too few cases).

[1] Race categories exclude persons of Hispanic ethnicity.

Note: See *supplemental note 4* for more information on the National Assessment of Educational Progress (NAEP).

Source: Mead, N., and Sandene, B. (2007). *The Nation's Report Card: Economics 2006* (NCES 2007-475), data from U.S. Department of Education, National Center for Education Statistics, NAEP Data Explorer.

Trends in the Achievement Gaps in Reading and Mathematics

Table 16-1. White-Black and White-Hispanic gaps in average reading and mathematics scores, by grade: Various years, 1990–2007

Subject, race/ethnicity,1 and grade	1990	1992	1994	1996	1998	2000	2002	2003	2005	2007
Reading										
White-Black gap Grade 4	—	32	38	—	32	34	30	31	29	27
Grade 8	—	30	30	—	26	—	27	28	28	27
White-Hispanic gap Grade 4	—	27	35	—	32	35	28	28	26	26
Grade 8	—	26	24	—	27	—	26	27	25	25
Mathematics										
White-Black gap Grade 4	32	35	—	34	—	31	—	27	26	26
Grade 8	33	40	—	41	—	40	—	35	34	32
White-Hispanic gap Grade 4	20	25	—	25	—	27	—	22	20	21
Grade 8	24	28	—	30	—	31	—	29	27	26

— Not available (tests not conducted in all grades for all years).

[1] Race categories exclude persons of Hispanic ethnicity.

Note: The score gap is determined by subtracting the average Black or Hispanic score, respectively, from the average White score. Testing accommodations (e.g., extended time, small group testing) for children with disabilities and limited-English-proficient students were not permitted from 1990 through 1994. Beginning in 2002, the National Assessment of Educational Progress (NAEP) national sample for grades 4 and 8 was obtained by aggregating the samples from each state, rather than by obtaining an independently selected national sample. As a consequence, the size of the national sample increased, and smaller differences between years or between types of students were found to be statistically significant than would have been detected in previous assessments. See *supplemental note 4* for more information on NAEP.

Source: U.S. Department of Education, National Center for Education Statistics, National Assessment of Educational Progress (NAEP), various years, 1990–2007 Reading and Mathematics Assessments, NAEP Data Explorer.

Reading and Mathematics Score Trends by Age

Table 17-1. Average reading scale scores on the long-term trend National Assessment of Educational Progress (NAEP), by age, sex, and race/ethnicity: Various years, 1971 through 2004

Age, sex, and race/ethnicity[1]	1971	1975	1980	1984	1988	1990	1992	1994	1996	1999	2004
9-year-olds											
Total	208	210	215	211	212	209	211	211	212	212	219
Sex											
Male	201	204	210	207	207	204	206	207	207	209	216
Female	214	216	220	214	216	215	215	215	218	215	221
Race/ethnicity White	214	217	221	218	218	217	218	218	220	221	226
Black	170	181	189	186	189	182	185	185	191	186	200
Hispanic	—	183	190	187	194	189	192	186	195	193	205
13-year-olds											
Total	255	256	258	257	257	257	260	258	258	259	259
Sex											
Male	250	250	254	253	252	251	254	251	251	254	254
Female	261	262	263	262	263	263	265	266	264	265	264
Race/ethnicity White	261	262	264	263	261	262	266	265	266	267	266
Black	222	226	233	236	243	241	238	234	234	238	244
Hispanic	—	232	237	240	240	238	239	235	238	244	242
17-year-olds											
Total	285	286	285	289	290	290	290	288	288	288	285
Sex											
Male	279	280	282	284	286	284	284	282	281	281	278
Female	291	291	289	294	294	296	296	295	295	295	292
Race/ethnicity White	291	293	293	295	295	297	297	296	295	295	293
Black	239	241	243	264	274	267	261	266	266	264	264
Hispanic	—	252	261	268	271	275	271	263	265	271	264

— Not available.

[1] Race categories exclude persons of Hispanic ethnicity.

Note: Includes public and private schools. Excludes persons not enrolled in school and those who were unable to be tested due to limited proficiency in English or a disability. Totals include other race/ethnicity categories not separately shown. The long-term trend NAEP scores range from 0 to 500 and have been evaluated at certain performance levels. Students at reading score level 150 are able to follow brief written directions and carry out simple, discrete reading tasks. Students at reading score level 200 are able to understand, combine ideas, and make inferences based on short uncomplicated passages about specific or sequentially related information. Students at reading score level 250 are able to search for specific information, interrelate ideas, and make generalizations about literature, science, and social studies materials. Students at reading score level 300 are able to find, understand, summarize, and explain relatively complicated literary and informational material. Students at reading score level 350 can extend and restructure the ideas presented and can synthesize and learn from specialized and complex texts.

Source: Perie, M., Moran, R., and Lutkus, A.D. (2005). *NAEP 2004 Trends in Academic Progress: Three Decades of Student Performance in Reading and Mathematics* (NCES 2005-464), figures 2-1, 3-1, 3-2, and 3-3, data from U.S. Department of Education, National Center for Education Statistics, National Assessment of Educational Progress (NAEP), various years, 1971–2004 Long-Term Trend Reading Assessment.

Table 17-2. Average mathematics scale scores on the long-term trend National Assessment of Educational Progress (NAEP), by age, sex, and race/ethnicity: Various years, 1973 through 2004

Age, sex, and race/ethnicity[1]	1973	1978	1982	1986	1990	1992	1994	1996	1999	2004
9-year-olds										
Total	219	219	219	222	230	230	231	231	232	241
Sex										
Male	218	217	217	222	229	231	232	233	233	243
Female	220	220	221	222	230	228	230	229	231	240
Race/ethnicity White	225	224	224	227	235	235	237	237	239	247
Black	190	192	195	202	208	208	212	212	211	224
Hispanic	202	203	204	205	214	212	210	215	213	230
13-year-olds										
Total	266	264	269	269	270	273	274	274	276	281
Sex										
Male	265	264	269	270	271	274	276	276	277	283
Female	267	265	268	268	270	272	273	272	274	279
Race/ethnicity White	274	272	274	274	276	279	281	281	283	288
Black	228	230	240	249	249	250	252	252	251	262
Hispanic	239	238	252	254	255	259	256	256	259	265
17-year-olds										
Total	304	300	298	302	305	307	306	307	308	307
Sex										
Male	309	304	301	305	306	309	309	310	310	308
Female	301	297	296	299	303	305	304	305	307	305
Race/ethnicity White	310	306	304	308	309	312	312	313	315	313
Black	270	268	272	279	289	286	286	286	283	285
Hispanic	277	276	277	283	284	292	291	292	293	289

[1] Race categories exclude persons of Hispanic ethnicity.

Note: Includes public and private schools. Excludes persons not enrolled in school and those who were unable to be tested due to limited proficiency in English or a disability. Totals include other race/ethnicity categories not separately shown. The long-term trend NAEP scores range from 0 to 500 and have been evaluated at certain performance levels. A score of 150 implies the knowledge of some basic addition and subtraction facts, and most students at this level can add 2-digit numbers without regrouping. They recognize simple situations in which addition and subtraction apply. A score of 200 implies considerable understanding of 2-digit numbers and knowledge of some basic multiplication and division facts. A score of 250 implies an initial understanding of the four basic operations. Students at this level can also compare information from graphs and charts and are developing an ability to analyze simple logical relations. A score of 300 implies an ability to compute decimals, simple fractions, and percents. Students at this level can identify geometric figures, measure lengths and angles, and calculate areas of rectangles. They are developing the skills to operate with signed numbers, exponents, and square roots. A score of 350 implies an ability to apply a range of reasoning skills to solve multistep problems. Students at this level can solve routine problems involving fractions and percents, recognize properties of basic geometric figures, and work with exponents and square roots.

Source: Perie, M., Moran, R., and Lutkus, A.D. (2005). *NAEP 2004 Trends in Academic Progress: Three Decades of Student Performance in Reading and Mathematics* (NCES 2005-464), figures 2-4, 3-5, 3-6, and 3-7, data from U.S. Department of Education, National Center for Education Statistics, National Assessment of Educational Progress (NAEP), various years, 1973–2004 Long-Term Trend Mathematics Assessment.

International Comparisons of Reading Literacy in Grade 4

Table 18-1. Average combined reading literacy scale scores of 4th-graders, by reading subscale and educational jurisdiction: 2006

Educational jurisdiction	Combined reading literacy	Literary subscale	Informational subscale
International average	500*	500*	500*
Alberta, Canada	560*	561*	556*
Austria	538	537	536
Belgium (Flemish)1	547	544	547*
Belgium (French)	500*	499*	498*
British Columbia, Canada	558*	559*	554*
Bulgaria	547	542	550*
Chinese Taipei	535	530*	538
Denmark	546	547	542
England	539	539	537
France	522*	516*	526*
Georgia	471*	476*	465*
Germany	548	549	544
Hong Kong, SAR2	564*	557*	568*
Hungary	551*	557*	541
Iceland	511*	514*	505*
Indonesia	405*	397*	418*
Iran, Islamic Republic of	421*	426*	420*
Israel	512*	516*	507*
Italy	551*	551*	549*
Kuwait	330*	340*	327*
Latvia	541	539	540
Lithuania	537	542	530
Luxembourg	557*	555*	557*
Macedonia	442*	439*	450*
Moldova	500*	492*	508*
Morocco	323*	317*	335*
Netherlands1	547	545	548*
New Zealand	532*	527*	534
Norway3	498*	501*	494*
Nova Scotia, Canada	542	543	539

Table 18-1. (Continued).

Educational jurisdiction	Combined reading literacy	Literary subscale	Informational subscale
Ontario, Canada	555*	555*	552*
Poland	519*	523*	515*
Qatar	353*	358*	356*
Quebec, Canada	533	529*	533
Romania	489*	493*	487*
Russian Federation	565*	561*	564*
Scotland1	527*	527*	527*
Singapore	558*	552*	563*
Slovak Republic	531*	533	527*
Slovenia	522*	519*	523*
South Africa	302*	299*	316*
Spain	513*	516*	508*
Sweden	549*	546	549*
Trinidad and Tobago	436*	434*	440*
United States1	540	541	537

* Significantly different from the U.S. average ($p < .05$).

[1] Met guidelines for sample participation rates only after replacement schools were included.

[2] Hong Kong SAR is a Special Administrative Region (SAR) of the People's Republic of China.

[3] Did not meet guidelines for sample participation rates after replacement schools were included.

Note: Results from the Progress in International Reading Literacy Study (PIRLS) assessment are reported on a combined reading literacy scale, which captures students' overall literacy skills, and two subscales that measure two types of purposes of reading: reading for literary purposes and reading for informational purposes. The combined reading literacy score is calculated on the basis of all the items in the assessment, whereas the subscale scores are calculated on the basis of the items making up each of the two subscales. Because the combined reading literacy scale and the two subscales are calculated separately using the properties of all of the items in the given scale or subscale, the combined reading literacy score is not the simple average of the two subscales.

Source: Baer, J., Baldi, S., Ayotte, K., and Green, P. (2007). *The Reading Literacy of U.S. Fourth-Grade Students in an International Context: Results From the 2001 and 2006 Progress in International Reading Literacy Study (PIRLS)* (NCES 2008-017), figure 3, data from the International Association for the Evaluation of Educational Achievement (IEA), Progress in International Reading Literacy Study (PIRLS), 2006.

Table 18-2. Average combined reading literacy scale scores of 4th-graders, by reading subscale and educational jurisdiction: 2001 and 2006

			Reading subscal			
	Combined reading literacy		Literary subscale		Informational subscale	
Educational jurisdiction	2001	2006	2001	2006	2001	2006
Bulgaria	550	547	550	542	551	550
England	553	539*	559	539*	546	537*
France	525	522	518	516	533	526*
Germany	539	548*	537	549*	538	544*
Hong Kong, SAR[1]	528	564*	518	557*	537	568*
Hungary	543	551*	548	557*	537	541
Iceland	512	511	520	514*	504	505
Iran, Islamic Republic of	414	421	421	426	408	420*
Israel	509	512	510	516	507	507
Italy	541	551*	543	551	536	549*
Kuwait	396	330*	394	340*	403	327*
Latvia	545	541	537	539	547	540*
Lithuania	543	537*	546	542	540	530*
Macedonia	442	442	441	439	445	450
Moldova	492	500	480	492*	505	508
Morocco	350	323*	347	317*	358	335
Netherlands[2]	554	547*	552	545*	553	548
New Zealand	529	532	531	527	525	534*
Norway[3]	499	498	506	501	492	494
Ontario, Canada	548	554	551	554	542	551*
Quebec, Canada	537	533	534	529	541	533*
Romania	512	489*	512	493*	512	487*
Russian Federation	528	565*	523	561*	531	564*
Scotland2	528	527	529	527	527	527
Singapore	528	558*	528	552*	527	563*
Slovak Republic	518	531*	512	533*	522	527
Slovenia	502	522*	499	519*	503	523*
Sweden	561	549*	559	546*	559	549*

* Significantly different from 2001 average ($p < .05$).

[1] Hong Kong SAR is a Special Administrative Region (SAR) of the People's Republic of China.

[2] Met guidelines for sample participation rates in 2006 only after replacement schools were included.

[3] Did not meet guidelines in 2006 for sample participation rates after replacement schools were included.

Note: Results from the Progress in International Reading Literacy Study (PIRLS) assessment are reported on a combined reading literacy scale, which captures students' overall literacy skills, and two subscales that measure two types of purposes of reading: reading for literary purposes and reading for informational purposes. The combined reading literacy score is calculated on the basis of all the items in the assessment, whereas the subscale scores are calculated on the basis of the items making up each of the two subscales. Because the combined reading literacy scale and the two subscales are calculated separately using the properties of all of the items in the given scale or subscale, the combined reading literacy score is not the simple average of the two subscales.

Source: Baer, J., Baldi, S., Ayotte, K., and Green, P. (2007). *The Reading Literacy of U.S. Fourth-Grade Students in an International Context: Results From the 2001 and 2006 Progress in International Reading Literacy Study (PIRLS)* (NCES 2008-017), table 2, data from the International Association for the Evaluation of Educational Achievement (IEA), Progress in International Reading Literacy Study (PIRLS), 2001 and 2006.

Table 18-3. Average combined reading literacy scale scores of 4th-graders, by reading subscale, sex, and educational jurisdiction: 2006

Reading subscale						
	Combined reading literacy		Literary subscale		Informational subscale	
Educational jurisdiction	Male	Female	Male	Female	Male	Female
International average	492	509*	491	509*	493	509*
Alberta, Canada	556	564*	556	567*	553	559*
Austria	533	543*	531	543*	533	540*
Belgium (Flemish)1	544	550*	541	547*	545	550*
Belgium (French)	497	502*	495	504*	497	499
British Columbia, Canada	554	562*	553	565*	551	556*
Bulgaria	537	558*	532	553*	542	558*
Chinese Taipei	529	542*	523	538*	534	543*
Denmark	539	553*	541	554*	536	547*
England	530	549*	528	550*	529	545*
France	516	527*	510	523*	521	531*
Georgia	463	480*	470	484*	457	474*
Germany	544	551*	544	554*	542	547*
Hong Kong, SAR2	559	569*	551	564*	564	572*
Hungary	548	554*	553	560*	539	543
Iceland	501	520*	504	525*	497	514*
Indonesia	395	415*	387	408*	409	427*
Iran, Islamic Republic of	414	429*	421	432	412	429*
Israel	506	520*	509	524*	502	513*
Italy	548	555*	548	556*	547	551
Kuwait	297	364*	310	372*	292	361*
Latvia	530	553*	529	550*	527	553*
Lithuania	528	546*	533	550*	521	539*
Luxembourg	556	559	552	557*	556	557
Macedonia	432	453*	429	449*	440	460*
Moldova	493	507*	486	499*	502	514*
Morocco	314	332*	310	326*	326	344*
Netherlands1	543	551*	541	548*	543	552*
New Zealand	520	544*	516	539*	522	545*
Norway3	489	508*	491	512*	486	502*
Nova Scotia, Canada	531	553*	534	552*	529	549*

Table 18-3. Continued

Reading subscale						
	Combined reading literacy		Literary subscale		Informational subscale	
Educational jurisdiction	Male	Female	Male	Female	Male	Female
Ontario, Canada	549	562*	549	562*	547	558*
Poland	511	528*	514	532*	507	523*
Qatar	335	372*	341	376*	339	374*
Quebec, Canada	527	539*	523	536*	528	539*
Romania	483	497*	485	501*	481	494*
Russian Federation	557	572*	554	568*	555	572*
Scotland1	516	538*	515	538*	517	537*
Singapore	550	567*	544	560*	555	572*
Slovak Republic	525	537*	527	539*	522	532*
Slovenia	512	532*	511	529*	514	533*
South Africa	283	319*	281	318*	299	332*
Spain	511	515	513	520*	508	508
Sweden	541	559*	536	557*	541	557*
Trinidad and Tobago	420	451*	419	450*	426	455*
United States1	535	545*	534	547*	532	542*

* Significantly different from the other sex ($p < .05$).
[1] Met guidelines for sample participation rates only after replacement schools were included.
[2] Hong Kong SAR is a Special Administrative Region (SAR) of the People's Republic of China.
[3] Did not meet guidelines for sample participation rates after replacement schools were included.

Note: Results from the Progress in International Reading Literacy Study (PIRLS) assessment are reported on a combined reading literacy scale, which captures students' overall literacy skills, and two subscales that measure two types of purposes of reading: reading for literary purposes and reading for informational purposes. The combined reading literacy score is calculated on the basis of all the items in the assessment, whereas the subscale scores are calculated on the basis of the items making up each of the two subscales. Because the combined reading literacy scale and the two subscales are calculated separately using the properties of all of the items in the given scale or subscale, the combined reading literacy score is not the simple average of the two subscales.

Source: Baer, J., Baldi, S., Ayotte, K., and Green, P. (2007). *The Reading Literacy of U.S. Fourth-Grade Students in an International Context: Results From the 2001 and 2006 Progress in International Reading Literacy Study (PIRLS)* (NCES 2008-017), tables R4 and R5, data from the International Association for the Evaluation of Educational Achievement (IEA), Progress in International Reading Literacy Study (PIRLS), 2006.

Table 18-4. Average combined reading literacy scale scores of U.S. 4th-graders, by reading subscale and race/ethnicity: 2006

		Reading subscale	
Race/ethnicity	Combined reading literacy	Literary subscale	Informational subscale
White	560	562	555
Black	503*	501*	505*
Hispanic	518*	517*	517*
Asian	567	569	561
American Indian/Alaska Native	468*	468*	472*
Other	573	568	571

* Significantly different from average score of White students ($p < .05$).

Note: Other includes students who were identified as Pacific Islander as well as those non-Hispanic students who were identified as belonging to multiple racial groups. Race categories exclude persons of Hispanic ethnicity. The United States met guidelines for sample participation rates only after replacement schools were included. Results from the Progress in International Reading Literacy Study (PIRLS) assessment are reported on a combined reading literacy scale, which captures students' overall literacy skills, and two subscales that measure two types of purposes of reading: reading for literary purposes and reading for informational purposes. The combined reading literacy score is calculated on the basis of all the items in the assessment, whereas the subscale scores are calculated on the basis of the items making up each of the two subscales. Because the combined reading literacy scale and the two subscales are calculated separately using the properties of all of the items in the given scale or subscale, the combined reading literacy score is not the simple average of the two subscales.

Source: Baer, J., Baldi, S., Ayotte, K., and Green, P. (2007). *The Reading Literacy of U.S. Fourth-Grade Students in an International Context: Results From the 2001 and 2006 Progress in International Reading Literacy Study (PIRLS)* (NCES 2008-017), table 3, data from the International Association for the Evaluation of Educational Achievement (IEA), Progress in International Reading Literacy Study (PIRLS), 2006.

International Comparisons of Science Literacy

Table 19-1. Average combined science literacy scale scores of 15-year-old students, by scientific skill subscale and country or jurisdiction: 2006

		Scientific skill subscale		
Country or jurisdiction	Combined science literacy score	Identifying scientific issues	Using scientific evidence	Explaining phenomena scientifically
OECD average	500*	499	499*	500*
OECD-member country				
Australia	527*	535*	531*	520*
Austria	511*	505*	505*	516*
Belgium	510*	515*	516*	503*
Canada	534*	532*	542*	531*
Czech Republic	513*	500	501	527*
Denmark	496	493	489	501*
Finland	563*	555*	567*	566*
France	495	499	511*	481
Germany	516*	510*	515*	519*
Greece	473*	469*	465*	476
Hungary	504*	483*	497	518*
Iceland	491	494	491	488
Ireland	508*	516*	506*	505*
Italy	475*	474*	467*	480
Japan	531*	522*	544*	527*
Korea, Republic of	522*	519*	538*	512*
Luxembourg	486	483*	492	483
Mexico	410*	421*	402*	406*
Netherlands	525*	533*	526*	522*
New Zealand	530*	536*	537*	522*
Norway	487	489	473*	495
Poland	498	483*	494	506*
Portugal	474*	486	472*	469*
Slovak Republic	488	475*	478	501*
Spain	488	489	485	490
Sweden	503*	499	496	510*
Switzerland	512*	515*	519*	508*
Turkey	424*	427*	417*	423*
United Kingdom	515*	514*	514*	517*
United States	489	492	489	486

Non-OECD-member jurisdiction				
Argentina	391*	395*	385*	386*
Azerbaijan	382*	353*	344*	412*
Brazil	390*	398*	378*	390*
Bulgaria	434*	427*	417*	444*
Chile	438*	444*	440*	432*
Chinese Taipei	532*	509*	532*	545*
Colombia	388*	402*	383*	379*
Croatia	493	494	490	492
Estonia	531*	516*	531*	541*
Hong Kong-China	542*	528*	542*	549*
Indonesia	393*	393*	386*	395*
Israel	454*	457*	460*	443*
Jordan	422*	409*	405*	438*
Kyrgyz Republic	322*	321*	288*	334*
Latvia	490	489	491	486
Liechtenstein	522*	522*	535*	516*
Lithuania	488	476*	487	494
Macao-China	511*	490	512*	520*
Montenegro, Republic of	412*	401*	407*	417*
Qatar	349*	352*	324*	356*
Romania	418*	409*	407*	426*
Russian Federation	479	463*	481	483
Serbia, Republic of	436*	431*	425*	441*
Slovenia	519*	517*	516*	523*
Thailand	421*	413*	423*	420*
Tunisia	386*	384*	382*	383*
Uruguay	428*	429*	429*	423*

* Significantly different from U.S. average ($p < .05$).

Note: The Organization for Economic Cooperation and Development (OECD) is an intergovernmental organization of 30 industrialized nations. The OECD average represents the average of the 30 member nations where each country is counted equally regardless of population size. The combined science scale and the three subscales are each computed separately. Therefore, the combined science scale score is not the average of the three subscale scores.

Source: Baldi, S., Jin, Y., Skewer, M., Green, P. J., and Herget, D. (2007). *Highlights From PISA 2006: Performance of U.S. 15-Year-Old Students in Science and Mathematics Literacy in an International Context* (NCES 2008-016), tables 2a–d, data from the Organization for Economic Cooperation and Development (OECD), Program for International Student Assessment (PISA), 2006.

Table 19-2. Average combined science literacy scale scores of 15-year-old students, by scientific skill subscale, sex, and country or jurisdiction: 2006

			Scientific skill subscale					
	Combined science literacy score		Identifying scientific issues		Using scientific evidence		Explaining phenomena scientifically	
Country or jurisdiction	Male	Female	Male	Female	Male	Female	Male	Female
OECD average	501*	499	490	508*	498	501*	508*	493
OECD-member country								
Australia	527	527	525	546*	530	533	527*	513
Austria	515	507	495	516*	509	500	526*	507
Belgium	511	510	508	523*	512	521	510*	494
Canada	536	532	525	539*	541	542	539*	522
Czech Republic	515	510	492	511*	501	500	537 *	516
Denmark	500*	491	488	499*	490	487	512 *	491
Finland	562	565	542	568*	564	571*	571*	562
France	497	494	491	507*	509	513	489*	474
Germany	519	512	502	518*	517	513	529*	508
Greece	468	479*	453	485*	456	475*	478	475
Hungary	507	501	477	489*	497	498	529*	507
Iceland	488	494	479	509*	487	495	491	485
Ireland	508	509	508	524*	503	509	510*	501
Italy	477	474	466	483*	466	468	487*	472
Japan	533	530	513	531*	543	545	535*	519
Korea, Republic of	521	523	508	530*	535	542	517	506
Luxembourg	491*	482	477	489*	493	490	495*	471
Mexico	413*	406	418	425*	404	401	415*	398
Netherlands	528*	521	527	539*	527	524	531*	512
New Zealand	528	532	525	547*	532	541	528*	517
Norway	484	489	478	501*	469	476	498	492
Poland	500	496	476	490*	492	495	514*	498

			Scientific skill subscale					
	Combined science literacy score		Identifying scientific issues		Using scientific evidence		Explaining phenomena scientifically	
Country or jurisdiction	Male	Female	Male	Female	Male	Female	Male	Female
Portugal	477	472	480	493*	473	471	477*	462
Slovak Republic	491	485	465	485*	478	478	512*	490
Spain	491	486	482	496*	484	485	499*	481
Sweden	504	503	491	507*	494	499	516*	504
Switzerland	514*	509	510	520*	520	517	517*	498
Turkey	418	430*	414	443*	410	426*	423	423
United Kingdom	520*	510	510	517*	517	510	527*	506
United States	489	489	484	500*	486	491	492*	480
Non-OECD-member jurisdiction Argentina	384	397*	381	408*	374	396*	387	386
Azerbaijan	379	386*	349	357*	342	347*	408	417*
Brazil	395*	386	394	402*	382*	375	400*	382
Bulgaria	426	443*	411	445*	404	430*	442	447
Chile	448*	426	445	443	447*	431	448*	414
Chinese Taipei	536	529	506	512	532	532	554*	535
Colombia	393	384	401	404	386	381	388*	371
Croatia	492	494	480	507*	488	493	498*	487
Estonia	530	533	504	528*	529	533	544	537
Hong Kong-China	546	539	520	535*	544	541	560*	539
Indonesia	399	387	397	389	388	383	403*	386
Israel	456	452	451	463	456	464	451*	436
Jordan	408	436*	393	425*	385	424*	427	448*
Kyrgyz Republic	319	325*	311	330*	280	295*	335	333
Latvia	486	493*	473	504*	484	497*	491*	481
Liechtenstein	516	527	508	534*	524	544	519	513
Lithuania	483	493*	463	489*	478	495*	499*	490
Macao-China	513	509	483	498*	512	511	527*	513

Table 19-2. (Continued).

			Scientific skill subscale					
	Combined science literacy score		Identifying scientific issues		Using scientific evidence		Explaining phenomena scientifically	
Country or jurisdiction	Male	Female	Male	Female	Male	Female	Male	Female
Montenegro, Republic of	411	413	393	409*	403	411*	421*	412
Qatar	334	365*	334	371*	307	341*	342	371*
Romania	417	419	401	418*	403	412	431*	421
Russian Federation	481	478	453	472*	478	483	493*	474
Serbia, Republic of	433	438	420	441*	419	431*	444	438
Slovenia	515	523*	504	530*	510	522*	528*	518
Thailand	411	428*	394	427*	409	433*	418	421
Tunisia	383	388	373	394*	377	387*	386	381
Uruguay	427	430	418	439*	425	433	429*	418

* Significantly higher score than other sex ($p < .05$).

Note: The Organization for Economic Cooperation and Development (OECD) is an intergovernmental organization of 30 industrialized nations. The OECD average represents the average of the 30 member nations where each country is counted equally regardless of population size. The combined science scale and the three subscales are each computed separately. Therefore, the combined science scale score is not the average of the three subscale scores.

Source: Baldi, S., Jin, Y., Skewer, M., Green, P. J., and Herget, D. (2007). *Highlights From PISA 2006: Performance of U.S. 15-Year-Old Students in Science and Mathematics Literacy in an International Context* (NCES 2008-016), figure 6, data from the Organization for Economic Cooperation and Development (OECD), Program for International Student Assessment (PISA), 2006.

Table 19-3. Average combined science literacy scale scores of OECD countries and U.S. 15-year-old students, by race/ethnicity: 2006

OECD average and U.S. racial/ethnic group	Combined science literacy score
OECD average	500
White	523*
Black	409*
Hispanic	439*
Asian	499
Native Hawaiian/Other Pacific Islander	483
American Indian/Alaska Native	436*
More than one race	501

* Significantly different from OECD average ($p < .05$).

Note: The Organization for Economic Cooperation and Development (OECD) is an intergovernmental organization of 30 industrialized nations. The OECD average represents the average of the 30 member nations where each country is counted equally regardless of population size. Race categories exclude persons of Hispanic ethnicity.

Source: Baldi, S., Jin, Y., Skewer, M., Green, P. J., and Herget, D. (2007). *Highlights From PISA 2006: Performance of U.S. 15-Year-Old Students in Science and Mathematics Literacy in an International Context* (NCES 2008-016), figure 7, data from the Organization for Economic Cooperation and Development (OECD), Program for International Student Assessment (PISA), 2006.

ANNUAL EARNINGS OF YOUNG ADULTS

Table 20-1. Median annual earnings of full-time, full-year wage and salary workers ages 25–34, by educational attainment, sex, and race/ethnicity: Selected years, 1980–2006; [In constant 2006 dollars]

Educational attainment, sex, and race/ethnicity[1]	1980	1985	1990	1995	2000	2005	2006
Race/ethnicity[1] and sex							
White	$38,200	$37,500	$37,000	$34,400	$37,900	$36,100	$37,400
Male	44,000	43,100	40,100	39,600	41,000	40,300	40,000
Female	29,400	31,900	30,900	30,400	33,900	33,000	34,000
Black	29,400	28,100	27,800	27,800	29,700	29,800	30,000
Male	34,000	31,900	29,300	30,400	33,900	29,900	30,000
Female	26,900	26,200	26,200	25,900	26,900	29,300	27,500
Hispanic	33,000	30,400	27,800	26,500	29,300	27,900	28,000
Male	36,700	33,700	30,100	27,500	30,400	28,900	29,000
Female	26,900	28,100	24,700	24,800	26,200	26,800	27,000
Male	—	—	37,4003	37,0003	48,0003	46,500	50,000
Female	—	—	33,4003	33,1003	41,0003	41,300	40,000
Pacific Islander	—	—	(3)	(3)	‡3	‡	30,000
American Indian/Alaska Native	—	—	30,900	26,500	28,100	31,000	27,000
More than one race	—	—	—	—	—	36,100	35,000
Male	—	—	—	—	—	38,200	35,000
Female	—	—	—	—	—	32,200	35,000
Other	36,700	37,100	‡	—	—	—	—
Male	42,800	41,200	‡	—	—	—	—
Female	30,600	32,000	‡	—	—	—	—

— Not available.

‡ Reporting standards not met (too few cases).

[1] Race categories exclude persons of Hispanic ethnicity. Estimates by sex for Pacific Islander, American Indian/Alaska Native, and More than one race subgroups did not meet reporting standards.

[2] Due to changes in categories across time, the category "some college" prior to 1992 is not comparable with "some college" from 1992 onwards. Prior to 1992, some college may include students who earned an associate's degree.

[3] From 1989 through 2002, data for Asians and Pacific Islanders were not reported separately; therefore, Pacific Islanders are included with Asians during this period.

Note: Earnings are presented in constant dollars by means of the Consumer Price Index (CPI) to eliminate inflationary factors and allow for direct comparison across years. See *supplemental note 11* for further discussion. *Full-year worker* refers to those who were employed 50 or more weeks during the previous year; *full-time worker* refers to those who were usually employed 35 or more hours per week. The Current Population Survey (CPS) questions used to obtain educational attainment were changed in 1992. In 1994, the survey instrument for the CPS was changed and weights were adjusted. See *supplemental note 2* for further discussion on both of these changes.

Source: U.S. Department of Commerce, Census Bureau, Current Population Survey (CPS), March and Annual Social and Economic Supplement, selected years, 1981–2007.

Table 20-2. Median annual earnings of full-time, full-year wage and salary workers ages 25–34, by race/ethnicity and educational attainment: Selected years, 1980–2006; [In constant 2006 dollars]

Race/ethnicity[1] and educational attainment	1980	1985	1990	1995	2000	2005	2006
White	$38,200	$37,500	$37,000	$34,400	$37,900	$36,100	$37,400
Less than high school	30,800	28,100	26,200	23,800	23,400	23,700	25,000
High school diploma or equivalent	35,100	33,700	30,900	29,100	32,200	31,000	30,000
Some college[2]	38,800	37,500	36,700	31,800	35,100	33,000	33,300
Associate's degree	—	—	—	34,400	37,500	36,100	35,000
Bachelor's degree or higher	44,000	46,900	46,300	45,000	46,800	46,500	45,000
Bachelor's degree	—	—	—	42,300	46,800	42,300	45,000
Master's degree or higher	—	—	—	52,900	52,700	51,600	50,000
Black	29,400	28,100	27,800	27,800	29,700	29,800	30,000
Less than high school	21,800	18,700	19,600	18,600	22,200	21,500	18,000
High school diploma or equivalent	29,400	26,200	24,500	23,800	24,600	23,700	25,000
Some college[2]	31,800	28,100	30,100	29,100	30,400	30,100	28,000
Associate's degree	—	—	—	29,100	29,300	28,900	29,000
Bachelor's degree or higher	36,700	37,500	38,600	36,400	41,000	40,300	40,000
Bachelor's degree	—	—	—	34,400	38,600	37,200	37,000
Master's degree or higher	—	—	—	45,000	50,300	45,400	50,000
Hispanic	33,000	30,400	27,800	26,500	29,300	27,900	28,000
Less than high school	29,300	24,400	21,700	20,600	21,300	21,500	20,800
High school diploma or equivalent	29,400	28,100	26,200	25,100	26,900	24,800	26,000
Some college[2]	36,700	35,600	30,900	26,500	31,600	33,000	30,000
Associate's degree	—	—	—	31,800	35,100	35,100	32,000
Bachelor's degree or higher	40,000	45,000	41,700	39,700	44,500	42,300	42,000
Bachelor's degree	—	—	—	38,100	42,100	41,300	40,000
Master's degree or higher	—	—	—	‡	‡	52,300	48,000
Asian	—	—	36,3003	34,4003	42,1003	41,300	45,000
Less than high school	—	—	‡3	‡3	‡3	‡	‡

Table 20-2. Continued

Race/ethnicity1 and educational attainment	1980	1985	1990	1995	2000	2005	2006
High school diploma or equivalent	—	—	25,5003	26,5003	29,3003	27,900	28,000
Some college[2]	—	—	30,9003	24,6003	32,8003	31,000	32,000
Associate's degree	—	—	—	26,5003	35,1003	36,100	36,000
Bachelor's degree or higher	—	—	46,3003	43,7003	58,5003	51,600	55,000
Bachelor's degree	—	—	—	40,3003	57,4003	51,600	50,000
Master's degree or higher	—	—	—	50,3003	62,0003	56,800	60,000
Pacific Islander	—	—	(3)	(3)	‡3	‡	30,000
American Indian/Alaska Native	—	—	30,900	26,500	28,100	31,000	27,000
More than one race	—	—	—	—	—	36,100	35,000
Other	$36,700	$37,100	‡	—	—	—	—
Less than high school	‡	‡	‡	—	—	—	—
High school diploma or equivalent	29,400	30,000	‡	—	—	—	—
Some college[2]	36,700	34,100	‡	—	—	—	—
Associate's degree	—	—	—	—	—	—	—
Bachelor's degree or higher	44,000	41,200	‡	—	—	—	—
Bachelor's degree	—	—	—	—	—	—	—
Master's degree or higher	—	—	—	—	—	—	—

— Not available.

‡ Reporting standards not met (too few cases).

[1] Race categories exclude persons of Hispanic ethnicity. Estimates for educational categories for Pacific Islander, American Indian/Alaska Native, and More than one race subgroups did not meet reporting standards.

[2] Due to changes in categories across time, the category "some college" prior to 1992 is not comparable with "some college" from 1992 onwards. Prior to 1992, some college may include students who earned an associate's degree.

[3] From 1989 through 2002, data for Asians and Pacific Islanders were not reported separately; therefore, Pacific Islanders are included with Asians during this period.

Note: Earnings are presented in constant dollars by means of the Consumer Price Index (CPI) to eliminate inflationary factors and allow for direct comparison across years. See *supplemental note 11* for further discussion. *Full-year worker* refers to those who were employed 50 or more weeks during the previous year; *full-time worker* refers to those who were usually employed 35 or more hours per week. The Current Population Survey (CPS) questions used to obtain educational attainment were changed in 1992. In 1994, the survey instrument for the CPS was changed and weights were adjusted. See *supplemental note 2* for further discussion on both of these changes.

Source: U.S. Department of Commerce, Census Bureau, Current Population Survey (CPS), March and Annual Social and Economic Supplement, selected years, 1981–2007.

PUBLIC HIGH SCHOOL GRADUATION RATES BY STATE

Table 21-1. Averaged freshman graduation rate for public high school students and number of graduates, by state: School years 2000–01 through 2004–05

	2000–01		2001–02		2002–03		2003–04		2004–05	
State	Averaged freshman graduation rate[1]	Total number of graduates[2]	Averaged freshman graduation rate[1]	Total number of graduates[2]	Averaged freshman graduationrate[1]	Total number of graduates[2]	Averaged freshman graduation rate[1]	Total number of graduates[2]	Averaged freshman graduation rate[1]	Total number of graduates[2]
United States	71.7	2,569,200	72.6	2,621,534	73.9	2,719,947	74.33	2,753,4383	74.7	2,799,250
Reporting 48 states and D.C.	†	†	†	†	†	†	75.0	2,548,128	†	†
Alabama	63.7	37,082	62.1	35,887	64.7	36,741	65.0	36,464	65.9	37,453
Alaska	68.0	6,812	65.9	6,945	68.0	7,297	67.2	7,236	64.1	6,909
Arizona	74.2	46,733	74.7	47,175	75.9	49,986	66.8	45,508	84.7	59,498
Arkansas	73.9	27,100	74.8	26,984	76.6	27,555	76.8	27,181	75.7	26,621
California	71.6	315,189	72.7	325,895	74.1	341,097	73.9	343,480	74.6	355,217
Colorado	73.2	39,241	74.7	40,760	76.4	42,379	78.7	44,777	76.7	44,532
Connecticut	77.5	30,388	79.7	32,327	80.9	33,667	80.7	34,573	80.9	35,515
Delaware	71.0	6,614	69.5	6,482	73.0	6,817	72.9	6,951	73.1	6,934
District of Columbia	60.2	2,808	68.4	3,090	59.6	2,725	68.2	3,031	68.8	2,781
Florida	61.2	111,112	63.4	119,537	66.7	127,484	66.4	131,418	64.6	133,318
Georgia	58.7	62,499	61.1	65,983	60.8	66,890	61.2	68,550	61.7	70,834
Hawaii	68.3	10,102	72.1	10,452	71.3	10,013	72.6	10,324	75.1	10,813
Idaho	79.6	15,941	79.3	15,874	81.4	15,858	81.5	15,547	81.0	15,768
Illinois	75.6	110,624	77.1	116,657	75.9	117,507	80.3	124,763	79.4	123,615
Indiana	72.1	56,172	73.1	56,722	75.5	57,897	73.5	56,008	73.2	55,444
Iowa	82.8	33,774	84.1	33,789	85.3	34,860	85.8	34,339	86.6	33,547
Kansas	76.5	29,360	77.1	29,541	76.9	29,963	77.9	30,155	79.2	30,355
Kentucky	69.8	36,957	69.8	36,337	71.7	37,654	73.0	37,787	75.9	38,399

Table 21-1. (Continued).

State	2000–01		2001–02		2002–03		2003–04		2004–05	
	Averaged freshman graduation rate[1]	Total number of graduates[2]	Averaged freshman graduation rate[1]	Total number of graduates[2]	Averaged freshman graduationrate[1]	Total number of graduates[2]	Averaged freshman graduation rate[1]	Total number of graduates[2]	Averaged freshman graduation rate[1]	Total number of graduates[2]
Louisiana	63.7	38,314	64.4	37,905	64.1	37,610	69.4	37,019	63.9	36,009
Maine	76.4	12,654	75.6	12,593	76.3	12,947	77.6	13,278	78.6	13,077
Maryland	78.7	49,222	79.7	50,881	79.2	51,864	79.5	52,870	79.3	54,170
Massachusetts	78.9	54,393	77.6	55,272	75.7	55,987	79.3	58,326	78.7	59,665
Michigan	75.4	96,515	72.9	95,001	74.0	100,301	72.5	98,823	73.0	101,582
Minnesota	83.6	56,581	83.9	57,440	84.8	59,432	84.7	59,096	85.9	58,391
Mississippi	59.7	23,748	61.2	23,740	62.7	23,810	62.7	23,735	63.3	23,523
Missouri	75.5	54,138	76.8	54,487	78.3	56,925	80.4	57,983	80.6	57,841
Montana	80.0	10,628	79.8	10,554	81.0	10,657	80.4	10,500	81.5	10,335
Nebraska	83.8	19,658	83.9	19,910	85.2	20,161	87.6	20,309	87.8	19,940
Nevada	70.0	15,127	71.9	16,270	72.3	16,378	57.4	15,201	55.8	15,740
New Hampshire	77.8	12,294	77.8	12,452	78.2	13,210	78.7	13,309	80.1	13,775
New Jersey	85.4	76,130	85.8	77,664	87.0	81,391	86.3	83,826	85.1	86,502
New Mexico	65.9	18,199	67.4	18,094	63.1	16,923	67.0	17,892	65.4	17,353
New York	61.5	141,884	60.5	140,139	60.9	143,818	60.94	142,5264	65.3	153,203
North Carolina	66.5	63,288	68.2	65,955	70.1	69,696	71.4	72,126	72.6	75,010
North Dakota	85.4	8,445	85.0	8,114	86.4	8,169	86.1	7,888	86.3	7,555
Ohio	76.5	111,281	77.5	110,608	79.0	115,762	81.3	119,029	80.2	116,702
Oklahoma	75.8	37,458	76.0	36,852	76.0	36,694	77.0	36,799	76.9	36,227
Oregon	68.3	29,939	71.0	31,153	73.7	32,587	74.2	32,958	74.2	32,602
Pennsylvania	79.0	114,436	80.2	114,943	81.7	119,933	82.2	123,474	82.5	124,758
Rhode Island	73.5	8,603	75.7	9,006	77.7	9,318	75.9	9,258	78.4	9,881
South Carolina	56.5	30,026	57.9	31,302	59.7	32,482	60.6	33,235	60.1	33,439
South Dakota	77.4	8,881	79.0	8,796	83.0	8,999	83.7	9,001	82.3	8,585
Tennessee	59.0	40,642	59.6	40,894	63.4	44,113	66.1	46,096	68.5	47,967

	2000–01		2001–02		2002–03		2003–04		2004–05	
State	Averaged freshman graduation rate[1]	Total number of graduates[2]	Averaged freshman graduation rate[1]	Total number of graduates[2]	Averaged freshman graduationrate[1]	Total number of graduates[2]	Averaged freshman graduation rate[1]	Total number of graduates[2]	Averaged freshman graduation rate[1]	Total number of graduates[2]
Texas	70.8	215,316	73.5	225,167	75.5	238,111	76.7	244,165	74.0	239,717
Utah	81.6	31,036	80.5	30,183	80.2	29,527	83.0	30,252	84.4	30,253
Vermont	80.2	6,856	82.0	7,083	83.6	6,970	85.4	7,100	86.5	7,152
Virginia	77.5	66,067	76.7	66,519	80.6	72,943	79.3	72,042	79.6	73,667
Washington	69.2	55,081	72.2	58,311	74.2	60,435	74.6	61,274	75.0	61,094
West Virginia	75.9	18,440	74.2	17,128	75.7	17,287	76.9	17,339	77.3	17,137
Wisconsin	83.3	59,341	84.8	60,575	85.8	63,272	85.84	62,7844	86.7	63,229
Wyoming	73.4	6,071	74.4	6,106	73.9	5,845	76.0	5,833	76.7	5,616

† Not applicable.

1 The rate is the number of graduates divided by the estimated count of freshmen 4 years earlier. The estimated averaged freshman enrollment count is the sum of the number of 8th-graders 5 years earlier, the number of 9th-graders 4 years earlier (because this is when current year seniors were freshmen), and the number of 10th-graders 3 years earlier, divided by 3. Enrollment counts include a proportional distribution of students not enrolled in a specific grade.

2 Graduates include only those who earned regular diplomas or diplomas for advanced academic achievement (e.g., honors diploma) as defined by the state or district.

3 The 2003–04 national estimates do not include data from two states with missing diploma counts: New York and Wisconsin.

4 To impute the number of graduates in these states in 2003–04, the 2002–03 averaged freshman graduation rates for Wisconsin and New York were applied to the average of the grade-specific enrollment data in the state for grade 8 in 1999–2000, grade 9 in 2000–01, and grade 10 in 2001–02.

Source: U.S. Department of Education, National Center for Education Statistics, Common Core of Data (CCD), "State Nonfiscal Survey of Public Elementary/Secondary Education," 1986–87 through 2005–06; and Seastrom, M., Hoffman, L., and Chapman, C. (2006). The Averaged Freshman Graduation Rate for Public High Schools From the Common Core of Data: School Years 2002–03 and 2003–04 (NCES 2006-606rev).

Students With Disabilities Exiting School With a Regular High School Diploma

Table 22-1. Number and percentage distribution of students ages 14–21 with disabilities served under Individuals with Disabilities Education Act (IDEA) (Part B) who exited school, by exit status: School years 1996–97 through 2005–06

Exit status	1996–97	1997–98	1998–99	1999–2000	2000–01	2001–02	2002–03	2003–04	2004–05	2005–06
Total, number	308,538	323,093	318,386	348,385	362,065	370,106	373,916	392,663	393,579	396,857
Total, percentage	100.0	100.0	100.0	100.0	100.0	100.0	100.0	100.0	100.0	100.0
Graduated with diploma	43.1	45.5	46.8	46.5	48.0	51.4	52.5	54.5	54.6	56.5
Received a certificate of attendance[1]	9.0	9.0	9.0	9.2	9.0	9.3	12.5	13.0	15.3	15.3
Reached maximum age[2]	0.9	0.9	1.0	1.5	1.4	1.0	1.0	1.0	1.3	1.4
Died	0.5	0.5	0.5	0.5	0.5	0.5	0.5	0.5	0.5	0.5
Dropped out[3]	46.4	44.0	42.6	42.3	41.2	37.8	33.6	31.1	28.3	26.2

[1] Students who exited an educational program and received a certificate of completion, modified diploma, or some similar document. This includes students who received a high school diploma, but did not meet the same standards for graduation as those for students without disabilities.

[2] Students may exit special education services by reaching the maximum age beginning at age 18, depending on state law or practice or order of any court.

[3] Defined as the total who were enrolled at some point in the reporting year, were not enrolled at the end of the reporting year, and did not exit for any of the other reasons described. For the purpose of calculating dropout rates, the Office of Special Education Programs (OSEP) counts as dropouts students who moved and were not known to continue.

Note: Data are from a cumulative 12-month reporting period. Detail may not sum to totals because of rounding. Estimates include students from the United States and other jurisdictions including American Samoa, Guam, Northern Marianas, Puerto Rico, Virgin Islands, and Bureau of Indian Education (BIE) schools.

Source: U.S. Department of Education, Office of Special Education Programs (OSEP), Data Analysis System (DANS), *Children with Disabilities Exiting Special Education, 2005–06* (OMB #1820-0521). Retrieved November 28, 2007, from https://www.ideadata.org/arc_toc8.asp#partbEX.

Students with Disabilities Exiting School with a Regular High School Diploma

Table 22-2. Number and percentage distribution of students ages 14–21 with disabilities served under Individuals with Disabilities Education Act (IDEA) (Part B) who exited school, by exit status, age, and type of disability: School year 2005–06

Age and type of disability	Total exiting special education	Graduated with diploma	Received a certificate of attendance[1]	Reached maximum age[2]	Died	Dropped out3
Total	396,857	56.5	15.3	1.4	0.5	26.2
Age 14	5,935	1.6	0.4	0.0	5.5	92.5
15	11,067	0.7	0.5	0.0	3.4	95.5
16	27,713	17.4	2.2	0.0	1.4	79.0
17	142,510	66.3	12.3	0.0	0.3	21.1
18	141,364	64.9	17.7	0.5	0.2	16.6
19	42,605	55.6	23.1	0.9	0.4	20.0
20	15,397	42.8	27.7	9.6	0.6	19.3
21	10,266	27.0	34.5	27.6	0.6	10.3
Disability Specific learning disability	236,135	61.6	12.5	0.5	0.3	25.1
Mental retardation	46,588	36.7	35.5	4.6	0.8	22.3
Emotional disturbance	47,519	43.4	9.9	1.2	0.5	44.9
Speech or language impairment	8,923	67.3	9.2	0.5	0.2	22.7
Multiple disabilities	8,251	43.8	25.6	8.3	3.6	18.7
Other health impairment	32,274	63.4	11.7	0.6	0.9	23.4
Hearing impairment4	4,674	68.7	16.5	1.2	0.3	13.4
Orthopedic impairment	3,455	61.7	19.2	3.8	3.6	11.7
Visual impairment	1,766	72.1	13.9	1.6	1.1	11.4
Autism	4,876	57.1	26.6	6.7	0.5	9.1
Deaf-blindness	150	65.3	14.0	8.7	3.3	8.7
Traumatic brain injury	2,246	65.0	16.5	2.9	0.8	14.8

[1] Students who exited an educational program and received a certificate of completion, modified diploma, or some similar document. This includes students who received a high school diploma, but did not meet the same standards for graduation as those for students without disabilities.

[2] Students may exit special education services by reaching the maximum age beginning at age 18, depending on state law or practice or order of any court.

[3] Defined as the total who were enrolled at some point in the reporting year, were not enrolled at the end of the reporting year, and did not exit for any of the other reasons described. For the purpose of calculating dropout rates, the Office of Special Education Programs (OSEP) counts as dropouts students who moved and were not known to continue.

[4] Includes deaf and hard-of-hearing.

Note: Data are from a cumulative 12-month reporting period. Detail may not sum to totals because of rounding. Estimates include students from the United States and other jurisdictions including American Samoa, Guam, Northern Marianas, Puerto Rico, Virgin Islands, and Bureau of Indian Education (BIE) schools.

Source: U.S. Department of Education, Office of Special Education Programs (OSEP), Data Analysis System (DANS), *Children with Disabilities Exiting Special Education, 2005–06* (OMB #1820-0521). Retrieved November 28, 2007, from https://www.ideadata.org/arc_toc8.asp#partbEX.

Table 22-3. Number and percentage of students ages 14–21 with disabilities served under Individuals with Disabilities Education Act (IDEA) (Part B) who exited school, by exit status and state or jurisdiction: School year 2005–06

State or jurisdiction	Exiting total[1]	Graduated with diploma	Received a certificate of attendance[2]	Dropped out[3]
Total	396,857	56.5	15.3	26.2
Alabama	5,974	24.1	37.7	36.3
Alaska	957	44.2	15.0	39.6
Arizona	4,490	50.4	0.0	46.4
Arkansas	3,950	78.8	1.3	19.3
California	33,352	59.6	5.4	32.5
Colorado	3,659	66.9	3.5	20.6
Connecticut	4,772	78.2	0.4	18.2
Delaware	826	66.6	6.3	25.8
District of Columbia	248	90.7	0.0	0.0
Florida	22,964	41.5	29.0	29.0
Georgia	11,192	30.9	36.6	32.1
Hawaii	1,401	82.7	4.6	3.4
Idaho	1,767	54.8	10.4	31.6
Illinois	34,559	72.5	1.5	24.5
Indiana	9,950	47.2	12.2	38.7
Iowa	5,340	69.4	2.7	26.3
Kansas	4,183	71.6	—	27.0
Kentucky	4,909	64.0	7.2	27.9
Louisiana	4,581	27.2	26.5	45.4
Maine	2,361	65.4	3.3	29.6
Maryland	6,541	58.3	9.2	29.7
Massachusetts	10,033	68.0	4.5	25.1
Michigan	7,647	72.9	1.2	25.3

Table 22-3. (Continued).

State or jurisdiction	Exiting total[1]	Graduated with diploma	Received a certificate of attendance[2]	Dropped out[3]
Minnesota	7,153	74.4	—	25.0
Mississippi	3,119	24.6	53.7	20.8
Missouri	9,007	69.7	0.3	27.6
Montana	1,273	68.7	0.5	30.3
Nebraska	2,373	74.3	1.3	19.3
Nevada	2,845	20.9	42.4	36.1
New Hampshire	3,223	51.9	1.1	46.5
New Jersey	17,670	74.5	0.0	23.7
New Mexico	2,511	55.7	26.2	18.0
New York	28,270	47.4	19.2	31.2
North Carolina	11,052	49.7	10.4	38.3
North Dakota	740	75.9	—	21.9
Ohio	15,965	36.8	44.6	11.5
Oklahoma	6,483	69.3	—	29.9
Oregon	4,478	44.6	16.3	32.9
Pennsylvania	17,296	89.3	0.6	9.5
Rhode Island	1,870	71.6	0.6	25.2
South Carolina	5,666	29.1	23.9	44.5
South Dakota	737	67.6	0.9	27.3
Tennessee	6,827	46.6	31.9	20.1
Texas	32,515	41.7	41.2	16.6
Utah	3,642	63.2	13.0	22.9
Vermont	900	65.9	1.4	30.1
Virginia	10,488	39.5	42.4	17.0
Washington	—	—	—	—
West Virginia	3,246	65.7	4.3	29.4
Wisconsin	7,791	74.8	2.4	20.4
Wyoming	734	61.7	2.3	33.8

State or jurisdiction	Exiting total[1]	Graduated with diploma	Received a certificate of attendance[2]	Dropped out[3]
BIE schools4	645	42.9	6.5	38.6
American Samoa	40	67.5	—	25.0
Guam	217	58.1	—	39.6
Northern Marianas	58	60.3	—	34.5
Puerto Rico	2,287	55.1	11.1	29.2
Virgin Islands	159	29.6	18.2	51.6

— Not available.

[1] Due to state-level data suppression, the national exiting total does not match the sum of the state exiting totals. Data for students who exited by reaching the maximum age or who died are not shown separately, but are included in the total.

[2] Students who exited an educational program and received a certificate of completion, modified diploma, or some similar document. This includes students who received a high school diploma, but did not meet the same standards for graduation as those for students without disabilities.

[3] Defined as the total who were enrolled at some point in the reporting year, were not enrolled at the end of the reporting year, and did not exit for any of the other reasons described. For the purpose of calculating dropout rates, the Office of Special Education Programs (OSEP) counts as dropouts students who moved and were not known to continue.

[4] Bureau of Indian Education schools.

Note: Data are from a cumulative 12-month reporting period. Estimates include students from the United States and other jurisdictions including American Samoa, Guam, Northern Marianas, Puerto Rico, Virgin Islands, and Bureau of Indian Education (BIE) schools.

Source: U.S. Department of Education, Office of Special Education Programs (OSEP), Data Analysis System (DANS), *Children with Disabilities Exiting Special Education, 2005–06* (OMB #1820-0521). Retrieved November 28, 2007, from https://www.ideadata.org/ arc_toc8.asp# partbEX.

Status Dropout Rates by Race/Ethnicity

Table 23-1. Status dropout rates of 16- through 24-year-olds, by race/ethnicity: October 1972–2006

Year	Total1	White	Black	Hispanic
1972	14.6	12.3	21.3	34.3
1973	14.1	11.6	22.2	33.5
1974	14.3	11.9	21.2	33.0
1975	13.9	11.4	22.9	29.2
1976	14.1	12.0	20.5	31.4
1977	14.1	11.9	19.8	33.0
1978	14.2	11.9	20.2	33.3
1979	14.6	12.0	21.1	33.8
1980	14.1	11.4	19.1	35.2
1981	13.9	11.4	18.4	33.2
1982	13.9	11.4	18.4	31.7
1983	13.7	11.2	18.0	31.6
1984	13.1	11.0	15.5	29.8
1985	12.6	10.4	15.2	27.6
1986	12.2	9.7	14.2	30.1
1987	12.7	10.4	14.1	28.6
1988	12.9	9.6	14.5	35.8
1989	12.6	9.4	13.9	33.0
1990	12.1	9.0	13.2	32.4
1991	12.5	8.9	13.6	35.3
1992	11.0	7.7	13.7	29.4
1993	11.0	7.9	13.6	27.5
1994	11.5	7.7	12.6	30.0
1995	12.0	8.6	12.1	30.0
1996	11.1	7.3	13.0	29.4

Year	Total1	White	Black	Hispanic
1997	11.0	7.6	13.4	25.3
1998	11.8	7.7	13.8	29.5
1999	11.2	7.3	12.6	28.6
2000	10.9	6.9	13.1	27.8
2001	10.7	7.3	10.9	27.0
2002	10.5	6.5	11.3	25.7
2003	9.9	6.3	10.9	23.5
2004	10.3	6.8	11.8	23.8
2005	9.4	6.0	10.4	22.4
2006	9.3	5.8	10.7	22.1

[1] Total includes other race/ethnicity categories not separately shown.

[2] Race categories exclude persons of Hispanic ethnicity. From 2003 onwards, respondents were able to identify as being more than one race, and the Black and White categories include individuals who considered themselves to be of only one race.

Note: The *status dropout rate* is the percentage of 16- through 24-year-olds who are not enrolled in high school and who lack a high school credential. A high school credential includes a high school diploma or equivalent credential such as a General Educational Development (GED) certificate. Estimates beginning in 1987 reflect new editing procedures for cases with missing data on school enrollment items. Estimates beginning in 1992 reflect new wording of the educational attainment item. Estimates beginning in 1994 reflect changes due to newly instituted computer-assisted interviewing. See *supplemental note 7* for more information on measures of student persistence and progress.

Source: U.S. Department of Commerce, Census Bureau, Current Population Survey (CPS), October Supplement, 1972–2006.

Status Dropout Rates by Race/Ethnicity

Table 23-2. Status dropout rates and number and percentage distribution of status dropouts ages 16–24, by selected characteristics: October 2006

		Number of status			
Characteristic	Status dropout rate (percent)	dropouts (in thousands)	Population (in thousands)	Percent of all status dropouts	Percent of population
Total	9.3	3,462	37,047	100.0	100.0
Sex					
Male	10.3	1,935	18,707	55.9	50.5
Female	8.3	1,527	18,340	44.1	49.5
Race/ethnicity[1] White	5.8	1,337	22,863	38.6	61.7
Black	10.7	565	5,260	16.3	14.2
Hispanic	22.1	1,421	6,439	41.0	17.4
Asian	3.7	53	1,444	1.5	3.9
Pacific Islander	‡	‡	105	‡	0.3
American Indian/Alaska Native	14.7	34	231	1.0	0.6
More than one race	7.0	49	703	1.4	1.9
Age 16	2.8	124	4,462	3.6	12.0
17	5.0	210	4,212	6.1	11.4
18	8.6	356	4,120	10.3	11.1
19	9.7	386	3,982	11.2	10.7
20–24	11.8	2,385	20,270	68.9	54.7
Immigration status Born outside the 50 states and the					
District of Columbia					
Hispanic	36.2	959	2,648	27.7	7.1
Non-Hispanic	6.6	126	1,898	3.6	5.1
First generation[2] Hispanic	12.3	270	2,196	7.8	5.9
Non-Hispanic	4.2	100	2,387	2.9	6.4
Second generation or mor[e3] Hispanic	12.1	193	1,595	5.6	4.3
Non-Hispanic	6.9	1,815	26,322	52.4	71.1
Region Northeast	6.5	426	6,523	12.3	17.6

Characteristic	Status dropout rate (percent)	Number of status dropouts (in thousands)	Population (in thousands)	Percent of all status dropouts	Percent of population
Midwest	6.1	515	8,390	14.9	22.6
South	11.7	1,577	13,467	45.6	36.4
West	10.9	945	8,666	27.3	23.4

‡ Reporting standards not met (too few cases).

[1] All racial/ethnic categories except "More than one race" are of persons who considered themselves as being of one race, with the exception of the Hispanic category, which consists of Hispanics of all races and racial combinations. Race categories exclude persons of Hispanic ethnicity.

[2] *First generation* describes an individual born in the 50 states or the District of Columbia with at least one parent born outside the 50 states or the District of Columbia.

[3] *Second generation or more* describes an individual born in the 50 states or the District of Columbia whose parents were both born inside the 50 states or the District of Columbia.

Note: The *status dropout rate* is the percentage of 16- through 24-year-olds who are not enrolled in high school and who lack a high school credential. See *supplemental note 7* for more information. A high school credential includes a high school diploma or equivalent credential such as a General Educational Development (GED) certificate. Detail may not sum to totals because of rounding.

Source: U.S. Department of Commerce, Census Bureau, Current Population Survey (CPS), October Supplement, 2006.

Immediate Transition to College

Table 24-1. Percentage of high school completers who were enrolled in college the October immediately following high school completion, by race/ethnicity and family income: 1972–2006

				Race/ethnicity[1]		Family income[2]				
Year	Total	White	Black	Hispanic	Gap between White and Black	Gap between White and Hispanic	Low	Middle	High	Gap between low and high
1972	49.2	49.7	44.6	45.0	5.1	4.7	26.1	45.2	63.8	37.7
1973	46.6	47.8	32.5	54.1	15.3	-6.3	20.3	40.9	64.4	44.1
1974	47.6	47.2	47.2	46.9	-0.1	0.3	—	—	—	—
1975	50.7	51.1	41.7	58.0	9.4	-6.9	31.2	46.2	64.5	33.3
1976	48.8	48.8	44.4	52.7	4.4	-3.9	39.1	40.5	63.0	23.8
1977	50.6	50.8	49.5	50.8	1.4	0.0	27.7	44.2	66.3	38.6
1978	50.1	50.5	46.4	42.0	4.1	8.5	31.4	44.3	64.0	32.6
1979	49.3	49.9	46.7	45.0	3.3	5.0	30.5	43.2	63.2	32.7
1980	49.3	49.8	42.7	52.3	7.1	-2.5	32.5	42.5	65.2	32.7
1981	53.9	54.9	42.7	52.1	12.2	2.8	33.6	49.2	67.6	34.0
1982	50.6	52.7	35.8	43.2	16.9	9.5	32.8	41.7	70.9	38.1
1983	52.7	55.0	38.2	54.2	16.9	0.8	34.6	45.2	70.3	35.8
1984	55.2	59.0	39.8	44.3	19.2	14.6	34.5	48.4	74.0	39.5
1985	57.7	60.1	42.2	51.0	17.9	9.0	40.2	50.6	74.6	34.3
1986	53.8	56.8	36.9	44.0	19.9	12.8	33.9	48.5	71.0	37.1
1987	56.8	58.6	52.2	33.5	6.4	25.0	36.9	50.0	73.8	36.9
1988	58.9	61.1	44.4	57.1	16.8	4.0	42.5	54.7	72.8	30.3
1989	59.6	60.7	53.4	55.1	7.3	5.6	48.1	55.4	70.7	22.6
1990	60.1	63.0	46.8	42.7	16.2	20.3	46.7	54.4	76.6	29.9
1991	62.5	65.4	46.4	57.2	19.0	8.2	39.5	58.4	78.2	38.8
1992	61.9	64.3	48.2	55.0	16.1	9.4	40.9	57.0	79.0	38.1

				Race/ethnicity[1]		Family income[2]				
Year	Total	White	Black	Hispanic	Gap between White and Black	Gap between White and Hispanic	Low	Middle	High	Gap between low and high
1993	62.6	62.9	55.6	62.2	7.3	0.7	50.4	56.9	79.3	28.9
1994	61.9	64.5	50.8	49.1	13.7	15.4	43.3	57.8	77.9	34.6
1995	61.9	64.3	51.2	53.7	13.1	10.6	34.2	56.0	83.5	49.2
1996	65.0	67.4	56.0	50.8	11.5	16.6	48.6	62.7	78.0	29.4
1997	67.0	68.2	58.5	65.6	9.6	2.6	57.0	60.7	82.2	25.2
1998	65.6	68.5	61.9	47.4	6.6	21.2	46.4	64.7	77.5	31.1
1999	62.9	66.3	58.9	42.3	7.4	24.0	49.4	59.4	76.1	26.7
2000	63.3	65.7	54.9	52.9	10.8	12.7	49.7	59.5	76.9	27.2
2001	61.7	64.2	54.6	51.7	9.5	12.5	43.8	56.3	79.9	36.1
2002	65.2	68.9	59.4	53.3	9.4	15.6	56.4	60.7	78.2	21.8
2003	63.9	66.2	57.5	58.6	8.7	7.6	52.8	57.6	80.1	27.3
2004	66.7	68.8	62.5	61.8	6.3	7.0	47.8	63.3	80.1	32.3
2005	68.6	73.2	55.7	54.0	17.5	19.2	53.5	65.1	81.2	27.6
2006	66.0	68.5	55.5	57.9	13.0	10.6	50.9	61.4	80.7	29.8

— Not available. Data on family income were not available in 1974.

[1] Included in the total but not shown separately are high school completers from other racial/ethnic groups. Race categories exclude persons of Hispanic ethnicity.

[2] *Low income* refers to the bottom 20 percent of all family incomes, *high income* refers to the top 20 percent of all family incomes, and *middle income* refers to the 60 percent in between. See *supplemental note 2* for further information.

Note: Includes those ages 16–24 completing high school in a given year. The Current Population Survey (CPS) questions about educational attainment were reworded in 1992. Before then, *high school completers* referred to those who had completed 12 years of schooling; beginning in 1992, the term referred to those who had received a high school diploma or equivalency certificate. In 1994, the survey methodology for the CPS was changed and weights were adjusted. See *supplemental note 2* for further information. Detail may not sum to totals because of rounding. Some estimates have been revised from previous publications.

Source: U.S. Department of Commerce, Census Bureau, Current Population Survey (CPS), October Supplement, 1972–2006.

IMMEDIATE TRANSITION TO COLLEGE

Table 24-2. Percentage of high school completers who were enrolled in college the October immediately following high school completion, by sex and type of institution: 1972–2006

Year	Total	2-year1	4-year1	Total	2-year1	4-year1
1972	52.7	—	—	46.0	—	—
1973	50.0	14.6	35.4	43.4	15.2	28.2
1974	49.4	16.6	32.8	45.9	13.9	32.0
1975	52.6	19.0	33.6	49.0	17.4	31.6
1976	47.2	14.5	32.7	50.3	16.6	33.8
1977	52.1	17.2	35.0	49.3	17.8	31.5
1978	51.1	15.6	35.5	49.3	18.3	31.0
1979	50.4	16.9	33.5	48.4	18.1	30.3
1980	46.7	17.1	29.7	51.8	21.6	30.2
1981	54.8	20.9	33.9	53.1	20.1	33.0
1982	49.1	17.5	31.6	52.0	20.6	31.4
1983	51.9	20.2	31.7	53.4	18.4	35.1
1984	56.0	17.7	38.4	54.5	21.0	33.5
1985	58.6	19.9	38.8	56.8	19.3	37.5
1986	55.8	21.3	34.5	51.9	17.3	34.6
1987	58.3	17.3	41.0	55.3	20.3	35.0
1988	57.1	21.3	35.8	60.7	22.4	38.3
1989	57.6	18.3	39.3	61.6	23.1	38.5
1990	58.0	19.6	38.4	62.2	20.6	41.6
1991	57.9	22.9	35.0	67.1	26.8	40.3
1992	60.0	22.1	37.8	63.8	23.9	40.0
1993	59.9	22.9	37.0	65.2	22.8	42.4
1994	60.6	23.0	37.5	63.2	19.1	44.1
1995	62.6	25.3	37.4	61.3	18.1	43.2
1996	60.1	21.5	38.5	69.7	24.6	45.1

Year	Total	2-year1	4-year1	Total	2-year1	4-year1
1997	63.6	21.4	42.2	70.3	24.1	46.2
1998	62.4	24.4	38.0	69.1	24.3	44.8
1999	61.4	21.0	40.5	64.4	21.1	43.3
2000	59.9	23.1	36.8	66.2	20.0	46.2
2001	59.7	18.6	41.1	63.6	20.7	42.9
2002	62.1	20.5	41.7	68.3	23.0	45.3
2003	61.2	21.9	39.3	66.5	21.0	45.5
2004	61.4	21.8	39.6	71.5	23.1	48.5
2005	66.5	24.7	41.8	70.4	23.4	47.0
2006	65.8	24.9	40.9	66.1	24.5	41.7

— Not available. Data on type of institution were not collected until 1973.

[1] From 1973 through 1986, due to a skip pattern in the Current Population Survey (CPS), about 3–9 percent of high school completers ages 16–24 who enrolled in college immediately were not asked the question about the type of institutions attended. Such respondents were assumed to have the same probability of enrolling at a 2- or 4-year institution as those who were asked the question.

Note: Includes those ages 16–24 completing high school in a given year. The Current Population Survey (CPS) questions about educational attainment were reworded in 1992. Before then, *high school completers* referred to those who had completed 12 years of schooling; beginning in 1992, the term referred to those who had received a high school diploma or equivalency certificate. In 1994, the survey methodology for the CPS was changed and weights were adjusted. See *supplemental note 2* for further information. Detail may not sum to totals because of rounding.

Source: U.S. Department of Commerce, Census Bureau, Current Population Survey (CPS), October Supplement, 1972–2006.

Table 24-3. Percentage of high school completers who were enrolled in college the October immediately following high school completion, by parents' education: 1992–2006

Year	Total	Less than high school	High school diploma or equivalent	Some college, including vocational/technical	Bachelor's degree or higher	Not available[1]
1992	61.9	33.1	55.5	67.5	81.3	38.0
1993	62.6	47.1	52.3	62.7	87.9	42.0
1994	61.9	43.0	49.9	65.0	82.5	43.1
1995	61.9	27.3	47.0	70.2	87.7	30.8
1996	65.0	45.0	56.1	66.6	85.2	45.6
1997	67.0	51.4	61.7	62.6	86.1	51.3
1998	65.6	49.8	57.2	67.7	82.3	50.1
1999	62.9	36.3	54.4	60.3	82.2	53.1
2000	63.3	44.4	51.8	63.8	81.2	50.5
2001	61.7	39.0	51.9	62.0	81.3	41.9
2002	65.2	43.3	51.9	65.9	82.6	58.7
2003	63.9	43.3	53.9	62.9	82.1	48.8
2004	66.7	40.2	53.8	67.0	85.9	53.6
2005	68.6	43.0	62.1	65.6	88.8	54.8
2006	66.0	43.0	56.1	67.0	78.2	54.6

[1] Information on parents' education was not available for those who did not live with their parents and were classified as a householder, and for those whose parents' educational attainment was not reported; about 9–14 percent of high school completers ages 16–24 were in this category for the period covered.

Note: Includes those ages 16–24 completing high school in a given year. *High school completers* referred to those who received a high school diploma or equivalency certificate. In 1994, the survey methodology for the CPS was changed and weights were adjusted. See *supplemental note 2* for further information, including the definition of parents' education. Some estimates have been revised from previous publications.

Source: U.S. Department of Commerce, Census Bureau, Current Population Survey (CPS), October Supplement, 1992–2006.

Table 25-1. Percentage of 25- to 29-year-olds who completed high school, by race/ethnicity and sex: March 1971–2007

		Total1			White			Black			Hispanic	
Year	Total	Male	Female	Total	Male	Female	Total	Male	Female	Total	Male	Female
1971	77.7	79.0	76.5	81.7	83.0	80.5	58.7	56.7	60.5	48.3	51.4	45.8
1972	79.8	80.5	79.2	83.4	84.1	82.7	64.1	61.7	66.0	47.5	47.0	48.0
1973	80.2	80.6	79.8	84.1	84.2	83.9	64.1	63.2	64.9	52.3	54.2	50.6
1974	81.9	83.1	80.8	85.5	86.0	85.0	68.3	71.5	65.8	54.1	55.8	52.5
1975	83.1	84.5	81.8	86.6	88.0	85.2	71.1	72.3	70.1	53.1	52.2	53.9
1976	84.7	86.0	83.5	87.7	89.0	86.4	74.0	72.8	74.9	58.1	57.7	58.4
1977	85.4	86.6	84.2	88.6	89.2	88.0	74.5	77.5	72.0	58.1	61.9	54.6
1978	85.3	86.0	84.6	88.5	88.8	88.2	77.4	78.7	76.3	56.6	58.5	54.7
1979	85.6	86.3	84.9	89.2	89.8	88.5	74.7	73.9	75.3	57.1	55.5	58.5
1980	85.4	85.4	85.5	89.2	89.1	89.2	76.7	74.7	78.3	58.0	57.0	58.9
1981	86.3	86.5	86.1	89.8	89.7	89.9	77.6	78.8	76.6	59.8	59.1	60.4
1982	86.2	86.3	86.1	89.1	89.1	89.1	81.0	80.5	81.5	60.9	60.7	61.2
1983	86.0	86.0	86.0	89.3	89.3	89.3	79.5	79.0	79.9	58.3	57.8	58.9
1984	85.9	85.6	86.3	89.4	89.4	89.4	79.0	75.9	81.7	58.6	56.8	60.2
1985	86.1	85.9	86.4	89.5	89.2	89.9	80.5	80.6	80.5	60.9	58.6	63.1
1986	86.1	85.9	86.4	89.6	88.8	90.4	83.5	86.4	81.0	59.1	58.2	60.0
1987	86.0	85.5	86.4	89.4	88.9	90.0	83.4	84.5	82.5	59.8	58.6	61.0
1988	85.9	84.7	87.0	89.7	88.4	90.9	80.9	80.8	80.9	62.3	59.9	64.9
1989	85.5	84.4	86.5	89.3	88.2	90.4	82.3	80.5	83.8	61.0	61.0	61.0
1990	85.7	84.4	87.0	90.1	88.6	91.7	81.7	81.4	82.0	58.2	56.6	59.9
1991	85.4	84.9	85.8	89.8	89.2	90.4	81.8	83.6	80.1	56.7	56.4	57.1
1992	86.3	86.1	86.5	90.7	90.2	91.1	80.9	82.7	79.3	60.9	61.1	60.6
1993	86.7	86.0	87.4	91.2	90.6	91.8	82.6	84.8	80.8	60.9	58.3	64.0
1994	86.1	84.5	87.6	91.1	90.0	92.3	84.1	82.7	85.3	60.3	58.0	63.0
1995	86.8	86.3	87.4	92.5	92.0	93.0	86.7	88.4	85.3	57.1	55.7	58.7

Table 25-1. (Continued).

		Total[1]			White			Black			Hispanic	
Year	Total	Male	Female	Total	Male	Female	Total	Male	Female	Total	Male	Female
1996	87.3	86.5	88.1	92.6	92.0	93.1	86.0	87.9	84.5	61.1	59.7	62.9
1997	87.4	85.8	88.9	92.9	91.7	94.0	86.9	85.8	87.8	61.8	59.2	64.9
1998	88.1	86.6	89.6	93.6	92.5	94.6	88.2	88.4	88.1	62.8	59.9	66.3
1999	87.8	86.1	89.5	93.0	91.9	94.1	88.7	88.2	89.2	61.6	57.4	66.0
2000	88.1	86.7	89.4	94.0	92.9	95.2	86.8	87.6	86.2	62.8	59.2	66.4
2001	87.7	86.9	88.6	93.3	93.0	93.6	87.0	87.5	86.7	63.2	59.4	67.2
2002	86.4	84.7	88.1	93.0	92.1	93.8	87.6	85.8	88.9	62.4	60.2	65.0
2003	86.5	84.9	88.2	93.7	92.8	94.5	88.5	87.4	89.4	61.7	59.6	64.2
2004	86.6	85.2	88.0	93.3	92.1	94.5	88.7	91.2	86.6	62.4	60.1	65.2
2005	86.1	84.9	87.3	92.8	91.8	93.8	86.9	86.6	87.3	63.3	63.2	63.3
2006	86.4	84.4	88.5	93.4	92.3	94.6	86.3	84.2	88.0	63.2	60.5	66.6
2007	87.0	84.9	89.1	93.5	92.7	94.2	87.7	87.4	87.9	65.0	60.5	70.7

[1] Included in the totals but not shown separately are estimates for those from other racial/ethnic categories.

Note: Prior to 1992, *high school completers* referred to those who completed 12 years of schooling; beginning in 1992, the term referred to those who received a high school diploma or equivalency certificate. In 1994, the survey instrument for the Current Population Survey (CPS) was changed and weights were adjusted. See *supplemental note 2* for further discussion. Some estimates are revised from previous publications. Race categories exclude persons of Hispanic ethnicity.

Source: U.S. Department of Commerce, Census Bureau, Current Population Survey (CPS), March Supplement, 1971–2007.

Table 25-2. Percentage of 25- to 29-year-olds who completed at least some college, by race/ethnicity and sex: March 1971–2007

		Totall			White			Black			Hispanic	
Year	Total	Male	Female	Total	Male	Female	Total	Male	Female	Total	Male	Female
1971	33.9	38.5	29.4	36.7	41.7	31.8	18.1	16.5	19.5	14.7	19.7	10.5!
1972	36.0	40.9	31.3	38.6	44.0	33.3	21.4	19.6	22.8	15.3	17.4	13.5
1973	36.3	41.4	31.4	39.2	44.6	33.7	21.5	21.2	21.8	16.6	21.4	12.4
1974	40.1	44.7	35.6	43.1	47.8	38.4	24.2	26.4	22.4	21.3	24.7	18.2
1975	41.6	47.4	36.0	44.3	50.4	38.3	27.5	29.7	25.8	21.8	26.3	17.6
1976	44.1	50.1	38.4	47.2	53.5	41.0	27.5	29.5	25.9	21.1	24.4	18.3
1977	45.5	50.3	40.8	48.6	53.4	43.7	31.1	34.3	28.5	23.8	26.5	21.5
1978	46.4	51.0	41.9	49.5	54.6	44.4	34.7	35.7	33.9	24.7	27.6	22.0
1979	46.3	49.8	42.9	49.6	53.3	45.9	31.2	30.2	32.0	25.1	28.2	22.3
1980	44.7	47.6	41.9	48.0	51.1	44.9	32.4	32.6	32.3	23.2	25.9	20.5
1981	43.2	45.6	40.9	46.0	48.5	43.5	33.0	33.9	32.3	23.6	24.6	22.7
1982	43.0	44.5	41.6	45.1	46.6	43.7	37.1	38.1	36.3	24.1	24.6	23.7
1983	43.5	44.8	42.2	46.1	47.7	44.4	33.0	33.2	32.9	25.0	23.8	26.3
1984	43.0	43.6	42.5	45.6	46.2	45.0	32.9	31.5	34.1	26.7	27.0	26.4
1985	43.7	44.2	43.3	46.4	46.8	46.0	34.4	34.2	34.5	26.9	26.9	27.0
1986	44.0	44.1	43.8	46.8	46.9	46.8	36.3	35.9	36.6	25.3	24.9	25.8
1987	43.6	43.1	44.0	46.0	45.7	46.2	35.9	32.4	38.8	26.7	27.1	26.2
1988	43.6	43.7	43.6	46.4	46.4	46.5	33.3	34.7	32.1	28.0	26.5	29.6
1989	43.8	43.9	43.7	47.2	47.1	47.2	34.6	34.0	35.1	27.0	27.3	26.7
1990	44.5	43.7	45.3	48.3	47.3	49.3	36.1	35.0	36.9	23.4	22.9	23.9
1991	45.3	44.4	46.2	49.3	48.8	49.9	35.3	32.0	38.2	23.9	23.1	24.8
1992	48.9	48.2	49.6	53.3	52.6	53.9	36.2	34.9	37.2	28.5	27.2	30.1
1993	51.0	49.5	52.5	55.6	54.7	56.6	40.0	37.0	42.5	29.7	26.9	33.1
1994	52.1	49.8	54.3	57.1	54.9	59.3	41.8	40.3	43.0	31.0	28.0	34.6
1995	54.1	52.3	55.8	59.8	57.5	62.1	45.1	45.3	44.8	28.7	26.7	30.9
1996	56.5	54.5	58.5	62.0	60.3	63.7	48.1	47.9	48.3	31.1	28.1	35.0
1997	57.1	54.9	59.4	63.3	61.3	65.3	46.6	43.0	49.6	33.3	30.7	36.4

Table 25-2. (Continued).

		Total1			White			Black			Hispanic	
Year	Total	Male	Female	Total	Male	Female	Total	Male	Female	Total	Male	Female
1998	57.8	54.6	61.0	64.1	61.3	66.9	49.9	46.8	52.6	32.5	29.3	36.3
1999	58.0	54.7	61.3	63.9	60.7	67.0	51.3	45.9	55.5	31.2	27.4	35.0
2000	58.3	55.1	61.5	64.1	60.5	67.7	52.7	50.4	54.6	32.8	29.0	36.6
2001	58.4	54.4	62.5	64.8	60.5	69.1	50.5	46.7	53.6	32.2	28.2	36.4
2002	58.0	54.5	61.6	65.8	62.0	69.5	53.4	51.8	54.6	30.9	28.3	34.1
2003	57.4	53.8	61.1	65.5	61.9	69.2	51.2	49.6	52.5	31.1	27.9	34.9
2004	57.3	53.4	61.3	64.7	60.8	68.6	51.9	49.3	54.0	32.3	27.9	37.7
2005	56.7	52.1	61.4	64.3	59.7	68.9	49.0	41.9	55.1	32.8	31.8	34.0
2006	57.8	53.3	62.4	66.3	62.1	70.4	49.9	44.8	54.3	31.7	28.3	35.9
2007	57.7	52.5	63.0	65.6	61.1	70.0	50.0	45.9	53.6	33.9	28.2	41.1

! Interpret data with caution (estimates are unstable).

[1] Included in the totals but not shown separately are estimates for those from other racial/ethnic categories.

Note: *Some college* also includes those with a bachelor's degree or higher. Prior to 1992, *some college* meant completing 1 or more years of college; beginning in 1992, the term meant completing any college at all. In 1994, the survey instrument for the Current Population Survey (CPS) was changed and weights were adjusted. See *supplemental note 2* for further discussion. Some estimates are revised from previous publications. Race categories exclude persons of Hispanic ethnicity.

Source: U.S. Department of Commerce, Census Bureau, Current Population Survey (CPS), March Supplement, 1971–2007.

Table 25-3. Percentage of 25- to 29-year-olds with a bachelor's degree or higher, by race/ethnicity and sex: March 1971–2007

		Total1			White			Black			Hispanic	
Year	Total	Male	Female	Total	Male	Female	Total	Male	Female	Total	Male	Female
1971	17.1	20.4	13.8	18.9	22.4	15.4	6.7	6.9	6.6	5.1!	8.0!	2.6!
1972	19.0	22.0	16.0	20.8	24.1	17.5	8.4	7.2	9.4	3.7!	4.5!	3.1!
1973	19.0	21.6	16.4	20.8	23.8	17.9	8.1	7.2	9.0	5.7	6.7!	4.8!
1974	20.7	23.9	17.6	23.2	26.7	19.7	7.9	8.7	7.2	5.5	4.9!	6.0!
1975	21.9	25.2	18.7	23.8	27.3	20.2	10.5	11.1	10.0	8.8	10.4	7.3
1976	23.7	27.5	20.1	25.7	29.8	21.6	13.0	12.0	13.9	7.3	10.3	4.7!
1977	24.0	27.0	21.1	26.4	29.7	23.1	12.6	12.8	12.5	6.7	7.1	6.3
1978	23.3	26.0	20.6	25.6	28.9	22.3	11.8	10.7	12.6	9.6	9.6	9.7
1979	23.1	25.8	20.5	25.5	28.4	22.6	12.4	13.2	11.8	7.3	7.9	6.8
1980	22.5	24.0	21.0	25.0	26.8	23.2	11.6	10.5	12.4	7.7	8.4	6.9
1981	21.3	23.1	19.6	23.6	25.5	21.7	11.6	12.1	11.1	7.5	8.6	6.5
1982	21.7	23.3	20.2	23.8	25.7	21.9	12.6	11.7	13.4	9.7	10.7	8.7
1983	22.5	23.9	21.1	24.5	26.2	22.7	12.9	13.1	12.7	10.4	9.6	11.1
1984	21.9	23.2	20.7	24.1	25.5	22.7	11.7	12.9	10.6	10.6	9.6	11.6
1985	22.2	23.1	21.3	24.4	25.5	23.3	11.6	10.3	12.6	11.1	10.9	11.2
1986	22.4	22.9	21.9	25.2	25.8	24.5	11.8	10.3	13.1	9.0	8.9	9.1
1987	22.0	22.3	21.7	24.6	24.9	24.4	11.5	11.8	11.2	8.7	9.2	8.2
1988	22.7	23.4	21.9	25.1	25.7	24.5	12.0	12.4	11.7	11.3	11.9	10.6
1989	23.4	23.9	22.9	26.3	26.9	25.8	12.6	12.1	13.1	10.1	9.6	10.6
1990	23.2	23.7	22.8	26.4	26.6	26.2	13.4	15.1	11.9	8.1	7.3	9.1
1991	23.2	23.0	23.4	26.7	26.5	26.9	11.0	11.5	10.5	9.2	8.1	10.4
1992	23.6	23.2	24.0	27.2	26.6	27.7	11.0	11.7	10.5	9.5	8.8	10.3
1993	23.7	23.4	23.9	27.2	27.2	27.1	13.3	12.5	13.9	8.3	7.1	9.8
1994	23.3	22.5	24.0	27.1	26.8	27.4	13.6	11.6	15.2	8.0	6.6	9.8
1995	24.7	24.5	24.9	28.8	28.4	29.2	15.4	17.4	13.7	8.9	7.8	10.1
1996	27.1	26.1	28.2	31.6	30.9	32.3	14.6	12.2	16.6	10.0	10.2	9.8
1997	27.8	26.3	29.3	32.6	31.2	34.1	14.2	11.8	16.3	11.0	9.6	12.7

Table 25-3. (Continued).

		Total1			White			Black			Hispanic	
Year	Total	Male	Female	Total	Male	Female	Total	Male	Female	Total	Male	Female
1998	27.3	25.6	29.0	32.3	30.5	34.2	15.8	14.3	17.0	10.4	9.5	11.3
1999	28.2	26.8	29.5	33.6	32.0	35.1	15.0	13.1	16.5	8.9	7.5	10.4
2000	29.1	27.9	30.1	34.0	32.3	35.8	17.8	18.4	17.4	9.7	8.3	11.0
2001	28.6	26.2	31.1	33.0	29.7	36.3	17.8	17.9	17.8	11.1	9.1	13.3
2002	29.3	26.9	31.8	35.9	32.6	39.2	18.0	17.9	18.1	8.9	8.3	9.7
2003	28.4	26.0	30.9	34.2	31.4	37.1	17.5	17.7	17.4	10.0	8.4	12.0
2004	28.7	26.1	31.4	34.5	31.4	37.5	17.1	13.5	20.0	10.9	9.6	12.4
2005	28.6	25.3	32.0	34.1	30.4	37.8	17.5	14.3	20.3	11.2	10.2	12.4
2006	28.4	25.3	31.6	34.3	31.4	37.2	18.7	15.2	21.7	9.5	6.9	12.8
2007	29.6	26.3	33.0	35.5	31.9	39.2	19.5	18.9	20.0	11.6	8.6	15.4

! Interpret data with caution (estimates are unstable).

[1] Included in the totals but not shown separately are estimates for those from other racial/ethnic categories.

Note: The Current Population Survey (CPS) questions used to obtain educational attainment were changed in 1992. In 1994, the survey instrument for the CPS was changed and weights were adjusted. See *supplemental note 2* for further discussion. Some estimates are revised from previous publications. Race categories exclude persons of Hispanic ethnicity.

Source: U.S. Department of Commerce, Census Bureau, Current Population Survey (CPS), March Supplement, 1971–2007.

Degrees Earned

Table 26-1. Number of degrees conferred by degree-granting institutions, by type of degree: 1990–91 through 2005–06

Academic year	Associate's	Bachelor's	Master's	First-professional1	Doctoral2
1990–91	481,720	1,094,538	337,168	71,948	39,294
1991–92	504,231	1,136,553	352,838	74,146	40,659
1992–93	514,756	1,165,178	369,585	75,387	42,132
1993–94	530,632	1,169,275	387,070	75,418	43,185
1994–95	539,691	1,160,134	397,629	75,800	44,446
1995–96	555,216	1,164,792	406,301	76,734	44,652
1996–97	571,226	1,172,879	419,401	78,730	45,876
1997–98	558,555	1,184,406	430,164	78,598	46,010
1998–99	559,954	1,200,303	439,986	78,439	44,077
1999–2000	564,933	1,237,875	457,056	80,057	44,808
2000–01	578,865	1,244,171	468,476	79,707	44,904
2001–02	595,133	1,291,900	482,118	80,698	44,160
2002–03	632,912	1,348,503	512,645	80,810	46,024
2003–04	665,301	1,399,542	558,940	83,041	48,378
2004–05	696,660	1,439,264	574,618	87,289	52,631
2005–06	713,066	1,485,242	594,065	87,655	56,067
Increase in the number of degrees conferred between 1990–91 and 2005–06	231,346	390,704	256,897	15,707	16,773
Increase in the number of degrees conferred between 1995–96 and 2005–06	157,850	320,450	187,764	10,921	11,415
Percentage change in the number of degrees conferred between 1990–91 and 2005–06	48.0	35.7	76.2	21.8	42.7

Table 26-1. (Continued).

Academic year	Associate's	Bachelor's	Master's	First-professional1	Doctoral2
Percentage change in the number of degrees conferred between 1995–96 and 2005–06	28.4	27.5	46.2	14.2	25.6

[1] An award that requires completion of a degree program that meets all of the following criteria: (1) completion of the academic requirements to begin practice in the profession; (2) at least 2 years of college work before entering the degree program; (3) a total of at least 6 academic years of college work to complete the degree program, including previously required college work plus the work required in the professional program itself. See glossary for a definition of first-professional degree.

[2] Includes Ph.D., Ed.D., and comparable degrees at the doctoral level. Excludes first-professional degrees, such as M.D., D.D.S., and law degrees.

Note: Detail in accompanying tables may not sum to totals shown here because of rounding.

Source: U.S. Department of Education, National Center for Education Statistics, 1990–91 through 2004–05 Integrated Postsecondary Education Data System, "Completions Survey" (IPEDS-C:90–99), and Fall 2000 through Fall 2006.

Table 26-2. Number and percentage distribution of degrees conferred by degree-granting institutions, by type of degree and racial/ethnic group: Academic years 1990–91, 1995–96, and 2005–06

	1990–91		1995–96		2005–06		Percent change		
Characteristic	Number	Percent of total	Number	Percent of total	Number	Percent of total	1990–91 to 1995–96	1995–96 to 2005–06	1990–91 to 2005–06
Associate's	481,720	100.0	555,216	100.0	713,066	100.0	15.3	28.4	48.0
White	391,264	81.2	426,106	76.7	485,297	68.1	8.9	13.9	24.0
Total minority	83,503	17.3	118,979	21.4	214,391	30.1	42.5	80.2	156.7
Black	38,835	8.1	52,014	9.4	89,784	12.6	33.9	72.6	131.2
Hispanic	25,540	5.3	38,254	6.9	80,854	11.3	49.8	111.4	216.6
Asian/Pacific Islander	15,257	3.2	23,138	4.2	35,201	4.9	51.7	52.1	130.7
American Indian/Alaska Native	3,871	0.8	5,573	1.0	8,552	1.2	44.0	53.5	120.9
Nonresident alien	6,953	1.4	10,131	1.8	13,378	1.9	45.7	32.1	92.4
Bachelor's	1,094,538	100.0	1,164,792	100.0	1,485,242	100.0	6.4	27.5	35.7
White	914,093	83.5	905,846	77.8	1,075,561	72.4	-0.9	18.7	17.7
Total minority	150,829	13.8	221,256	19.0	363,324	24.5	46.7	64.2	140.9
Black	66,375	6.1	91,496	7.9	142,420	9.6	37.8	55.7	114.6
Hispanic	37,342	3.4	58,351	5.0	107,588	7.2	56.3	84.4	188.1
Asian/Pacific Islander	42,529	3.9	64,433	5.5	102,376	6.9	51.5	58.9	140.7
American Indian/Alaska Native	4,583	0.4	6,976	0.6	10,940	0.7	52.2	56.8	138.7
Nonresident alien	29,616	2.7	37,690	3.2	46,357	3.1	27.3	23.0	56.5
Master's	337,168	100.0	406,301	100.0	594,065	100.0	20.5	46.2	76.2
White	261,232	77.5	298,133	73.4	393,357	66.2	14.1	31.9	50.6
Total minority	38,331	11.4	60,258	14.8	128,947	21.7	57.2	114.0	236.4
Black	16,616	4.9	25,822	6.4	58,976	9.9	55.4	128.4	254.9
Hispanic	8,887	2.6	14,442	3.6	32,438	5.5	62.5	124.6	265.0
Asian/Pacific Islander	11,650	3.5	18,216	4.5	34,029	5.7	56.4	86.8	192.1
American Indian/Alaska Native	1,178	0.3	1,778	0.4	3,504	0.6	50.9	97.1	197.5
Nonresident alien	37,605	11.2	47,910	11.8	71,761	12.1	27.4	49.8	90.8
First-professional1	71,948	100.0	76,734	100.0	87,655	100.0	6.7	14.2	21.8
White	60,631	84.3	59,525	77.6	63,590	72.5	-1.8	6.8	4.9

Table 26-2. (Continued).

Characteristic	1990–91 Number	1990–91 Percent of total	1995–96 Number	1995–96 Percent of total	2005–06 Number	2005–06 Percent of total	Percent change 1990–91 to 1995–96	Percent change 1995–96 to 2005–06	Percent change 1990–91 to 2005–06
Total minority	10,231	14.2	15,587	20.3	22,024	25.1	52.4	41.3	115.3
Black	3,588	5.0	5,022	6.5	6,223	7.1	40.0	23.9	73.4
Hispanic	2,547	3.5	3,475	4.5	4,446	5.1	36.4	27.9	74.6
Asian/Pacific Islander	3,835	5.3	6,627	8.6	10,645	12.1	72.8	60.6	177.6
American Indian/Alaska Native	261	0.4	463	0.6	710	0.8	77.4	53.3	172.0
Nonresident alien	1,086	1.5	1,622	2.1	2,041	2.3	49.4	25.8	87.9
Doctoral2	39,294	100.0	44,652	100.0	56,067	100.0	13.6	25.6	42.7
White	25,855	65.8	27,773	62.2	31,601	56.4	7.4	13.8	22.2
Total minority	3,615	9.2	5,429	12.2	8,491	15.1	50.2	56.4	134.9
Black	1,248	3.2	1,632	3.7	3,122	5.6	30.8	91.3	150.2
Hispanic	757	1.9	997	2.2	1,882	3.4	31.7	88.8	148.6
Asian/Pacific Islander	1,504	3.8	2,641	5.9	3,257	5.8	75.6	23.3	116.6
American Indian/Alaska Native	106	0.3	159	0.4	230	0.4	50.0	44.7	117.0
Nonresident alien	9,824	25.0	11,450	25.6	15,975	28.5	16.6	39.5	62.6

[1] An award that requires completion of a degree program that meets all of the following criteria: (1) completion of the academic requirements to begin practice in the profession; (2) at least 2 years of college work before entering the degree program; (3) a total of at least 6 academic years of college work to complete the degree program, including previously required college work plus the work required in the professional program itself. See glossary for a definition of first-professional degree.

[2] Includes Ph.D., Ed.D., and comparable degrees at the doctoral level. Excludes first-professional degrees, such as M.D., D.D.S., and law degrees.

Note: Reported racial/ethnic distributions of students by type of degree, field of degree, and sex were used to estimate race/ethnicity for students whose race/ethnicity was not reported. Race categories exclude persons of Hispanic ethnicity. Nonresident aliens are shown separately because information about their race/ethnicity is not available. Detail may not sum to totals because of rounding.

Source: U.S. Department of Education, National Center for Education Statistics, 1990–91 through 2004–05 Integrated Postsecondary Education Data System, "Completions Survey" (IPEDS-C:90–99), and Fall 2000 through Fall 2006.

Degrees Earned by Women

Table 27-1. Number and percentage of bachelor's, master's, and doctoral degrees women earned, percent change in the number of degrees women earned, and change in the percentage of degrees women earned, by field of study: Academic years 1990–91, 1995–96, and 2005–06

	1990–91		1995–96		2005–06			
Field of study	Number	Percent of total	Number	Percent of total	Number	Percent of total	Percent change in the number of degrees earned between 1995–96 and 2005–06	Change in percentage points between 1995–96 and 2005–06
Bachelor's degrees Total1	590,493	53.9	642,338	55.1	854,642	57.5	33.1	2.4
Health professions and related clinical sciences	50,256	83.9	70,145	81.5	79,059	86.0	12.7	4.5
Education	87,390	78.9	79,170	75.1	84,790	79.1	7.1	3.9
Psychology	42,588	72.6	53,580	73.0	68,269	77.5	27.4	4.5
English language and literature/letters	34,173	66.9	32,921	65.9	37,780	68.6	14.8	2.6
Communication, journalism, and related programs	32,241	60.8	28,305	58.8	48,794	63.4	72.4	4.7
Biological and biomedical sciences	20,019	50.8	31,968	52.6	42,527	61.5	33.0	8.9
Visual and performing arts	26,425	62.6	29,170	59.2	51,180	61.4	75.5	2.3
Social sciences and history	56,406	45.1	60,607	47.9	80,686	50.0	33.1	2.0
Business	117,608	47.2	110,078	48.6	158,359	49.8	43.9	1.2
Agriculture and natural resources	4,292	32.7	7,894	36.8	10,990	47.7	39.2	10.8
Mathematics and statistics	6,813	47.3	5,866	46.1	6,655	45.1	13.5	-1.1
Physical sciences and science technologies	5,164	31.6	7,061	36.0	8,487	41.8	20.2	5.8
Computer and information sciences and support services	7,388	29.4	6,749	27.5	9,775	20.6	44.8	-7.0
Engineering and engineering technologies	11,269	14.1	12,656	16.2	14,597	17.9	15.3	1.7
Master's degrees Total1	180,686	53.6	227,220	55.9	356,169	60.0	56.8	4.0

Table 27-1. (Continued).

	1990–91		1995–96		2005–06			
Field of study	Number	Percent of total	Number	Percent of total	Number	Percent of total	Percent change in the number of degrees earned between 1995–96 and 2005–06	Change in percentage points between 1995–96 and 2005–06
Psychology	8,020	70.7	11,062	73.0	15,691	79.4	41.8	6.4
Health professions and related clinical sciences	16,931	79.3	26,903	79.3	40,750	79.3	51.5	#
Education	66,904	76.6	79,981	76.2	133,920	76.7	67.4	0.5
Communication, journalism, and related programs	2,616	60.5	3,408	61.3	5,134	66.3	50.6	5.0
English language and literature/letters	4,581	67.5	4,930	64.4	5,985	67.7	21.4	3.3
Biological and biomedical sciences	2,400	50.0	3,364	51.4	5,027	57.9	49.4	6.5
Visual and performing arts	4,827	55.8	5,919	57.6	7,729	57.1	30.6	-0.5
Social sciences and history	5,217	42.6	6,919	46.1	8,954	51.6	29.4	5.5
Agriculture and natural resources	1,135	34.4	1,909	41.9	2,360	50.9	23.6	8.9
Business	27,372	35.0	35,154	37.6	62,856	42.9	78.8	5.4
Mathematics and statistics	1,453	40.9	1,473	40.3	2,018	42.7	37.0	2.3
Physical sciences and science technologies	1,458	27.6	1,864	32.1	2,354	39.8	26.3	7.7
Computer and information sciences and support services	2,761	29.6	2,850	26.9	4,585	26.9	60.9	-0.1
Engineering and engineering technologies	3,670	14.4	5,018	17.3	7,864	23.5	56.7	6.1
Doctoral degrees Total1	14,538	37.0	17,811	39.9	27,433	48.9	54.0	9.0
Psychology	2,412	61.3	2,761	66.7	3,574	72.6	29.4	6.0
Health professions and related clinical sciences	885	57.7	996	60.3	5,169	72.5	419.0	12.2
Education	3,575	57.8	3,842	61.5	4,920	64.9	28.1	3.4
English language and literature/letters	587	55.6	860	61.6	744	59.3	-13.5	-2.3

	1990–91		1995–96		2005–06			
Field of study	Number	Percent of total	Number	Percent of total	Number	Percent of total	Percent change in the number of degrees earned between 1995–96 and 2005–06	Change in percentage points between 1995–96 and 2005–06
Communication, journalism, and related programs	122	44.9	155	44.9	257	55.4	65.8	10.5
Visual and performing arts	372	44.4	543	50.9	744	53.8	37.0	2.9
Biological and biomedical sciences	1,487	36.9	2,106	41.8	2,842	49.2	34.9	7.4
Social sciences and history	1,056	35.1	1,421	37.8	1,696	43.3	19.4	5.5
Agriculture and natural resources	232	19.6	333	26.4	484	40.5	45.3	14.1
Business	309	26.1	394	28.8	662	38.7	68.0	9.8
Physical sciences and science technologies	831	19.6	1,033	22.9	1,346	30.0	30.3	7.1
Mathematics and statistics	188	19.2	239	20.6	382	29.5	59.8	8.9
Computer and information sciences and support services	92	13.6	126	14.5	307	21.7	143.7	7.2
Engineering and engineering technologies	496	9.3	808	12.6	1,508	20.2	86.6	7.6

Rounds to zero.

[1] Includes other fields not shown separately.

Note: See *supplemental note 10* for more information on fields of study. Figures are based on data from Title IV degree-granting institutions. See *supplemental note 9* for more information. The shaded sections show fields in which women earned at least 50 percent of the degrees in 2005–06. Calculations are based on unrounded numbers. Detail may not sum to totals because of rounding.

Source: U.S. Department of Education, National Center for Education Statistics (NCES). *Digest of Education Statistics, 2007* (NCES 2008-022), tables 258, 286, 288, 290–294, 296, 299–301, 303, 305, and 307, data from U.S. Department of Education, NCES, 1990–91, 1995–96, and 2005–06 Integrated Postsecondary Education Data System, "Completions Survey" (IPEDS-C:91–96), and IPEDS, Fall 2006.

Table 28-1. Percentage of public schools experiencing at least one incident and reporting at least one incident that occurred at school to the police, by type of incident: School years 1999–2000, 2003–04, and 2005–06

	Experienced various types of incidents			Reported to police		
Type of incident	1999–2000	2003–04	2005–06	1999–2000	2003–04	2005–06
Total	86.4	88.5	85.7	62.5	65.2	60.9
Violent incidents	71.4	81.4	77.7	36.0	43.6	37.7
Physical attack or fight without a weapon	63.7	76.7	74.3	25.8	35.6	29.2
Threat of physical attack without a weapon	52.2	53.0	52.2	18.9	21.0	19.7
Serious violent incidents	19.7	18.3	17.1	14.8	13.3	12.6
Rape or attempted rape	0.7	0.8	0.3	0.6	0.8	0.3
Sexual battery other than rape	2.5	3.0	2.8	2.3	2.6	2.6
Physical attack or fight with a weapon	5.2	4.0	3.0	3.9	2.8	2.2
Threat of physical attack with a weapon	11.1	8.6	8.8	8.5	6.0	5.9
Robbery with a weapon	0.5!	0.6	0.4	0.3!	0.6	0.4
Robbery without a weapon	5.3	6.3	6.4	3.4	4.2	4.9
Theft/larceny1	45.6	46.0	46.0	28.5	30.5	27.9
Other incidents	72.7	64.0	68.2	52.0	50.0	50.6
Possession of a firearm/explosive device	5.5	6.1	7.2	4.5	4.9	5.5
Possession of a knife or sharp object2	42.6	15.9	42.8	23.0	12.1	25.0
Distribution of illegal drugs	12.3	12.9	—	11.4	12.4	—
Possession or use of alcohol or illegal drugs	26.6	29.3	—	22.2	26.0	—
Distribution, possession, or use of illegal drugs	—	—	25.9	—	—	22.8
Distribution, possession, or use of alcohol	—	—	16.2	—	—	11.6
Student sexual harassment of other students	36.3	—	—	14.7	—	—
Vandalism	51.4	51.4	50.5	32.7	34.3	31.9

— Not available.

! Interpret data with caution (estimates are unstable).

[1] Theft/larceny (taking things worth over $10 without personal confrontation) was defined for respondents as "the unlawful taking of another person's property without personal confrontation, threat, violence, or bodily harm. Included are pocket picking, stealing a purse or backpack (if left unattended or no force was used to take it from owner), theft from a building, theft from a motor vehicle or of motor vehicle parts or accessories, theft of bicycles, theft from vending machines, and all other types of thefts."

[2] The questionnaire wording for possession of a knife or sharp object differed among survey administrations. In 1999–2000 and 2005–06, the question asked about possession of a knife or sharp object. In 2003–04, the question was changed to refer to possession of a knife or sharp object with intent to harm.

Note: "At school" was defined for respondents to include activities that happen in school buildings, on school grounds, on school buses, and at places that hold school-sponsored events or activities. Respondents were instructed to respond only for those times that were during normal school hours or when school activities or events were in session. Reported crimes are computed by dividing the number of public schools that reported crimes to the police by all public schools, including those that did not report experiencing crime. For more information, please see *supplemental note 3*.

Source: U.S. Department of Education, National Center for Education Statistics, 1999–2000, 2003–04, and 2005–06 School Survey on Crime and Safety (SSOCS), 2000, 2004, and 2006.

Table 28-2. Percentage of public schools experiencing at least one incident and reporting at least one incident that occurred at school to the police, by type of incident and selected school characteristics: School year 2005–06

	Violent incidents[1]		Serious violent incidents[2]		Theft[3]		Other[4]	
School characteristic	Experienced	Reported	Experienced	Reported	Experienced	Reported	Experienced	Reported
Total	77.7	37.7	17.1	12.6	46.0	27.9	68.2	50.6
School level5								
Primary	67.3	18.7	11.0	6.2	27.8	12.5	54.8	34.1
Middle	94.4	63.1	25.2	19.7	68.7	43.3	87.8	72.6
High school	95.2	77.3	31.8	29.5	85.6	67.6	93.6	86.9
Combined	83.5	46.2	17.4	13.2	54.9	33.9	75.0	55.3
Enrollment size								
Less than 300	63.7	26.6	11.4	8.4	29.6	14.1	53.2	36.4
300–499	77.3	24.8	11.7	6.1	37.2	18.5	63.4	39.6
500–999	82.1	43.1	19.2	14.1	52.1	32.1	74.2	57.2
1,000 or more	96.5	78.4	37.2	34.1	85.8	69.4	95.1	89.7
Locale6								
City	82.5	39.9	23.2	17.4	47.2	30.3	73.1	54.6
Suburban	78.2	35.3	15.4	11.5	47.0	29.7	71.0	52.5
Town	81.7	41.8	16.6	12.1	51.0	32.3	70.1	56.4
Rural	71.9	35.9	14.4	10.0	42.1	22.1	61.5	44.1
Percent minority enrollment7								
Less than 5 percent	71.6	32.8	13.1	7.3	42.8	21.9	62.4	41.4
5 to 20 percent	73.5	34.7	15.7	11.5	43.4	26.8	63.4	45.2
20 to 50 percent	79.7	39.3	16.6	12.1	47.9	30.0	71.5	52.0
50 percent or more	82.9	42.7	21.6	17.4	48.4	30.9	71.9	59.0
Percent of students eligible for free								
or reduced-price lunch								
0–20 percent	68.0	30.8	12.5	9.4	45.9	28.5	61.7	44.0
21–50 percent	79.7	40.0	19.2	13.0	52.5	31.6	72.3	50.8
More than 50 percent	81.4	39.5	18.0	14.0	41.0	24.7	68.5	54.0

[1] Violent incidents include serious violent incidents (rape or attempted rape, sexual battery other than rape, physical attack or fight with a weapon, threat of physical attack with a weapon, and robbery with or without a weapon), physical attack or fight without a weapon, and threat of physical attack without a weapon.

[2] Serious violent incidents include rape or attempted rape, sexual battery other than rape, physical attack or fight with a weapon, threat of physical attack with a weapon, and robbery with or without a weapon.

[3] Theft/larceny (taking things worth over $10 without personal confrontation) was defined for respondents as “the unlawful taking of another person’s property without personal confrontation, threat, violence, or bodily harm. Included are pocket picking, stealing a purse or backpack (if left unattended or no force was used to take it from owner), theft from a building, theft from a motor vehicle or of motor vehicle parts or accessories, theft of bicycles, theft from vending machines, and all other types of thefts.”

[4] Other incidents include possession of a firearm or explosive device, possession of a knife or sharp object, distribution, possession, or use of illegal drugs or alcohol, and vandalism.

[5] Primary schools are defined as schools in which the lowest grade is not higher than grade 3 and the highest grade is not higher than grade 8. Middle schools are defined as schools in which the lowest grade is not lower than grade 4 and the highest grade is not higher than grade 9. High schools are defined as schools in which the lowest grade is not lower than grade 9. Combined schools include all other combinations of grades, including K–12 schools.

[6] Estimates are based on the 2006 urban-centric locale codes and may differ from previously published figures. Excludes 52 schools without information on locale. See *supplemental note 1* for more information.

[7] These estimates exclude data from the 73 schools that did not report estimates of student race/ethnicity.

Note: “At school” was defined for respondents to include activities that happen in school buildings, on school grounds, on school buses, and at places that hold school-sponsored events or activities. Respondents were instructed to respond only for those times that were during normal school hours or when school activities or events were in session. Reported crimes are computed by dividing the number of public schools that reported crimes to the police by all public schools, including those that did not report experiencing crime. For more information, please see *supplemental note 3*.

Source: U.S. Department of Education, National Center for Education Statistics, 2005–06 School Survey on Crime and Safety (SSOCS), 2006.

Poverty Concentration in Public Schools by Locale and Race/Ethnicity

Table 29-1. Number and percentage distribution of public elementary and secondary students, by percentage of students in school eligible for free or reduced-price lunch, locale, and race/ethnicity: School year 2005–06

Locale and race/ethnicity	Number eligible for free or reduced-price lunch	10 percent or less	11–25 percent	26–50 percent	51–75 percent	More than 75 percent
Total1	47,190,246	14.3	19.5	29.8	21.3	15.1
White	27,196,646	19.1	26.1	34.5	16.3	4.0
Black	7,887,387	4.2	8.7	24.2	30.5	32.4
Hispanic	9,140,172	7.0	8.9	21.6	28.5	34.1
Asian/Pacific Islander	2,086,658	24.3	21.8	26.5	17.2	10.2
American Indian/Alaska Native	560,053	5.4	11.8	27.8	30.6	24.3
City1	13,420,920	8.8	11.9	23.8	25.0	30.5
White	4,695,316	13.1	22.4	34.7	20.6	9.2
Black	3,650,628	2.7	4.7	18.4	29.9	44.2
Hispanic	4,038,790	6.7	5.1	15.9	26.4	45.9
Asian/Pacific Islander	830,330	20.5	16.5	24.4	21.4	17.1
American Indian/Alaska Native	111,639	5.4	13.3	27.8	26.4	27.1
Suburban1	17,081,489	23.9	25.3	26.3	15.3	9.2
White	10,120,962	32.7	31.8	25.3	8.3	1.9
Black	2,470,871	7.2	14.8	31.8	27.3	18.8
Hispanic	3,287,008	7.8	13.2	25.5	28.1	25.4
Asian/Pacific Islander	957,859	30.1	25.3	25.1	13.8	5.8
American Indian/Alaska Native	95,073	12.5	25.6	35.2	18.5	8.2
Town1	6,149,758	5.2	16.8	40.1	27.5	10.3
White	4,335,316	5.9	21.3	45.7	23.3	3.7
Black	690,920	1.2	4.2	23.0	40.7	30.8
Hispanic	866,261	4.8	5.7	25.8	37.3	26.3

Locale and race/ethnicity	Number eligible for free or reduced-price lunch	10 percent or less	11–25 percent	26–50 percent	51–75 percent	More than 75 percent
Asian/Pacific Islander	106,049	5.5	16.6	48.3	22.0	7.7
American Indian/Alaska Native	118,647	2.7	9.5	32.7	37.3	17.8
Rural1	10,538,079	11.3	21.2	36.9	22.7	8.0
White	8,045,052	12.7	23.6	39.8	20.2	3.6
Black	1,074,968	3.8	11.2	27.2	33.1	24.8
Hispanic	948,113	7.3	13.1	28.4	30.5	20.7
Asian/Pacific Islander	192,420	22.5	29.9	30.6	13.5	3.5
American Indian/Alaska Native	234,694	3.8	6.7	22.4	34.2	32.9

[1] Includes other racial/ethnic groups not separately shown.

Note: The National School Lunch Program is a federally assisted meal program. To be eligible, a student must be from a household with an income at or below 130 percent of the poverty threshold for free lunch or between 130 percent and 185 percent of the poverty threshold for reduced-price lunch. Approximately 10,745 public schools (or 11 percent) did not report information on the number of students eligible for free or reduced-price school lunch. For details on Census-defined areas and poverty thresholds, see *supplemental note 1*. Race categories exclude persons of Hispanic ethnicity. Detail may not sum to totals because of rounding.

Source: U.S. Department of Education, National Center for Education Statistics, Common Core of Data (CCD), "Public Elementary/Secondary School Universe Survey," 2005–06.

Concentration of Public School Enrollment by Locale and Race/Ethnicity

Table 30-1. Percentage distribution of public elementary and secondary school students of each racial/ethnic group, by percent minority enrollment in school, locale, and race/ethnicity: School year 2005–06

			Percent minority enrollment		
		Less than 25	25–49 50–74		75 percent or
Locale and race/ethnicity	Total	percent	percent percent		more
Total	100.0	42.1	20.8	14.1	22.9
White	100.0	65.2	22.6	9.1	3.2
Black	100.0	9.1	19.1	21.7	50.1
Hispanic	100.0	8.3	15.2	20.1	56.4
Asian/Pacific Islander	100.0	20.9	25.9	22.0	31.3
American Indian/Alaska Native	100.0	24.7	27.1	19.0	29.2
City	100.0	14.6	20.3	19.9	45.3
White	100.0	34.9	35.4	20.6	9.1
Black	100.0	3.0	11.9	19.2	66.0
Hispanic	100.0	2.6	9.4	17.8	70.3
Asian/Pacific Islander	100.0	8.5	21.7	26.2	43.7
American Indian/Alaska Native	100.0	17.1	26.8	29.1	27.1
Suburban	100.0	43.6	23.1	13.7	19.6
White	100.0	64.2	24.4	8.6	2.9
Black	100.0	11.9	21.5	22.4	44.2
Hispanic	100.0	9.5	17.5	21.2	51.9
Asian/Pacific Islander	100.0	26.5	30.0	19.9	23.7
American Indian/Alaska Native	100.0	37.6	34.7	14.2	13.4
Town	100.0	57.5	20.0	12.5	10.0
White	100.0	73.9	17.9	6.8	1.4
Black	100.0	15.5	28.2	29.5	26.8
Hispanic	100.0	15.8	22.2	26.0	35.9
Asian/Pacific Islander	100.0	36.6	19.6	15.7	28.1
American Indian/Alaska Native	100.0	29.1	31.7	19.7	19.6
Rural	100.0	66.0	18.3	8.3	7.4
White	100.0	79.5	15.2	4.2	1.0
Black	100.0	19.3	32.0	23.9	24.8

			Percent minority enrollment		
		Less than 25	25–49 50–74		75 percent or
Locale and race/ethnicity	Total	percent	percent percent		more
Hispanic	100.0	22.1	25.5	21.2	31.2
Asian/Pacific Islander	100.0	37.6	26.9	17.7	17.9
American Indian/Alaska Native	100.0	21.1	22.1	15.8	41.0

Note: Minority enrollment includes Black, Hispanic, Asian/Pacific Islander, and American Indian/Alaska Native students. Race categories exclude persons of Hispanic ethnicity. For details on Census-defined areas, see *supplemental note 1*. Detail may not sum to totals because of rounding.

Source: U.S. Department of Education, National Center for Education Statistics, Common Core of Data (CCD), "Public Elementary/Secondary School Universe Survey," 2005–06.

Table 30-2. Percentage distribution of public elementary and secondary school students of each racial/ethnic group, by percent Black enrollment in school, locale, and race/ethnicity: School year 2005–06

			Percent Black enrollment		
		Less than 25	25–49 50–74		75 percent or
Locale and race/ethnicity	Total	percent	percent percent		more
Total	100.0	78.2	11.4 4.7		5.7
White	100.0	89.5	8.1	2.0	0.4
Black	100.0	27.5	24.0	17.3	31.2
Hispanic	100.0	85.5	10.6	2.9	0.9
Asian/Pacific Islander	100.0	86.4	10.3	2.5	0.8
American Indian/Alaska Native	100.0	91.7	5.9	1.7	0.7
City	100.0	63.6	16.0	7.9	12.5
White	100.0	78.3	15.9	4.7	1.2
Black	100.0	18.8	20.9	17.9	42.4
Hispanic	100.0	82.9	12.2	3.7	1.3
Asian/Pacific Islander	100.0	81.4	13.6	3.7	1.2
American Indian/Alaska Native	100.0	81.9	11.9	4.1	2.1
Suburban	100.0	82.2	10.4	3.8	3.6
White	100.0	91.7	6.8	1.3	0.2
Black	100.0	36.4	25.0	15.9	22.6
Hispanic	100.0	85.0	11.3	2.9	0.8
Asian/Pacific Islander	100.0	88.8	8.7	1.9	0.6
American Indian/Alaska Native	100.0	88.7	8.0	2.1	1.2
Town	100.0	84.8	8.6	3.9	2.7
White	100.0	91.3	6.5	1.9	0.3
Black	100.0	30.2	27.4	20.6	21.7
Hispanic	100.0	93.8	4.9	1.1	0.3
Asian/Pacific Islander	100.0	92.8	5.2	1.5	0.5
American Indian/Alaska Native	100.0	94.0	4.8	1.1	0.2
Rural	100.0	86.4	8.7	2.7	2.2
White	100.0	92.4	6.2	1.2	0.2
Black	100.0	34.7	30.1	16.1	19.1
Hispanic	100.0	91.0	7.2	1.3	0.4

			Percent Black enrollment		
		Less than 25	25–49 50–74		75 percent or
Locale and race/ethnicity	Total	percent	percent percent		more
Asian/Pacific Islander	100.0	91.8	6.7	1.2	0.3
American Indian/Alaska Native	100.0	96.2	2.8	0.8	0.2

Note: Race categories exclude persons of Hispanic ethnicity. For details on Census-defined areas, see *supplemental note 1*. Detail may not sum to totals because of rounding.

Source: U.S. Department of Education, National Center for Education Statistics, Common Core of Data (CCD), "Public Elementary/Secondary School Universe Survey," 2005–06.

Table 30-3. Percentage distribution of public elementary and secondary school students of each racial/ethnic group, by percent Hispanic enrollment in school, locale, and race/ethnicity: School year 2005–06

			Percent Hispanic enrollment		
		Less than 25	25–49 50–74		75 percent or
Locale and race/ethnicity	Total	percent	percent percent		more
Total	100.0	74.3	11.5 7.0		7.2
White	100.0	89.6	7.5	2.3	0.6
Black	100.0	81.2	11.8	5.4	1.6
Hispanic	100.0	23.1	21.5	22.3	33.1
Asian/Pacific Islander	100.0	71.1	18.0	8.0	3.0
American Indian/Alaska Native	100.0	83.4	9.7	4.8	2.1
City	100.0	58.6	15.3	12.1	13.9
White	100.0	78.8	14.1	5.4	1.7
Black	100.0	79.2	11.9	6.7	2.2
Hispanic	100.0	15.1	18.7	25.1	41.1
Asian/Pacific Islander	100.0	63.4	20.8	11.4	4.4
American Indian/Alaska Native	100.0	61.0	19.7	12.9	6.4
Suburban	100.0	74.3	13.1	6.5	6.0
White	100.0	89.4	8.1	2.0	0.5
Black	100.0	76.3	16.1	6.1	1.5
Hispanic	100.0	26.5	24.6	21.0	27.9
Asian/Pacific Islander	100.0	73.4	18.4	6.2	2.0
American Indian/Alaska Native	100.0	76.2	14.1	6.8	2.8
Town	100.0	82.0	8.7	4.7	4.6
White	100.0	91.1	6.3	2.1	0.5
Black	100.0	90.8	6.7	1.9	0.5
Hispanic	100.0	28.3	22.1	20.6	29.0
Asian/Pacific Islander	100.0	85.1	7.1	4.3	3.4
American Indian/Alaska Native	100.0	87.7	8.7	2.6	1.0
Rural	100.0	89.9	5.6	2.4	2.1
White	100.0	95.3	3.7	0.9	0.2
Black	100.0	92.8	5.2	1.8	0.3

			Percent Hispanic enrollment		
		Less than 25	25–49 50–74		75 percent or
Locale and race/ethnicity	Total	percent	percent percent		more
Hispanic	100.0	40.5	22.1	16.4	21.0
Asian/Pacific Islander	100.0	85.6	9.9	3.6	0.9
American Indian/Alaska Native	100.0	94.5	3.8	1.4	0.4

Note: Race categories exclude persons of Hispanic ethnicity. For details on Census-defined areas, see *supplemental note 1*. Detail may not sum to totals because of rounding.

Source: U.S. Department of Education, National Center for Education Statistics, Common Core of Data (CCD), “Public Elementary/Secondary School Universe Survey,” 2005–06.

Table 30-4. Percentage distribution of public elementary and secondary school students of each racial/ethnic group, by percent White enrollment in school, locale, and race/ethnicity: School year 2005–06

Locale and race/ethnicity	Total	Percent White enrollment			
		Less than 25 percent	25–49 percent	50–74 percent	75 percent or more
Total	100.0	23.4	14.3	21.0	41.3
White	100.0	3.3	9.4	23.1	64.1
Black	100.0	50.9	21.6	18.8	8.7
Hispanic	100.0	57.2	20.0	14.8	8.0
Asian/Pacific Islander	100.0	32.5	22.1	25.6	19.8
American Indian/Alaska Native	100.0	29.4	19.0	27.4	24.2
City	100.0	46.1	19.9	20.1	13.9
White	100.0	9.6	21.1	35.7	33.6
Black	100.0	66.8	19.0	11.5	2.8
Hispanic	100.0	71.0	17.4	9.1	2.4
Asian/Pacific Islander	100.0	45.2	25.8	21.1	7.9
American Indian/Alaska Native	100.0	27.5	29.1	27.0	16.4
Suburban	100.0	20.2	14.1	23.3	42.5
White	100.0	3.1	9.1	25.0	62.8
Black	100.0	45.3	22.3	21.0	11.5
Hispanic	100.0	53.0	21.2	16.8	9.0
Asian/Pacific Islander	100.0	24.8	20.3	29.9	25.1
American Indian/Alaska Native	100.0	13.9	14.6	34.8	36.7
Town	100.0	10.2	12.5	20.6	56.6
White	100.0	1.5	6.9	18.6	73.0
Black	100.0	27.1	29.7	28.4	14.9
Hispanic	100.0	36.7	25.6	22.5	15.2
Asian/Pacific Islander	100.0	28.4	16.0	19.7	35.8
American Indian/Alaska Native	100.0	19.7	19.5	32.3	28.6
Rural	100.0	7.5	8.5	18.6	65.4

			Percent White enrollment		
		Less than 25	25–49 50–74		75 percent or
Locale and race/ethnicity	Total	percent	percent percent		more
White	100.0	1.0	4.4	15.6	79.0
Black	100.0	25.1	24.0	32.1	18.8
Hispanic	100.0	31.6	21.4	25.4	21.6
Asian/Pacific Islander	100.0	18.4	18.4	26.7	36.6
American Indian/Alaska Native	100.0	41.0	15.8	22.3	20.9

Note: Race categories exclude persons of Hispanic ethnicity. For details on Census-defined areas, see *supplemental note 1*. Detail may not sum to totals because of rounding.

Source: U.S. Department of Education, National Center for Education Statistics, Common Core of Data (CCD), "Public Elementary/Secondary School Universe Survey," 2005–06.

Teacher Turnover

Table 31-1. Number of 1987–88, 1990–91, 1993–94, 1999–2000, and 2003–04 public and private K–12 teachers who did not teach in the same school the following school year, by turnover category and reason for leaving

			Percent White enrollment		
		Less than 25	25–49 50–74		75 percent or
Locale and race/ethnicity	Total	percent	percent percent		more
Total	100.0	23.4	14.3 21.0		41.3
White	100.0	3.3	9.4	23.1	64.1
Black	100.0	50.9	21.6	18.8	8.7
Hispanic	100.0	57.2	20.0	14.8	8.0
Asian/Pacific Islander	100.0	32.5	22.1	25.6	19.8
American Indian/Alaska Native	100.0	29.4	19.0	27.4	24.2
City	100.0	46.1	19.9	20.1	13.9
White	100.0	9.6	21.1	35.7	33.6
Black	100.0	66.8	19.0	11.5	2.8
Hispanic	100.0	71.0	17.4	9.1	2.4
Asian/Pacific Islander	100.0	45.2	25.8	21.1	7.9
American Indian/Alaska Native	100.0	27.5	29.1	27.0	16.4
Suburban	100.0	20.2	14.1	23.3	42.5
White	100.0	3.1	9.1	25.0	62.8
Black	100.0	45.3	22.3	21.0	11.5
Hispanic	100.0	53.0	21.2	16.8	9.0
Asian/Pacific Islander	100.0	24.8	20.3	29.9	25.1
American Indian/Alaska Native	100.0	13.9	14.6	34.8	36.7
Town	100.0	10.2	12.5	20.6	56.6
White	100.0	1.5	6.9	18.6	73.0
Black	100.0	27.1	29.7	28.4	14.9
Hispanic	100.0	36.7	25.6	22.5	15.2
Asian/Pacific Islander	100.0	28.4	16.0	19.7	35.8
American Indian/Alaska Native	100.0	19.7	19.5	32.3	28.6
Rural	100.0	7.5	8.5	18.6	65.4
White	100.0	1.0	4.4	15.6	79.0
Black	100.0	25.1	24.0	32.1	18.8

			Percent White enrollment		
		Less than 25	25–49 50–74		75 percent or
Locale and race/ethnicity	Total	percent	percent percent		more
Hispanic	100.0	31.6	21.4	25.4	21.6
Asian/Pacific Islander	100.0	18.4	18.4	26.7	36.6
American Indian/Alaska Native	100.0	41.0	15.8	22.3	20.9

[1] Leavers in this category left teaching for a variety of personal reasons, ranging from "starting their own business" to becoming "a member of a contemplative religious community." However, the most common reason reported by leavers who left for "other" reasons was to take a year-long sabbatical or leave of absence from teaching.

Note: Schools and Staffing Survey (SASS) teachers who died or left the country are excluded. Retired category includes all teachers who reported retiring between the SASS and Teacher Follow-up Survey (TFS) school year including those 45 years old or younger who were excluded in earlier estimates. Detail may not sum to totals because of rounding.

Source: U.S. Department of Education, National Center for Education Statistics, Teacher Follow-up Survey (TFS), "Current Teacher Data File" and "Former Teacher Data File," 1988–89, 1991–92, 1994–95, 2000–01, and 2004–05.

Table 31-2. Percentage distribution of 1987–88, 1990–91, 1993–94, 1999–2000, and 2003–04 public and private K–12 teachers who did not teach in the same school the following school year, by turnover category and reason for leaving

Turnover category and reason for leaving	1987–88	1990–91	1993–94	1999–2000	2003–04
Total turnover at the end of the year	14.5	13.2	14.2	15.9	16.9
Transfers at the end of the year	8.1	7.2	7.0	7.8	7.8
Leavers	6.4	6.0	7.3	8.1	9.0
Took other job	2.4	1.9	3.1	3.7	3.8
Pursued further education	0.4	0.5	0.3	0.3	0.3
Left for family reasons	1.8	1.1	1.2	1.4	1.2
Retired	1.3	1.6	1.7	1.9	2.4
Other1	0.5	0.9	1.0	0.8	1.3

[1] Leavers in this category left teaching for a variety of personal reasons, ranging from "starting their own business" to becoming "a member of a contemplative religious community." However, the most common reason reported by leavers who left for "other" reasons was to take a year-long sabbatical or leave of absence from teaching.

Note: Denominator used to calculate the percentage is the weighted number of Schools and Staffing Survey (SASS) teachers surveyed during the Teacher Follow-up Survey (TFS) year; SASS teachers who died or left the country are excluded. Retired category includes all teachers who reported retiring between the SASS and TFS year, including those 45 years old and younger who were excluded in earlier estimates. Detail may not sum to totals because of rounding.

Source: U.S. Department of Education, National Center for Education Statistics, Teacher Follow-up Survey (TFS), "Current Teacher Data File" and "Former Teacher Data File," 1988–89, 1991–92, 1994–95, 2000–01, and 2004–05.

Table 31-3. Percentage of 1987–88, 1990–91, 1993–94, 1999–2000, and 2003–04 public K–12 teachers who did not teach in the same school the following school year, by poverty level of school and the reason teachers left

	1987–88		1990–91[1]		1993–94		1999–2000		2003–04	
Reason teachers left	High-poverty	Low-poverty	High-poverty	Low-poverty	High-poverty	Low-poverty	High-poverty	Low-poverty	High-poverty	Low-poverty
Total turnover	14.9	11.9	15.9	10.1	17.3	12.6	18.4	14.0	21.1	14.2
Transferred to another school	8.7	6.2	10.4	5.7	9.7	5.9	10.0	5.7	10.6	6.4
Took other job	3.2	2.1	1.9	1.0	3.3	2.0	3.1	4.2	3.5	3.9
Pursued further education	0.3	0.4	0.8!	0.3	0.2	0.1	0.5	0.3	0.5	0.3!
Left for family reasons	0.4	1.7	0.1	1.1	0.6	1.4	0.4	1.2	2.6!	0.7!
Retired	1.6	1.0	1.7	1.4	2.1	2.4	3.1	2.0	2.4	2.6
Other	0.7	0.5	0.9	0.7	1.4	0.7	1.4	0.6!	1.5	0.4

! Interpret data with caution (estimates are unstable).

[1] High- and low-poverty schools can only be identified in 1990–91 based on the percentage of students who receive free or reduced-price lunches and not on the percentage *eligible* to receive free or reduced-price lunches.

Note: Schools were considered high poverty if 75 percent or more of their students were eligible for free or reduced-price lunch, and low poverty if less than 15 percent of their students were eligible. Public schools for which data are missing or that do not participate in the program were excluded. Estimates for 1999–2000 have been revised. Denominator used to calculate the percentage is the weighted number of Schools and Staffing Survey (SASS) teachers surveyed during the Teacher Follow-up Survey (TFS) year; SASS teachers who died or left the country are excluded. Retired category includes all teachers who reported retiring between the SASS and TFS year, including those 45 years old and younger who were excluded in earlier estimates. Detail may not sum to totals because of rounding.

Source: U.S. Department of Education, National Center for Education Statistics, Schools and Staffing Survey (SASS), "Public School Data File," 1987–88, 1990–91, 1993–94, 1999–2000, and 2003–04, "Charter School Data File," 1999–2000, and Teacher Follow-up Survey (TFS), "Current Teacher Data File" and "Former Teacher Data File," 1988–89, 1991–92, 1994–95, 2000–01, and 2004–05.

Public School Staff

Table 32-1. Number and percentage distribution of staff employed in public schools, by staff type and school characteristics: School year 2003–04

		Professional instructional staff					
School characteristic	Total staff	Total	Principals[1]	Teachers	Instructional coordinators and supervisors	Librarians/library media specialists	School counselors
Total	5,514,300	64.3	2.7	57.3	0.9	1.3	2.0
Instructional level							
Elementary	2,803,300	61.8	2.5	55.5	1.0	1.5	1.4
Middle	948,800	67.0	3.0	59.5	0.9	1.3	2.3
Secondary	1,448,900	68.2	3.0	60.2	0.9	1.1	2.9
Combined	313,300	60.5	3.1	53.4	0.7	1.3	2.0
School type							
Regular	4,979,900	64.6	2.7	57.7	0.9	1.4	2.0
Special emphasis5	317,100	65.1	2.8	57.6	1.6	1.2	1.9
Special education	60,300	45.6	2.3	40.5	1.1	0.6	1.2
Vocational/technical	47,700	66.8	3.7	58.4	1.0	0.6	3.1
Alternative	109,400	58.1	5.5	47.5	1.0	0.9	3.3
Enrollment size							
Less than 300	754,000	58.3	3.5	50.0	0.7	1.9	2.1
300–499	1,300,400	62.3	2.6	55.4	1.0	1.6	1.7
500–999	2,181,200	65.0	2.6	58.5	0.9	1.2	1.8
1,000–1,499	656,600	68.4	2.7	61.3	0.9	1.0	2.4
1,500 or more	622,100	68.8	2.5	61.7	0.9	0.8	2.8
Percentage of students approved for free or reduced-price lunch 10 percent or less	740,500	67.1	2.4	60.2	1.1	1.3	2.1

		Professional instructional staff					
School characteristic	Total staff	Total	Principals[1]	Teachers	Instructional coordinators and supervisors	Librarians/library media specialists	School counselors
11–25 percent	1,064,100	65.7	2.6	58.8	0.7	1.4	2.1
26–50 percent	1,548,200	64.1	2.7	57.2	0.6	1.4	2.1
51–75 percent	1,085,400	63.4	2.8	56.5	0.9	1.4	1.8
More than 75 percent	959,900	61.9	2.8	54.7	1.4	1.2	1.7
Region							
Northeast	1,112,800	64.8	2.3	57.9	1.4	1.2	2.0
Midwest	1,303,200	63.5	2.7	56.7	0.8	1.5	1.9
South	2,055,100	65.1	2.9	58.0	0.8	1.4	2.1
West	1,043,200	63.3	2.9	56.2	0.9	1.3	1.9
Locale							
City	1,585,000	64.9	2.8	57.6	1.3	1.2	1.9
Suburban	1,907,900	65.3	2.5	58.5	1.0	1.3	2.0
Town	782,800	63.4	2.7	56.8	0.6	1.4	2.0
Rural	1,238,600	62.6	2.9	55.5	0.5	1.6	2.1

		Student services professional staff					Aides			
School characteristic	Total staff	Total	Nurses	Social workers and psychologists	Speech therapists	Other professional staff	Total	Special needs aides[2]	Other aides[3]	Other staff[4]
Total	5,514,300	5.1	1.2	1.4	1.3	1.1	12.7	6.0	6.7	18.0
Instructional level										
Elementary	2,803,300	6.0	1.3	1.6	1.8	1.3	15.9	6.6	9.3	16.2
Middle	948,800	4.4	1.1	1.4	1.0	0.8	10.3	6.3	4.0	18.3
Secondary	1,448,900	3.5	0.9	1.2	0.6	0.8	7.8	4.6	3.3	20.5
Combined	313,300	5.9	1.3	1.6	1.4	1.6	13.2	6.6	6.6	20.5
School type										
Regular	4,979,900	4.8	1.2	1.4	1.3	1.0	12.6	6.0	6.7	18.0
Special emphasis[5]	317,100	5.4	1.0	1.5	1.2	1.6	12.2	5.5	6.7	17.3
Special education	60,300	13.7	2.3	4.1	3.0	4.3	23.8	18.6	5.2!	16.9
Vocational/technical	47,700	5.6	1.2	1.2	0.6	2.7	7.0	2.7	4.4	20.5

Alternative	109,400	10.1	1.9	3.8	1.2	3.3	12.7	4.5	8.2	19.2
Enrollment size										
Less than 300	754,000	7.8	1.8	2.2	1.9	1.8	15.1	6.9	8.2	18.9
300–499	1,300,400	5.9	1.4	1.7	1.7	1.2	14.4	6.0	8.4	17.4
500–999	2,181,200	4.8	1.1	1.3	1.3	1.0	13.2	6.4	6.7	17.0
1,000–1,499	656,600	3.5	0.8	1.1	0.8	0.9	9.0	4.8	4.2	19.0
1,500 or more	622,100	2.7	0.6	0.9	0.5	0.7	8.3	4.9	3.4	20.1
Percentage of students approved										
for free or reduced-price lunch										
10 percent or less	740,500	4.9	1.1	1.5	1.2	1.0	11.3	6.0	5.3	16.7
11–25 percent	1,064,100	4.7	1.1	1.4	1.2	1.0	11.5	5.6	5.9	18.1
26–50 percent	1,548,200	4.8	1.2	1.3	1.3	0.9	12.9	6.4	6.5	18.2
51–75 percent	1,085,400	5.1	1.2	1.4	1.4	1.1	13.3	5.8	7.6	18.2
More than 75 percent	959,900	5.7	1.2	1.6	1.4	1.4	14.2	6.2	7.9	18.3
Region										
Northeast	1,112,800	5.6	1.4	1.8	1.3	1.1	12.8	5.8	7.0	16.8
		Student services professional staff					Aides			
School characteristic	Total staff	Total	Nurses	Social workers and psychologists	Speech therapists	Other professional staff	Total	Special needs aides[2]	Other aides[3]	Other staff[4]
Midwest	1,303,200	5.6	1.2	1.9	1.5	1.1	12.7	6.3	6.4	18.1
South	2,055,100	4.5	1.1	1.0	1.2	1.1	11.7	4.8	6.9	18.7
West	1,043,200	5.0	1.1	1.5	1.3	1.0	14.4	8.2	6.1	17.4
Locale										
City	1,585,000	5.2	1.1	1.6	1.2	1.2	12.3	6.1	6.1	17.7
Suburban	1,907,900	5.0	1.1	1.5	1.3	1.1	12.4	6.3	6.1	17.2
Town	782,800	5.1	1.2	1.4	1.3	1.1	13.4	5.8	7.6	18.0
Rural	1,238,600	4.9	1.3	1.2	1.4	0.9	13.1	5.5	7.6	19.4

! Interpret with caution (estimates are unstable).

[1] Includes principals, vice principals, and assistant principals.

[2] Includes English as a second language (ESL)/bilingual aides, and special education instructional and noninstructional aides.

[3] Includes all other aides: regular Title I aides, library media center instructional and noninstructional aides, and other classroom instructional and noninstructional aides.

[4] Includes secretaries and other support staff; food service personnel; custodial, maintenance, and security personnel; and other employees not reported above.

[5] Includes schools with a special program emphasis, such as science/math schools, performing arts schools, talented/gifted schools, foreign language immersion schools, etc.

Note: Estimates are for both full- and part-time staff. Full-time-equivalent calculations were completed for part-time staff within each staff category. Elementary schools are defined as schools with at least one grade lower than 5 and no grade higher than 8. Middle schools are defined as schools with no grade lower than 5 and no grade higher than 8. Secondary schools are defined as schools with no grade lower than 7 and at least one grade higher than 8. Combined schools have at least one grade lower than 7 and at least one grade higher than 8; schools with only ungraded classes are also included in combined schools. Detail may not sum to totals because of rounding. See *supplemental note 3* for more information on the Schools and Staffing Survey (SASS).

Source: U.S. Department of Education, National Center for Education Statistics, Schools and Staffing Survey (SASS), "Public School Data File," 2003–04.

Table 32-2. Average number of students per staff member employed in public schools with such staff, by staff type and school characteristics: School year 2003–04

		Professional instructional staff					
School characteristic	Total staff	Total	Principals[1]	Teachers	Instructional coordinators and supervisors	Librarians/ library media specialists	School counselors
Total	8.6	13.3	312.4	15.0	387.4	574.7	373.0
Instructional level							
Elementary	8.1	13.1	327.3	14.6	342.6	475.4	448.6
Middle	9.1	13.5	301.4	15.2	429.1	662.5	373.4
Secondary	9.7	14.2	319.2	16.0	466.1	801.0	315.9
Combined	6.6	10.9	208.5	12.3	327.5	414.3	294.5
School type Regular	8.6	13.4	323.3	15.0	403.0	573.1	380.3
Special emphasis[5]	9.0	13.8	315.7	15.6	338.5	686.7	428.7
Special education	2.8	6.1	110.9	6.9	104.5!	229.2!	143.5!
Vocational/technical	11.3	16.9	306.9	19.4	402.7	767.5	332.0
Alternative	6.7	11.5	117.1	14.1	171.6	312.4	141.6
Enrollment size							
Less than 300	5.6	9.6	153.6	11.2	176.7	217.6	195.4
300–499	7.6	12.1	288.0	13.7	273.8	401.8	368.2
500–999	8.9	13.8	344.3	15.3	411.8	658.7	434.2
1,000–1,499	10.1	14.8	373.1	16.5	496.2	937.4	389.6
1,500 or more	11.4	16.6	449.6	18.5	641.2	1,366.0	392.9
Percentage of students approved for free or reduced-price lunch 10 percent or less	9.3	13.9	384.0	15.5	364.7	683.5	363.7
11–25 percent	9.1	13.9	347.9	15.5	437.7	628.3	383.0
26–50 percent	8.5	13.2	308.3	14.8	441.5	545.7	366.4
51–75 percent	8.2	12.9	285.7	14.5	394.0	519.0	376.1
More than 75 percent	7.9	12.8	278.7	14.5	337.1	548.4	393.0
Region Northeast	7.4	11.4	316.4	12.7	289.5	563.4	320.6
Midwest	8.3	13.0	307.0	14.6	389.3	508.9	352.8
South	8.4	12.9	289.9	14.5	447.4	583.4	386.2
West	10.6	16.7	358.5	18.8	439.7	659.7	430.4
Locale							
		Professional instructional staff					

School characteristic	Total staff	Total	Principals[1]	Teachers	Instructional coordinators and supervisors	Librarians/ library media specialists	School counselors
City	9.0	13.8	313.4	15.5	381.8	656.6	391.1
Suburban	9.0	13.9	356.9	15.5	373.7	662.2	385.7
Town	8.1	12.7	296.6	14.2	411.5	509.3	358.4
Rural	7.7	12.3	261.2	13.9	431.4	429.6	341.1

		Student services professional staff					Aides			
School characteristic	Total staff	Total	Nurses	Social workers and psychol ogists	Speech therapists	Other profession al staff	Total	Special needs aides[2]	Other aides	Other staff[4]
Total	8.6	165.6	617.2	464.4	574.4	318.7	66.2	123.5	117.4	47.6
Instructional level										
Elementary	8.1	133.3	520.8	403.6	439.4	264.2	50.0	107.0	82.3	49.7
Middle	9.1	203.1	714.1	517.6	781.9	433.6	86.4	126.5	199.9	49.4
Secondary	9.7	264.6	886.9	658.7	1,173.1	495.1	119.1	182.8	259.0	46.7
Combined	6.6	101.8	371.3	214.6	354.4	135.4	47.5	72.6	85.6	31.6
School type Regular	8.6	176.0	638.4	499.9	587.8	355.1	67.3	127.4	119.3	47.9
Special emphasis[5]	9.0	165.5	739.0	491.1	674.4	301.5	72.6	137.3	125.9	51.9
Special education	2.8	17.0	88.5	51.4	75.1	39.8	11.1	10.2	27.2!	16.3
Vocational/technical	11.3	158.9	563.2	375.5	804.7	209.4	114.1	187.9	137.4	55.1
Alternative	6.7	51.3	191.0	109.9	242.6	91.9	43.1	78.4	54.8	32.8
Enrollment size										
Less than 300	5.6	66.8	224.4	156.0	229.5	107.9	34.2	58.4	57.7	29.4
300–499	7.6	124.1	444.3	339.7	412.5	231.3	51.5	106.1	81.2	43.4
500–999	8.9	186.1	718.8	530.2	619.0	375.4	66.7	125.0	121.8	52.3
1,000–1,499	10.1	277.7	1,081.9	795.1	1,087.8	503.5	110.0	179.9	217.0	53.1
1,500 or more	11.4	416.6	1,546.0	1,106.1	1,978.3	788.4	136.9	213.2	319.4	56.1
Percentage of students approved for free or reduced-price lunch 10 percent or less	9.3	187.3	723.4	538.3	669.5	412.2	81.4	137.3	158.2	55.7
11–25 percent	9.1	189.4	698.9	550.6	668.8	365.8	78.2	140.8	143.4	50.1
26–50 percent	8.5	172.0	599.8	472.1	554.4	321.8	65.1	118.7	120.0	46.3

51–75 percent	8.2	157.3	580.5	448.5	529.6	297.8	59.9	118.8	98.2	44.9
More than 75 percent	7.9	135.8	554.2	367.1	511.6	258.2	54.3	111.3	92.4	43.2
Region Northeast	7.4	131.1	525.6	382.3	505.0	296.2	56.1	100.4	96.8	43.7
Midwest	8.3	143.1	566.0	367.7	494.0	287.7	63.5	111.3	116.9	45.5
South	8.4	183.3	642.5	530.8	602.1	318.3	70.1	149.8	111.8	44.6
West	10.6	207.1	753.0	634.4	705.5	388.2	72.4	122.1	155.7	60.4
Locale										
		Student services professional staff					Aides			
School characteristic	Total staff	Total	Nurses	Social workers and psychol ogists	Speech therapists	Other profession al staff	Total	Special needs aides[2]	Other aides	Other staff[4]
City	9.0	170.4	684.9	481.4	655.2	322.8	71.2	127.2	132.6	50.3
Suburban	9.0	176.2	688.1	516.4	633.1	365.7	71.5	125.3	136.3	52.2
Town	8.1	154.0	562.9	406.9	511.7	265.9	58.7	117.8	96.8	44.6
Rural	7.7	149.9	480.5	381.7	439.7	267.4	57.2	118.5	91.7	39.7

! Interpret with caution (estimates are unstable).

[1] Includes principals, vice principals, and assistant principals.

[2] Includes English as a second language (ESL)/bilingual aides, and special education instructional and noninstructional aides.

[3] Includes all other aides: regular Title I aides, library media center instructional and noninstructional aides, and other classroom instructional and noninstructional aides.

[4] Includes secretaries and other support staff; food service personnel; custodial, maintenance, and security personnel; and other employees not reported above.

[5] Includes schools with a special program emphasis, such as science/math schools, performing arts schools, talented/gifted schools, foreign language immersion schools, etc.

Note: Estimates are for both full- and part-time staff. Full-time-equivalent calculations were completed for part-time staff within each staff category. Data for each staff category are derived from schools with staff members in those categories. Not all schools have each type of staff member. Elementary schools are defined as schools with at least one grade lower than 5 and no grade higher than 8. Middle schools are defined as schools with no grade lower than 5 and no grade higher than 8. Secondary schools are defined as schools with no grade lower than 7 and at least one grade higher than 8. Combined schools have at least one grade lower than 7 and at least one grade higher than 8; schools with only ungraded classes are also included in combined schools. See *supplemental note 3* for more information on the Schools and Staffing Survey (SASS).

Source: U.S. Department of Education, National Center for Education Statistics, Schools and Staffing Survey (SASS), “Public School Data File,” 2003–04.

Table 32-3. Percentage of public schools with staff, by staff type and school characteristics: School year 2003–04

Professional instructional staff					
School characteristic Total	Principals1 97	Teachers 100	Instructional coordinators and supervisors 35	Librarians/ library media specialists 82	School counselors 80
Instructional level					
Elementary	98	100	36	84	74
Middle	98	100	36	93	94
Secondary	96	100	33	75	88
Combined	94	100	23	61	69
School type Regular	98	100	35	87	82
Special emphasis[5]	99	100	53	84	83
Special education	88	100	30	35	40
Vocational/technical	98	100	28	28	87
Alternative	85	100	18	17	50
Enrollment size					
Less than 300	93	100	20	61	67
300–499	99	100	37	87	81
500–999	100	100	41	91	85
1,000–1,499	99	100	46	94	94
1,500 or more	99	100	52	98	97
Percentage of students approved for free or reduced-price lunch 10 percent or less	99	100	38	91	74
11–25 percent	98	100	30	91	86
26–50 percent	98	100	28	85	84
51–75 percent	97	100	35	81	79
More than 75 percent	97	100	49	75	76
Region Northeast	99	100	43	89	83
Midwest	98	100	30	80	75
South	98	100	36	87	91
West	96	100	32	69	66
Locale					
City	98	100	48	79	76
Suburban	99	100	40	87	78
Town	97	100	26	77	81
Rural	95	100	22	80	83

	Student services professional staff					Aides			
School characteristic	Total	Nurses	Social workers and psychologists	Speech therapists	Other professional staff	Total	Special needs aides[2]	Other aides[3]	Other staff[4]
Total	95	80	71	84	38	95	80	87	99
Instructional level									
Elementary	97	83	74	94	40	98	84	93	100
Middle	98	88	78	87	37	97	86	86	100
Secondary	91	74	67	62	34	87	71	75	98
Combined	80	57	46	59	30	89	68	76	97
School type Regular	96	83	73	88	37	97	84	91	100
Special emphasis[5]	96	81	76	85	53	96	79	89	100
Special education	94	70	72	80	60	92	75	46	96
Vocational/technical	70	49	25	26	41	62	37	46	100
Alternative	76	45	60	30	31	66	36	55	93
Enrollment size									
Less than 300	87	64	57	69	32	87	65	78	98
300–499	97	84	74	90	36	98	83	90	100
500–999	99	89	78	91	43	98	90	92	100
1,000–1,499	97	86	83	89	42	98	86	91	99
1,500 or more	99	88	88	88	46	100	91	94	99
Percentage of students approved for free or reduced-price lunch 10 percent or less	98	88	87	89	39	97	86	89	99
11–25 percent	97	82	79	88	40	97	84	90	99
26–50 percent	95	82	67	84	33	97	84	90	100
51–75 percent	96	79	70	87	39	96	79	89	100
More than 75 percent	96	81	71	84	43	92	78	85	99
Region Northeast	99	96	87	90	45	97	77	90	99
Midwest	93	75	75	82	34	95	79	87	99
South	96	82	56	84	39	95	80	88	99
West	92	72	79	81	35	92	85	84	98
Locale									

(Continued).

	Student services professional staff					Aides			
School characteristic	Total	Nurses	Social workers and psychologists	Speech therapists	Other professional staff	Total	Special needs aides[2]	Other aides[3]	Other staff[4]
City	97	84	81	86	44	95	81	87	99
Suburban	98	84	83	91	44	97	84	90	99
Town	93	78	65	80	34	94	78	87	99
Rural	91	74	55	77	28	93	77	85	99

[1] Includes principals, vice principals, and assistant principals.

[2] Includes English as a second language (ESL)/bilingual aides, and special education instructional and noninstructional aides.

[3] Includes all other aides: regular Title I aides, library media center instructional and noninstructional aides, and other classroom instructional and noninstructional aides.

[4] Includes secretaries and other support staff; food service personnel; custodial, maintenance, and security personnel; and other employees not reported above.

[5] Includes schools with a special program emphasis, such as science/math schools, performing arts schools, talented/gifted schools, foreign language immersion schools, etc.

Note: Estimates are for both full- and part-time staff. Full-time-equivalent calculations were completed for part-time staff within each staff category. Measures in this table are intended to reveal how many schools have access to staff. Elementary schools are defined as schools with at least one grade lower than 5 and no grade higher than 8. Middle schools are defined as schools with no grade lower than 5 and no grade higher than 8. Secondary schools are defined as schools with no grade lower than 7 and at least one grade higher than 8. Combined schools have at least one grade lower than 7 and at least one grade higher than 8; schools with only ungraded classes are also included in combined schools. See *supplemental note 3* for more information on the Schools and Staffing Survey (SASS).

Source: U.S. Department of Education, National Center for Education Statistics, Schools and Staffing Survey (SASS), "Public School Data File," 2003–04.

Student/Teacher Ratios in Public Elementary and Secondary Schools

Table 33-1. Student/teacher ratios in public schools, by type, level, and enrollment of school: Selected years, fall 1990–2005

					Year				
Type, level, and enrollment of school	1990	1992	1994	1996	1998	2000	2002	2004	2005
All schools	17.4	17.7	17.7	17.6	16.9	16.4	16.2	16.2	16.0
Regular schools	17.6	17.8	17.8	17.7	17.0	16.5	16.3	16.3	16.1
Elementary schools	18.2	18.1	18.0	17.9	17.0	16.5	16.2	16.0	15.8
Under 300	16.0	15.9	15.7	15.6	15.1	14.4	13.9	13.7	13.6
300–499	17.6	17.5	17.5	17.2	16.4	15.8	15.5	15.3	15.2
500–999	18.8	18.7	18.5	18.3	17.4	16.9	16.7	16.5	16.3
1,000–1,499	19.5	19.7	19.6	19.4	18.4	18.1	18.0	17.7	17.2
1,500 or more	19.9	20.3	20.4	21.2	19.9	20.5	20.3	20.5	19.6
Secondary schools	16.7	17.4	17.6	17.6	17.1	16.7	16.8	16.9	16.8
Under 300	12.3	12.3	12.7	12.7	12.5	12.0	12.0	12.0	12.2
300–499	14.9	15.3	15.7	15.5	15.1	14.5	14.4	14.7	14.6
500–999	16.1	16.7	16.8	16.7	16.2	15.8	15.8	15.9	15.8
1,000–1,499	17.2	17.9	17.9	17.9	17.2	16.8	16.9	17.0	16.8
1,500 or more	19.3	20.0	19.9	20.0	19.3	18.9	18.8	19.0	18.8
Combined schools	15.8	15.8	16.1	15.7	14.6	14.9	15.2	15.2	15.3
Under 300	11.0	10.9	11.3	10.0	10.4	10.4	10.8	10.3	11.1
300–499	14.8	14.5	14.4	14.6	14.1	13.9	14.1	14.2	14.5
500–999	16.7	15.8	16.5	16.6	15.6	15.9	16.2	15.9	15.9
1,000–1,499	17.8	18.5	18.1	17.9	17.2	17.6	18.1	17.6	16.7
1,500 or more	19.0	19.8	20.0	19.6	18.9	20.0	20.7	19.4	20.7
Alternative	14.2	16.5	18.0	16.6	16.4	15.2	14.9	14.4	14.0
Special education	6.5	7.0	6.9	7.4	7.3	7.0	7.0	7.4	6.2
Vocational	13.0	13.0	12.9	12.9	13.1	12.7	9.9	11.5	12.0

Note: The student/teacher ratio is determined by dividing the total number of full-time-equivalent teachers into the total fall enrollment. Regular schools include all schools except special education schools, vocational schools, and alternative schools. Combined schools include both elementary and secondary grades. Charter schools can be of any school type. This analysis excludes schools that did not report both enrollment and teacher data. See *supplemental note 3* for more information about the Common Core of Data (CCD).

Source: U.S. Department of Education, National Center for Education Statistics, Common Core of Data (CCD), "Public Elementary/Secondary School Universe Survey," 1990–91 through 2005–06.

Changes in Sources of Public School Revenue

Table 34-1. Total revenue for public elementary and secondary schools, by region and revenue source: Selected years, 1989–90 to 2004–05; [Billions of constant 2006–07 dollars]

Region and revenue source	1989–90	1991–92	1993–94	1995–96	1997–98	1999–2000	2001–02	2003–04	2004–05
United States Total	$335.3	$346.5	$363.2	$380.1	$411.4	$449.7	$480.6	$506.8	$519.4
Federal	20.4	22.9	25.6	25.2	28.0	32.7	38.0	46.0	47.7
State	157.9	160.7	164.0	180.6	199.0	222.6	236.6	238.5	243.4
Local	156.9	162.9	173.6	174.3	184.4	194.4	206.0	222.4	228.3
From property taxes	120.4	126.8	136.5	134.5	140.3	150.4	161.6	176.2	178.8
From other sources	36.6	36.1	37.1	39.8	44.0	44.0	44.4	46.2	49.5
Northeast									
Total	82.4	84.2	86.8	89.7	93.3	102.1	109.1	118.0	122.8
Federal	3.8	4.3	4.6	4.5	4.7	5.6	6.4	8.1	8.2
State	33.1	33.2	33.3	34.8	36.3	43.7	48.4	48.8	51.2
Local	45.4	46.6	48.9	50.5	52.3	52.8	54.2	61.1	63.3
From property taxes	40.1	41.4	43.7	44.7	46.4	46.3	47.9	54.1	56.0
From other sources	5.3	5.2	5.2	5.8	5.9	6.5	6.4	7.0	7.3
Midwest									
Total	78.8	81.8	87.4	92.1	99.7	106.4	113.3	117.0	118.3
Federal	4.2	4.8	5.2	5.3	6.0	6.8	7.8	9.2	9.6
State	31.2	31.0	34.1	43.0	47.0	51.1	55.2	55.9	55.0
Local	43.4	45.9	48.1	43.8	46.7	48.5	50.3	52.0	53.7
From property taxes	35.4	37.7	40.2	35.5	37.2	38.3	40.2	42.6	43.7
From other sources	7.9	8.3	7.9	8.3	9.5	10.2	10.2	9.3	10.0
South									
Total	103.8	107.3	113.4	120.3	130.4	143.8	151.6	159.3	164.8
Federal	7.6	8.4	9.5	9.2	10.4	12.0	14.0	16.7	17.5

Table 34-1. (Continued).

Region and revenue source	1989–90	1991–92	1993–94	1995–96	1997–98	1999–2000	2001–02	2003–04	2004–05
State	51.0	52.0	54.5	58.9	64.3	71.7	71.8	72.3	73.2
Local	45.2	47.0	49.4	52.2	55.7	60.2	65.8	70.4	74.1
From property taxes	28.1	30.3	31.3	33.4	34.9	41.9	47.2	49.9	51.9
From other sources	17.1	16.6	18.0	18.8	20.8	18.2	18.7	20.5	22.2
West									
Total	70.3	73.2	75.7	78.1	88.0	97.4	106.6	112.5	113.6
Federal	4.8	5.4	6.2	6.3	7.0	8.3	9.8	12.0	12.4
State	42.6	44.4	42.2	44.0	51.3	56.2	61.2	61.5	64.0
Local	22.9	23.4	27.3	27.8	29.7	32.9	35.6	38.9	37.2
From property taxes	16.7	17.4	21.3	20.9	21.8	23.8	26.4	29.6	27.1
From other sources	6.2	6.0	6.0	6.9	7.9	9.1	9.2	9.4	10.1

Note: Detail may not sum to totals because of rounding. Estimates are revised from previous publications. Revenues are in constant 2006–07 dollars, adjusted using the Consumer Price Index (CPI). See *supplemental note 11* for information about the CPI and also information about revenue types. *Supplemental note 1* identifies the states in each region. See *supplemental note 3* for more information about the Common Core of Data (CCD).

Source: U.S. Department of Education, National Center for Education Statistics, Common Core of Data (CCD), “National Public Education Financial Survey,” 1989–90 to 2004–05.

Table 34-2. Percentage distribution of total revenue for public elementary and secondary schools, by region and revenue source: Selected years, 1989–90 to 2004–05

United States Total	100.0	100.0	100.0	100.0	100.0	100.0	100.0	100.0	100.0
Federal	6.1	6.6	7.1	6.6	6.8	7.3	7.9	9.1	9.2
State	47.1	46.4	45.2	47.5	48.4	49.5	49.2	47.1	46.9
Local	46.8	47.0	47.8	45.9	44.8	43.2	42.9	43.9	44.0
From property taxes	35.9	36.6	37.6	35.4	34.1	33.4	33.6	34.8	34.4
From other sources	10.9	10.4	10.2	10.5	10.7	9.8	9.2	9.1	9.5
Northeast Total	100.0	100.0	100.0	100.0	100.0	100.0	100.0	100.0	100.0
Federal	4.6	5.1	5.3	5.0	5.0	5.4	5.9	6.9	6.7
State	40.2	39.5	38.4	38.7	38.9	42.8	44.4	41.4	41.7
Local	55.1	55.4	56.3	56.3	56.0	51.7	49.7	51.8	51.6
From property taxes	48.7	49.2	50.3	49.8	49.8	45.4	43.9	45.8	45.7
From other sources	6.5	6.2	6.0	6.5	6.3	6.3	5.8	5.9	5.9
Midwest Total	100.0	100.0	100.0	100.0	100.0	100.0	100.0	100.0	100.0
Federal	5.4	5.9	6.0	5.7	6.0	6.4	6.9	7.8	8.1
State	39.6	37.9	39.0	46.7	47.2	48.0	48.7	47.8	46.5
Local	55.0	56.2	55.0	47.6	46.9	45.6	44.4	44.4	45.4
From property taxes	45.0	46.1	46.0	38.6	37.4	36.0	35.5	36.4	37.0
From other sources	10.1	10.1	9.0	9.0	9.5	9.6	9.0	8.0	8.4
South Total	100.0	100.0	100.0	100.0	100.0	100.0	100.0	100.0	100.0
Federal	7.3	7.8	8.4	7.6	8.0	8.3	9.2	10.5	10.6
State	49.1	48.5	48.0	49.0	49.3	49.8	47.3	45.4	44.4
Local	43.6	43.8	43.5	43.4	42.7	41.8	43.4	44.2	45.0
From property taxes	27.1	28.3	27.6	27.7	26.8	29.1	31.1	31.3	31.5
From other sources	16.5	15.5	15.9	15.7	15.9	12.7	12.3	12.9	13.4
West Total	100.0	100.0	100.0	100.0	100.0	100.0	100.0	100.0	100.0
Federal	6.8	7.3	8.2	8.1	7.9	8.6	9.2	10.7	10.9
State	60.6	60.7	55.7	56.3	58.3	57.6	57.4	54.7	56.4
Local	32.6	32.0	36.1	35.6	33.7	33.8	33.4	34.6	32.7
United States Total	100.0	100.0	100.0	100.0	100.0	100.0	100.0	100.0	100.0
From property taxes	23.8	23.8	28.1	26.8	24.7	24.5	24.8	26.3	23.9
From other sources	8.8	8.2	8.0	8.8	9.0	9.3	8.6	8.3	8.9

Note: Detail may not sum to totals because of rounding. Estimates are revised from previous publications. *Supplemental note 1* identifies the states in each region. See *supplemental note 11* for further information about revenue types. See *supplemental note 3* for more information about the Common Core of Data (CCD).

Source: U.S. Department of Education, National Center for Education Statistics, Common Core of Data (CCD), "National Public Education Financial Survey," 1989–90 to 2004–05.

Public Elementary and Secondary Expenditures by Type and Function

Table 35-1. Total expenditures per student in fall enrollment in public elementary and secondary schools, percentage distribution of current expenditures, and percentage change of total expenditures, by type and function: School years 1989–90 through 2004–05

Type and function	Expenditures [in constant 2006–07 dollars]			Percentage distribution of current expenditures			Percentage change		
	1989–90	1996–97	2004–05	1989–90	1996–97	2004–05	1989–90 to 1996–97	1996–97 to 2004–05	1989–90 to 2004–05
Total expenditures	$8,437	$8,820	$10,892	†	†	†	5	23	29
Current expenditures1	7,464	7,609	9,266	100	100	100	2	22	24
Salaries	4,896	4,930	5,701	66	65	62	1	16	16
Employee benefits	1,246	1,327	1,787	17	17	19	7	35	43
Purchased services	616	649	869	8	9	9	5	34	41
Supplies	557	574	738	7	8	8	3	29	32
Tuition and other	149	130	170	2	2	2	-13	31	14
Capital outlay	705	885	1,169	†	†	†	26	32	66
Interest on school debt	150	194	290	†	†	†	30	49	94
Other2	118	131	167	†	†	†	11	28	41

† Not applicable.

[1] Categories include estimated data for food services and enterprise operations for 1989–90 by subfunction because those data were not collected for that year.

[2] Includes expenditures for adult education, community colleges, private school programs funded by local and state education agencies, and community services.

Note: Detail may not sum to totals because of rounding. Estimates are revised from previous editions. Expenditures are in constant 2006–07 dollars, adjusted using the Consumer Price Index (CPI). See *supplemental note 11* for information about this index and about classifications of expenditures for elementary and secondary education. See *supplemental note 3* for more information about the Common Core of Data (CCD).

Source: U.S. Department of Education, National Center for Education Statistics, Common Core of Data (CCD), "National Public Education Financial Survey," 1989–90 through 2004–05.

Table 35-2. Current expenditures per student in fall enrollment in public elementary and secondary schools, percentage distribution of current expenditures, and percentage change of current expenditures, by function and subfunction: School years 1989–90 through 2004–05

	Expenditures [in constant 2006–07 dollars]			Percentage distribution of current expenditures			Percentage change		
Function and subfunction	1989–90	1996–97	2004–05	1989–90	1996–97	2004–05	1989–90 to 1996–97	1996–97 to 2004–05	1989–90 to 2004–05
Current expenditures	$7,464	$7,609	$9,266	100	100	100	2	22	24
Instruction	4,503	4,708	5,666	60	62	61	5	20	26
Salaries	3,345	3,413	3,902	45	45	42	2	14	17
Employee benefits	821	901	1,200	11	12	13	10	33	46
Purchased services	101	121	196	1	2	2	19	62	94
Supplies	170	201	265	2	3	3	19	32	56
Tuition and other	66	72	103	1	1	1	9	43	57
Administration	648	608	713	9	8	8	-6	17	10
Salaries	428	413	462	6	5	5	-4	12	8
Employee benefits	113	112	144	2	1	2	-1	28	27
Purchased services	65	58	77	1	1	1	-11	33	19
Supplies	14	13	14	#	#	#	-6	8	2
Tuition and other	28	12	15	#	#	#	-56	22	-46
Student and staff support[1]	835	890	1,235	11	12	13	7	39	48
Salaries	544	564	736	7	7	8	4	30	35
Employee benefits	145	154	229	2	2	2	6	49	58
Purchased services	70	95	170	1	1	2	36	79	143
Supplies	49	49	66	1	1	1	1	36	36
Tuition and other	27	27	32	#	#	#	3	18	21
Operation and maintenance	803	756	892	11	10	10	-6	18	11
Transportation	318	310	381	4	4	4	-3	23	20
Food services	322	317	358	4	4	4	-1	13	11
Enterprise operations	34	20	21	#	#	#	-41	4	-39

Rounds to zero.

[1] Includes expenditures for student support, other instructional staff, and other support services.

Note: Detail may not sum to totals because of rounding. Estimates are revised from previous editions. Expenditures are in constant 2006–07 dollars, adjusted using the Consumer Price Index (CPI). See *supplemental note 11* for information about this index and about classifications of expenditures for elementary and secondary education. See *supplemental note 3* for more information about the Common Core of Data (CCD).

Source: U.S. Department of Education, National Center for Education Statistics, Common Core of Data (CCD), "National Public Education Financial Survey," 1989–90 through 2004–05.

Table 36-1. Variation and percentage distribution of variation in instruction expenditures per student in unified public elementary and secondary school districts, by source of variation for unadjusted estimates and for estimates adjusted for geographic cost differences: 1989–90 to 2004–05

	Theil coefficient1			Percentage distribution		
School year	Total	Between-state component	component	Total	Between-state component	Within-state component
Not adjusted for geographic						
cost differences						
1989–90	0.0448	0.0322	0.0125	100.0	72.0	28.0
1990–91	0.0469	0.0346	0.0123	100.0	73.8	26.2
1991–92	0.0434	0.0320	0.0115	100.0	73.6	26.4
1992–93	0.0437	0.0324	0.0113	100.0	74.2	25.8
1993–94	0.0405	0.0301	0.0104	100.0	74.3	25.7
1994–95	0.0389	0.0288	0.0100	100.0	74.2	25.8
1995–96	0.0373	0.0279	0.0094	100.0	74.8	25.2
1996–97	0.0349	0.0257	0.0092	100.0	73.7	26.3
1997–98	0.0332	0.0246	0.0086	100.0	74.0	26.0
1998–99	0.0335	0.0249	0.0087	100.0	74.2	25.8
1999–2000	0.0337	0.0253	0.0085	100.0	74.9	25.1
2000–01	0.0370	0.0280	0.0090	100.0	75.7	24.3
2001–02	0.0373	0.0283	0.0089	100.0	76.1	23.9
2002–03	0.0391	0.0303	0.0088	100.0	77.6	22.4
2003–04	0.0420	0.0327	0.0093	100.0	77.9	22.1
2004–05	0.0455	0.0358	0.0097	100.0	78.7	21.3
Adjusted for geographic cost differences[2]						
1997–98	0.0258	0.0147	0.0111	100.0	56.9	43.1
1998–99	0.0260	0.0151	0.0110	100.0	57.9	42.1
1999–2000	0.0252	0.0151	0.0101	100.0	59.8	40.2

	Theil coefficient1			Percentage distribution		
School year	Total	Between-state component	component	Total	Between-state component	Within-state component
2000–01	0.0266	0.0161	0.0105	100.0	60.4	39.6
2001–02	0.0277	0.0168	0.0108	100.0	60.9	39.1
2002–03	0.0290	0.0180	0.0110	100.0	62.2	37.8
2003–04	0.0313	0.0204	0.0109	100.0	65.3	34.7
2004–05	0.0342	0.0226	0.0117	100.0	65.9	34.1

[1] The *Theil coefficient* measures variation for groups within a set (i.e., states within the country) and indicates relative variation and any differences that may exist among them. It can be decomposed into components measuring between-state and within-state variation in expenditures per student. It has a minimum value of zero and increasing values indicate increases in the variation, with a maximum value of 1.0. See *supplemental note 11* for more information.

[2] The NCES Comparable Wage Index (CWI) was used to adjust for geographic cost differences for 1997–98, the first year that it is available, through 2004–05. For more details on the CWI, see *supplemental note 11*.

Note: Detail may not sum to totals because of rounding. Public elementary and secondary unified districts are those districts that serve both elementary and secondary grades. In 2004–05, approximately 91 percent of all public elementary and secondary school students were enrolled in unified school districts.

Source: U.S. Department of Education, National Center for Education Statistics (NCES), Common Core of Data (CCD), "NCES Longitudinal School District Fiscal-Nonfiscal (FNF) File, Fiscal Years 1990 to 2002"; "School District Finance Survey (Form F-33)," 2002–03 to 2004–05; and NCES Comparable Wage Index Files, "School District CWI."

PUBLIC ELEMENTARY AND SECONDARY EXPENDITURES BY DISTRICT POVERTY

Table 37-1. Current expenditures per student at fall enrollment in public school districts, by district poverty category: Various years, 1997–98 to 2004–05

	Current expenditures per student							
District poverty category[1]	1997–98	1999–2000	2000–01	2001–02	2002–03	2003–04	2004–05	Percent change from 1997–98 to 2004–05
	Unadjusted dollars							
Total	$6,023	$6,727	$7,200	$7,541	$7,870	$8,135	$8,539	42.0
Low	6,552	7,207	7,713	8,126	8,477	8,833	9,241	41.0
Middle low	5,853	6,604	7,032	7,345	7,640	7,862	8,191	40.0
Middle	5,620	6,194	6,601	6,952	7,214	7,453	7,726	37.0
Middle high	5,608	6,440	6,876	7,212	7,420	7,709	8,058	44.0
High	6,482	7,181	7,782	8,075	8,606	8,858	9,482	46.0
	In constant 2006–07 dollars, not adjusted for geographic cost differences2							
Total	$7,602	$8,111	$8,395	$8,639	$8,822	$8,924	$9,094	19.6
Low	8,269	8,690	8,993	9,310	9,503	9,690	9,841	19.0
Middle low	7,388	7,963	8,199	8,414	8,564	8,625	8,723	18.1
Middle	7,094	7,469	7,696	7,965	8,087	8,176	8,228	16.0
Middle high	7,077	7,766	8,017	8,262	8,318	8,456	8,581	21.2
High	8,181	8,659	9,073	9,251	9,647	9,718	10,098	23.4
	In constant 2006–07 dollars and adjusted for geographic cost differences[2, 3]							
Total	$7,602	$8,111	$8,395	$8,639	$8,822	$8,924	$9,094	19.6
Low	7,818	8,261	8,520	8,764	8,967	9,166	9,263	18.5
Middle low	7,362	7,944	8,119	8,342	8,476	8,530	8,652	17.5
Middle	7,388	7,757	7,973	8,248	8,414	8,471	8,536	15.5
Middle high	7,559	8,140	8,441	8,673	8,777	8,908	9,083	20.2
High	7,848	8,422	8,897	9,147	9,444	9,531	9,892	26.0

[1] District poverty was determined by ranking school districts by the percentage of related children ages 5–17 from families with an income below the poverty threshold to all district children ages 5–17, and then dividing these districts into five categories with equal proportions of the total enrollment. The low-poverty district category consists of the 20 percent of students in districts with the lowest percentages of poor school-age children. Conversely, the high-

poverty district category consists of the 20 percent of students in districts with the highest percentages of poor school-age children. See *supplemental note 1* for further information on poverty.

[2] Current expenditures have been adjusted for the effects of inflation using the Consumer Price Index (CPI) and are in constant 2006–07 dollars. See *supplemental note 11* for information about the CPI.

[3] The NCES Comparable Wage Index (CWI) was used to adjust for geographic cost of living differences. For more details on the CWI, see *supplemental note 11*.

Note: Data are for regular districts, elementary/secondary combined districts, and separate elementary or secondary districts. They exclude Department of Defense districts and Bureau of Indian Education districts. See *supplemental note 1* for further information about the accounting terms used in this indicator.

Source: U.S. Department of Commerce, Census Bureau, “Small Area Income and Poverty Estimates,” 1997–98 and 1999–2000 to 2004–05; and U.S. Department of Education, National Center for Education Statistics (NCES), Common Core of Data (CCD), “School District Finance Survey (Form F-33),” 1997–98 and 1999–2000 to 2004–05, and NCES Comparable Wage Index Files, ”2005 School District CWI.”

Table 37-2. Current expenditures per student at fall enrollment in public school districts, by community type and district poverty category: 2004–05

District poverty category[1]	Total	City	Suburban	Town	Rural
	In constant 2006–07 dollars, not adjusted for geographic cost differences[2]				
Total	$9,094	$9,416	$9,321	$8,333	$8,589
Low	9,841	8,591	10,227	8,792	9,315
Middle low	8,723	8,455	8,914	8,478	8,626
Middle	8,228	8,259	8,096	8,274	8,380
Middle high	8,581	8,586	9,136	8,212	8,260
High	10,098	10,630	10,508	8,215	8,562
	In constant 2006–07 dollars and adjusted for geographic cost differences[2, 3]				
Total	$9,094	$9,092	$8,862	$9,430	$9,426
Low	9,263	7,932	9,455	9,060	9,335
Middle low	8,652	8,153	8,490	9,256	9,239
Middle	8,536	8,333	7,992	9,442	9,234
Middle high	9,083	8,765	8,868	9,578	9,541
High	9,892	9,901	9,965	9,596	10,044

[1] District poverty was determined by ranking school districts by the percentage of related children ages 5–17 from families with an income below the poverty threshold to all district children ages 5–17, and then dividing these districts into five categories with equal proportions of the total enrollment. The low-poverty district category consists of the 20 percent of students in districts with the lowest percentages of poor school-age children. Conversely, the high-poverty district category consists of the 20 percent of students in districts with the highest percentages of poor school-age children. See *supplemental note 1* for further information on poverty.

[2] Current expenditures have been adjusted for the effects of inflation using the Consumer Price Index (CPI) and are in constant 2006–07 dollars. See *supplemental note 11* for information about the CPI.

[3] The NCES Comparable Wage Index (CWI) was used to adjust for geographic cost of living differences. For more details on the CWI, see *supplemental note 11*.

Note: Data are for regular districts, elementary/secondary combined districts, and separate elementary or secondary districts. They exclude Department of Defense districts and Bureau of Indian Education districts. See *supplemental note 1* for information about community types.

Source: U.S. Department of Commerce, Census Bureau, “Small Area Income and Poverty Estimates,” 2004–05; and U.S. Department of Education, National Center for Education Statistics (NCES), Common Core of Data (CCD), “Local Education Agency Universe Survey,” 2003–04, “School District Finance Survey (Form F-33),” 2004–05, and NCES Comparable Wage Index Files, “2005 School District CWI.”

Table 37-3. Percentage distribution of fall enrollment in public school districts, by community type and district poverty category: 2004–05

District poverty category1 Total	Total 100.0	City 31.5	Suburban 37.7	Town 12.6	Rural 18.2
Low	100.0	10.0	68.8	5.6	15.7
Middle low	100.0	17.3	50.8	13.1	18.9
Middle	100.0	25.9	37.2	14.5	22.4
Middle high	100.0	35.2	24.5	18.8	21.5
High	100.0	69.3	7.2	11.2	12.4

[1] District poverty was determined by ranking school districts by the percentage of related children ages 5–17 from families with an income below the poverty threshold to all district children ages 5–17, and then dividing these districts into five categories with equal proportions of the total enrollment. The low-poverty district category consists of the 20 percent of students in districts with the lowest percentages of poor school-age children. Conversely, the high-poverty district category consists of the 20 percent of students in districts with the highest percentages of poor school-age children. See *supplemental note 1* for further information on poverty.

Note: Detail may not sum to total because of rounding. Data are for regular districts, elementary/secondary combined districts, and separate elementary or secondary districts. They exclude Department of Defense districts and Bureau of Indian Education districts. See *supplemental note 1* for information about community types.

Source: U.S. Department of Commerce, Census Bureau, "Small Area Income and Poverty Estimates," 2004–05; and U.S. Department of Education, National Center for Education Statistics (NCES), Common Core of Data (CCD), "Local Education Agency Universe Survey," 2003–04 and "School District Finance Survey (Form F-33)," 2004–05.

International Comparisons of Expenditures for Education

Table 38-1. Annual expenditures on public and private institutions per student and as a percentage of gross domestic product (GDP) in OECD countries, by level of education: 2004

	Expenditures per student[1]		Expenditures as a percentage of GDP			
Country	Elementary and secondary[2]	Post-secondary[3]	Elementary and secondary[2]	Post-secondary[3]	Total4	GDP per capita
OECD average	$6,604	$11,418	3.8	1.4	5.8	$28,442
Australia	6,911	14,036	4.2	1.6	5.9	30,875
Austria	8,938	13,959	3.7	1.2	5.4	33,235
Belgium	7,310	11,842	4.1	1.2	6.1	31,975
Canada[5,6]	6,482	19,992	3.6	2.4	5.9	32,413
Czech Republic	4,030	6,752	3.2	1.1	4.9	19,426
Denmark	8,492	15,225	4.3	1.8	7.2	32,335
Finland	6,660	12,505	3.9	1.8	6.1	29,833
France	7,262	10,668	4.1	1.3	6.1	29,006
Germany	6,983	12,255	3.5	1.1	5.2	29,916
Greece	4,931	5,593	2.2	1.1	3.4	27,691
Hungary6	3,833	7,095	3.5	1.1	5.6	16,519
Iceland	8,138	8,881	5.4	1.2	8.0	33,271
Ireland	6,034	10,211	3.4	1.2	4.6	36,536
Italy6	7,741	7,723	3.4	0.9	4.9	27,744
Japan	7,105	12,193	2.9	1.3	4.8	28,930
Korea	5,550	7,068	4.4	2.3	7.2	20,723
Luxembourg[6,7]	15,157	†	—	†	†	64,843!
Mexico	1,789	5,778	4.3	1.3	6.4	10,145
Netherlands	6,914	13,846	3.4	1.3	5.1	33,571
New Zealand	5,815	8,866	5.0	1.4	6.9	24,834
Norway	9,772	14,997	4.2	1.4	6.2	41,880
Poland[6]	2,998	4,412	3.8	1.5	6.0	13,089
Portugal[6]	5,400	7,741	3.8	1.0	5.4	19,324

Slovak Republic	2,562	6,535	3.0	1.1	4.8	14,651
Spain	5,892	9,378	3.0	1.2	4.7	26,018
Sweden	7,744	16,218	4.5	1.8	6.7	31,072
Switzerland6	10,378	21,966	4.5	1.6	6.2	34,740
Turkey6	1,262	—	3.1	1.0	4.1	7,212
United Kingdom	6,656	11,484	4.4	1.1	5.9	31,780
United States	9,368	22,476	4.1	2.9	7.4	39,660

— Not available.

† Not applicable.

! Interpret data with caution (estimates are unstable).

[1] Per student expenditures are calculated based on public and private full-time-equivalent (FTE) enrollment figures for the 2003–04 school year and on current expenditures and capital outlays from both public and private sources where data are available.

[2] Includes postsecondary nontertiary data (International Standard Classification of Education [ISCED] level 4) for Australia, Austria, Belgium, Czech Republic, Denmark, Finland, France, Germany, Greece, Hungary, Iceland, Ireland, Japan, Netherlands, New Zealand, Norway, Poland, Slovak Republic, Spain, Sweden, Switzerland, and the United Kingdom. Also includes preprimary data (ISCED level 0) for Canada, Greece, and Luxembourg.

[3] Includes all tertiary-level data (ISCED levels 5A, 5B, and 6). Also, includes postsecondary nontertiary data for Canada, Denmark, Iceland, and Japan.

[4] Total includes elementary/secondary, postsecondary, and postsecondary nontertiary expenditures with the exception of Italy, Korea, Luxembourg, Mexico, Portugal, Turkey, and the United States where data for postsecondary nontertiary are either not applicable or not available.

[5] Data are for 2002.

[6] Public institutions only.

[7] Luxembourg data are excluded from percentages because of anomalies with respect to their GDP per capita data (large revenues from international finance institutions distort the wealth of the population). Luxembourg has no postsecondary institutions.

Note: Education expenditures are from public and private revenue sources. Private sources include payments from households for school-based expenses such as tuition, transportation fees, book rentals, or food services, as well as funds raised by institutions through endowments or returns on investments. Purchasing power parity (PPP) indices are used to convert other currencies to U.S. dollars. Within-country consumer price indices are used to adjust the PPP indices to account for inflation because the fiscal year has a different starting date in different countries. See *supplemental note 5* for more information on ISCED levels.

Source: Organization for Economic Cooperation and Development (OECD), Center for Educational Research and Innovation. (2007). *Education at a Glance: OECD Indicators, 2007*, tables B1.1b, B2.1, and X2.1.

UNDERGRADUATE FIELDS OF STUDY

Table 39-1. Number of associate's degrees awarded by degree-granting institutions, percentage of total, and percent change, by selected fields of study: Academic years 1990–91, 1995–96, and 2005–06

	1990–91		1995–96		2005–06		Percent change		
Field of study	Number	Percent of total	Number	Percent of total	Numbe	Percent of total	1990–91 to 1995–96	1995–96 to 2005–06	1990–91 to 2005–06
Total1	481,720	100.0	555,216	100.0	713,066	100.0	15.3	28.4	48.0
Liberal arts and sciences, general studies, and humanities	142,722	29.6	174,970	31.5	244,689	34.3	22.6	39.8	71.4
Health professions and related clinical sciences	71,921	14.9	104,775	18.9	134,931	18.9	45.7	28.8	87.6
Business	98,018	20.3	98,665	17.8	114,095	16.0	0.7	15.6	16.4
Engineering and engineering technologies	46,638	9.7	42,605	7.7	32,623	4.6	-8.6	-23.4	-30.1
Computer and information sciences and support services	11,533	2.4	12,500	2.3	31,246	4.4	8.4	150.0	170.9
Security and protective services	13,564	2.8	19,196	3.5	26,425	3.7	41.5	37.7	94.8
Visual and performing arts	9,126	1.9	13,534	2.4	21,754	3.1	48.3	60.7	138.4
Multi/interdisciplinary studies	7,458	1.5	8,619	1.6	14,473	2.0	15.6	67.9	94.1
Education	7,928	1.6	9,809	1.8	14,475	2.0	23.7	47.6	82.6
Mechanics and repairers	7,613	1.6	12,519	2.3	14,454	2.0	64.4	15.5	89.9
Legal professions and studies	7,341	1.5	11,916	2.1	10,509	1.5	62.3	-11.8	43.2
Family and consumer sciences/human sciences	7,764	1.6	7,651	1.4	9,488	1.3	-1.5	24.0	22.2
Agriculture and natural resources	4,910	1.0	6,182	1.1	6,168	0.9	25.9	-0.2	25.6
Social sciences and history	2,505	0.5	4,021	0.7	6,730	0.9	60.5	67.4	168.7
Communications and communications technologies	4,984	1.0	4,994	0.9	6,009	0.8	0.2	20.3	20.6
Public administration and social services	2,779	0.6	4,218	0.8	4,415	0.6	51.8	4.7	58.9
Physical sciences and science technologies	2,091	0.4	2,612	0.5	2,902	0.4	24.9	11.1	38.8
Precision production trades	1,632	0.3	1,727	0.3	1,977	0.3	5.8	14.5	21.1
Psychology	997	0.2	1,583	0.3	1,944	0.3	58.8	22.8	95.0

	1990–91		1995–96		2005–06		Percent change		
Field of study	Number	Percent of total	Number	Percent of total	Numbe	Percent of total	1990–91 to 1995–96	1995–96 to 2005–06	1990–91 to 2005–06
Biological and biomedical sciences	1,121	0.2	2,049	0.4	1,827	0.3	82.8	-10.8	63.0
Transportation and material moving workers	2,609	0.5	1,551	0.3	1,472	0.2	-40.6	-5.1	-43.6
Foreign languages, literatures, and linguistics	555	0.1	1,612	0.3	1,161	0.2	190.5	-28.0	109.2

[1] Includes other fields not shown separately.

Note: See *supplemental note 10* for more information on fields of study. The new *Classification of Instructional Programs* was initiated in 2002–03. Estimates for earlier years have been reclassified when necessary to conform to the new taxonomy. See *supplemental note 9* for information on the Classification of Postsecondary Education Institutions. See *supplemental note 3* for more information about the Integrated Postsecondary Education Data System (IPEDS). Detail may not sum to totals because of rounding.

Source: U.S. Department of Education, National Center for Education Statistics (NCES). *Digest of Education Statistics, 2007* (NCES 2008-022), table 259, data from U.S. Department of Education, NCES, 1990–91, 1995–96, and 2005–06 Integrated Postsecondary Education Data System, "Completions Survey" (IPEDS-C:91 and 96), and Fall 2006.

Table 39-2. Number of bachelor's degrees awarded by degree-granting institutions, percentage of total, and percent change, by selected fields of study: Academic years 1990–91, 1995–96, and 2005–06

	1990–91		1995–96		2005–06		Percent change		
Field of study	Number	Percent of total	Number	Percent of total	Number	Percent of total	1990–91 to 1995–96	1995–96 to 2005–06	1990–91 to 2005–06
Total1	1,094,538	100.0	1,164,792	100.0	1,485,242	100.0	6.4	27.5	35.7
Business	249,165	22.8	226,623	19.5	318,042	21.4	-9.0	40.3	27.6
Social sciences and history	125,107	11.4	126,479	10.9	161,485	10.9	1.1	27.7	29.1
Education	110,807	10.1	105,384	9.0	107,238	7.2	-4.9	1.8	-3.2
Health professions and related clinical sciences	59,875	5.5	86,087	7.4	91,973	6.2	43.8	6.8	53.6
Psychology	58,655	5.4	73,416	6.3	88,134	5.9	25.2	20.0	50.3
Visual and performing arts	42,186	3.9	49,296	4.2	83,297	5.6	16.9	69.0	97.5
Engineering and engineering technologies	79,751	7.3	78,086	6.7	81,610	5.5	-2.1	4.5	2.3
Communication, journalism, and related programs	51,650	4.7	47,320	4.1	73,955	5.0	-8.4	56.3	43.2
Biological and biomedical sciences	39,377	3.6	60,750	5.2	69,178	4.7	54.3	13.9	75.7
English language and literature/letters	51,064	4.7	49,928	4.3	55,096	3.7	-2.2	10.4	7.9
Computer and information sciences and support services	25,159	2.3	24,506	2.1	47,480	3.2	-2.6	93.7	88.7
Liberal arts and sciences, general studies, and humanities	30,526	2.8	33,997	2.9	44,898	3.0	11.4	32.1	47.1
Security and protective services	16,806	1.5	24,810	2.1	35,319	2.4	47.6	42.4	110.2
Multi/interdisciplinary studies	17,879	1.6	27,149	2.3	32,012	2.2	51.8	17.9	79.0
Parks, recreation, leisure and fitness studies	4,315	0.4	12,974	1.1	25,490	1.7	200.7	96.5	490.7
Agriculture and natural resources	13,124	1.2	21,425	1.8	23,053	1.6	63.3	7.6	75.7
Public administration and social services	14,350	1.3	19,849	1.7	21,986	1.5	38.3	10.8	53.2
Family and consumer sciences/human sciences	13,920	1.3	14,353	1.2	20,775	1.4	3.1	44.7	49.2

	1990–91		1995–96		2005–06		Percent change		
Field of study	Number	Percent of total	Number	Percent of total	Number	Percent of total	1990–91 to 1995–96	1995–96 to 2005–06	1990–91 to 2005–06
Physical sciences and science technologies	16,334	1.5	19,627	1.7	20,318	1.4	20.2	3.5	24.4
Foreign languages, literatures, and linguistics	13,937	1.3	14,832	1.3	19,410	1.3	6.4	30.9	39.3
Mathematics and statistics	14,393	1.3	12,713	1.1	14,770	1.0	-11.7	16.2	2.6
Philosophy and religious studies	7,423	0.7	7,541	0.6	11,985	0.8	1.6	58.9	61.5

[1] Includes other fields not shown separately.

Note: See *supplemental note 10* for more information on fields of study. The new *Classification of Instructional Programs* was initiated in 2002–03. Estimates for earlier years have been reclassified when necessary to conform to the new taxonomy. See *supplemental note 9* for information on the Classification of Postsecondary Education Institutions. See *supplemental note 3* for more information about the Integrated Postsecondary Education Data System (IPEDS). Detail may not sum to totals because of rounding.

Source: U.S. Department of Education, National Center for Education Statistics (NCES). *Digest of Education Statistics, 2007* (NCES 2008-022), table 261, data from U.S. Department of Education, NCES, 1990–91, 1995–96, and 2005–06 Integrated Postsecondary Education Data System, "Completions Survey" (IPEDS-C:91 and 96), and Fall 2006.

GRADUATE FIELDS OF STUDY

Table 40-1. Number of master's, doctoral, and first-professional degrees awarded by degree-granting institutions, percentage of total, and percent change, by selected fields of study: Academic years 1990–91, 1995–96, and 2005–06

	1990–91		1995–96		2005–06		Percent change		
Field of study	Number	Percent of total	Number	Percent of total	Number	Percent of total	1990–91 to 1995–96	1995–96 to 2005–06	1990–91 to 2005–06
Doctoral degrees[2] Total[1]	337,168	100.0	406,301	100.0	594,065	100.0	20.5	46.2	76.2
Education	87,352	25.9	104,936	25.8	174,620	29.4	20.1	66.4	99.9
Business	78,255	23.2	93,554	23.0	146,406	24.6	19.6	56.5	87.1
Health professions and related clinical sciences	21,354	6.3	33,920	8.3	51,380	8.6	58.8	51.5	140.6
Engineering and engineering technologies	25,450	7.5	28,946	7.1	33,530	5.6	13.7	15.8	31.7
Public administration and social services	17,905	5.3	24,229	6.0	30,510	5.1	35.3	25.9	70.4
Psychology	11,349	3.4	15,152	3.7	19,770	3.3	33.5	30.5	74.2
Social sciences and history	12,233	3.6	15,012	3.7	17,369	2.9	22.7	15.7	42.0
Computer and information sciences and support services	9,324	2.8	10,579	2.6	17,055	2.9	13.5	61.2	82.9
Visual and performing arts	8,657	2.6	10,280	2.5	13,530	2.3	18.7	31.6	56.3
English language and literature/ letters	6,784	2.0	7,657	1.9	8,845	1.5	12.9	15.5	30.4
Biological and biomedical sciences	4,796	1.4	6,544	1.6	8,681	1.5	36.4	32.7	81.0
Communication, journalism, and related programs	4,123	1.2	5,080	1.3	7,244	1.2	23.2	42.6	75.7
Library science	4,763	1.4	5,099	1.3	6,448	1.1	7.1	26.5	35.4
Theology and religious vocations	4,803	1.4	5,030	1.2	6,092	1.0	4.7	21.1	26.8
Physical sciences and science technologies	5,281	1.6	5,807	1.4	5,922	1.0	10.0	2.0	12.1
Architecture and related services	3,490	1.0	3,993	1.0	5,743	1.0	14.4	43.8	64.6
Mathematics and statistics	3,549	1.1	3,651	0.9	4,730	0.8	2.9	29.6	33.3

	1990–91		1995–96		2005–06		Percent change		
Field of study	Number	Percent of total	Number	Percent of total	Number	Percent of total	1990–91 to 1995–96	1995–96 to 2005–06	1990–91 to 2005–06
Agriculture and natural resources	3,295	1.0	4,551	1.1	4,640	0.8	38.1	2.0	40.8
Doctoral degrees[2]									
Total1	39,294	100.0	44,652	100.0	56,067	100.0	13.6	25.6	42.7
Education	6,189	15.8	6,246	14.0	7,584	13.5	0.9	21.4	22.5
Engineering and engineering									
technologies	5,330	13.6	6,431	14.4	7,471	13.3	20.7	16.2	40.2
Health professions and related									
clinical sciences	1,534	3.9	1,651	3.7	7,128	12.7	7.6	331.7	364.7
Biological and biomedical sciences	4,034	10.3	5,035	11.3	5,775	10.3	24.8	14.7	43.2
Psychology	3,932	10.0	4,141	9.3	4,921	8.8	5.3	18.8	25.2
Physical sciences and science									
technologies	4,248	10.8	4,512	10.1	4,489	8.0	6.2	-0.5	5.7
Social sciences and history	3,012	7.7	3,760	8.4	3,914	7.0	24.8	4.1	29.9
Business	1,185	3.0	1,366	3.1	1,711	3.1	15.3	25.3	44.4
Theology and religious vocations	1,076	2.7	1,517	3.4	1,429	2.5	41.0	-5.8	32.8
Computer and information									
sciences and support services	676	1.7	869	1.9	1,416	2.5	28.6	62.9	109.5
Visual and performing arts	838	2.1	1,067	2.4	1,383	2.5	27.3	29.6	65.0
Mathematics and statistics	978	2.5	1,158	2.6	1,293	2.3	18.4	11.7	32.2
English language and literature/									
letters	1,056	2.7	1,395	3.1	1,254	2.2	32.1	-10.1	18.8
Agriculture and natural resources	1,185	3.0	1,259	2.8	1,194	2.1	6.2	-5.2	0.8
Foreign languages, literatures, and									
linguistics	889	2.3	1,020	2.3	1,074	1.9	14.7	5.3	20.8
Multi/interdisciplinary studies	424	1.1	764	1.7	987	1.8	80.2	29.2	132.8
First-professional degrees[3]									
Total1	71,948	100.0	76,734	100.0	87,655	100.0	6.7	14.2	21.8
Law	37,945	52.7	39,828	51.9	43,440	49.6	5.0	9.1	14.5
Medicine	15,043	20.9	15,341	20.0	15,455	17.6	2.0	0.7	2.7
Pharmacy	1,244	1.7	2,555	3.3	9,292	10.6	105.4	263.7	646.9
Theology	5,695	7.9	5,879	7.7	5,666	6.5	3.2	-3.6	-0.5

Table 40-1. (Continued).

	1990–91		1995–96		2005–06		Percent change		
Field of study	Number	Percent of total	Number	Percent of total	Number	Percent of total	1990–91 to 1995–96	1995–96 to 2005–06	1990–91 to 2005–06
Dentistry	3,699	5.1	3,697	4.8	4,389	5.0	-0.1	18.7	18.7
Osteopathic	1,459	2.0	1,895	2.5	2,718	3.1	29.9	43.4	86.3
Chiropractic	2,640	3.7	3,379	4.4	2,564	2.9	28.0	-24.1	-2.9
Veterinary medicine	2,032	2.8	2,109	2.7	2,370	2.7	3.8	12.4	16.6
Optometry	1,115	1.5	1,231	1.6	1,198	1.4	10.4	-2.7	7.4

[1] Includes other fields not shown separately.

[2] Includes Ph.D., Ed.D., and comparable degrees at the doctoral level.

[3] An award that requires completion of a degree program that meets all of the following criteria: (1) completion of the academic requirements to begin practice in the profession; (2) at least 2 years of college work before entering the degree program; and (3) a total of at least 6 academic years of college work to complete the degree program, including previously required college work plus the work required in the professional program itself. See glossary for a complete list of first-professional degrees.

Note: See *supplemental note 10* for more information on fields of study. The new *Classification of Instructional Programs* was initiated in 2002–03. Estimates for earlier years have been reclassified when necessary to conform to the new taxonomy. See *supplemental note 9* for information on the Classification of Postsecondary Education Institutions. See *supplemental note 3* for more information about the Integrated Postsecondary Education Data System (IPEDS). Detail may not sum to totals because of rounding.

Source: U.S. Department of Education, National Center for Education Statistics (NCES). *Digest of Education Statistics, 2007* (NCES 2008-022), tables 262, 263 and 270, data from U.S. Department of Education, NCES, 1990–91, 1995–96, and 2005–06 Integrated Postsecondary Education Data System, "Completions Survey" (IPEDS-C:91 and 96), and Fall 2006.

Degrees Conferred by Public and Private Institutions

Table 41-1. Number and percentage distribution of degrees conferred by degree-granting institutions, by level of degree and control of institution: 1995–96 through 2005–06

	Number of degrees conferred					Percentage distribution of degrees conferred				
			Private					Private		
Level of degree and academic year	Total	Public	Total	Not-forprofit	Forprofit	Total	Public	Total	Not-for-profit	For-profit
Associate's 1995–96	555,216	454,291	100,925	50,678	50,247	100.0	81.8	18.2	9.1	9.0
1996–97	571,226	465,494	105,732	49,168	56,564	100.0	81.5	18.5	8.6	9.9
1997–98	558,555	455,084	103,471	47,625	55,846	100.0	81.5	18.5	8.5	10.0
1998–99	559,954	448,334	111,620	47,611	64,009	100.0	80.1	19.9	8.5	11.4
1999–2000	564,933	448,446	116,487	46,337	70,150	100.0	79.4	20.6	8.2	12.4
2000–01	578,865	456,487	122,378	45,711	76,667	100.0	78.9	21.1	7.9	13.2
2001–02	595,133	471,660	123,473	45,761	77,712	100.0	79.3	20.7	7.7	13.1
2002–03	634,016	498,279	135,737	46,183	89,554	100.0	78.6	21.4	7.3	14.1
2003–04	665,301	524,875	140,426	45,759	94,667	100.0	78.9	21.1	6.9	14.2
2004–05	696,660	547,519	149,141	45,344	103,797	100.0	78.6	21.4	6.5	14.9
2005–06	713,066	557,134	155,932	46,442	109,490	100.0	78.1	21.9	6.5	15.4
Bachelor's 1995–96	1,164,792	774,070	390,722	379,916	10,806	100.0	66.5	33.5	32.6	0.9
1996–97	1,172,879	776,677	396,202	384,086	12,116	100.0	66.2	33.8	32.7	1.0
1997–98	1,184,406	784,296	400,110	386,455	13,655	100.0	66.2	33.8	32.6	1.2
1998–99	1,200,303	790,287	410,016	393,680	16,336	100.0	65.8	34.2	32.8	1.4
1999–2000	1,237,875	810,855	427,020	406,958	20,062	100.0	65.5	34.5	32.9	1.6
2000–01	1,244,171	812,438	431,733	408,701	23,032	100.0	65.3	34.7	32.8	1.9
2001–02	1,291,900	841,180	450,720	424,322	26,398	100.0	65.1	34.9	32.8	2.0
2002–03	1,348,811	875,596	473,215	442,060	31,155	100.0	64.9	35.1	32.8	2.3
2003–04	1,399,542	905,718	493,824	451,518	42,306	100.0	64.7	35.3	32.3	3.0
2004–05	1,439,264	932,443	506,821	457,963	48,858	100.0	64.8	35.2	31.8	3.4
2005–06	1,485,242	955,369	529,873	467,836	62,037	100.0	64.3	35.7	31.5	4.2

Table 41-1. (Continued).

Master's										
1995–96	406,301	227,179	179,122	175,263	3,859	100.0	55.9	44.1	43.1	0.9
1996–97	419,401	233,237	186,164	181,104	5,060	100.0	55.6	44.4	43.2	1.2
1997–98	430,164	235,922	194,242	188,175	6,067	100.0	54.8	45.2	43.7	1.4
1998–99	439,986	238,501	201,485	192,152	9,333	100.0	54.2	45.8	43.7	2.1
1999–2000	457,056	243,157	213,899	203,591	10,308	100.0	53.2	46.8	44.5	2.3
2000–01	468,476	246,054	222,422	210,789	11,633	100.0	52.5	47.5	45.0	2.5
2001–02	482,118	249,820	232,298	218,034	14,264	100.0	51.8	48.2	45.2	3.0
2002–03	513,339	265,643	247,696	232,709	14,987	100.0	51.7	48.3	45.3	2.9
2003–04	558,940	285,138	273,802	245,562	28,240	100.0	51.0	49.0	43.9	5.1
2004–05	574,618	291,505	283,113	248,031	35,082	100.0	50.7	49.3	43.2	6.1
2005–06	594,065	293,517	300,548	255,424	45,124	100.0	49.4	50.6	43.0	7.6
First-professional										
1995–96	76,734	29,882	46,852	46,532	320	100.0	38.9	61.1	60.6	0.4
1996–97	78,730	31,243	47,487	47,029	458	100.0	39.7	60.3	59.7	0.6
1997–98	78,598	31,233	47,365	47,018	347	100.0	39.7	60.3	59.8	0.4
1998–99	78,439	31,693	46,746	46,315	431	100.0	40.4	59.6	59.0	0.5
1999–2000	80,057	32,247	47,810	47,301	509	100.0	40.3	59.7	59.1	0.6
2000–01	79,707	32,633	47,074	46,828	246	100.0	40.9	59.1	58.8	0.3
2001–02	80,698	33,439	47,259	47,020	239	100.0	41.4	58.6	58.3	0.3
2002–03	80,897	33,549	47,348	47,116	232	100.0	41.5	58.5	58.2	0.3
2003–04	83,041	34,499	48,542	48,278	264	100.0	41.5	58.5	58.1	0.3
2004–05	87,289	35,768	51,521	51,259	262	100.0	41.0	59.0	58.7	0.3
2005–06	87,655	36,269	51,386	50,902	484	100.0	41.4	58.6	58.1	0.6
Doctoral 1995–96	44,652	29,516	15,136	14,853	283	100.0	66.1	33.9	33.3	0.6
1996–97	45,876	29,838	16,038	15,694	344	100.0	65.0	35.0	34.2	0.7
1997–98	46,010	29,715	16,295	15,944	351	100.0	64.6	35.4	34.7	0.8
1998–99	44,077	28,134	15,943	15,501	442	100.0	63.8	36.2	35.2	1.0
1999–2000	44,808	28,408	16,400	15,800	600	100.0	63.4	36.6	35.3	1.3
2000–01	44,904	28,187	16,717	15,920	797	100.0	62.8	37.2	35.5	1.8
2001–02	44,160	27,622	16,538	15,882	656	100.0	62.5	37.5	36.0	1.5
2002–03	46,042	28,062	17,980	17,138	842	100.0	60.9	39.1	37.2	1.8

	Number of degrees conferred					Percentage distribution of degrees conferred				
			Private					Private		
Level of degree and academic year	Total	Public	Total	Not-forprofit	Forprofit	Total	Public	Total	Not-for-profit	For-profit
2003–04	48,378	29,706	18,672	17,501	1,171	100.0	61.4	38.6	36.2	2.4
2004–05	52,631	31,743	20,888	19,552	1,336	100.0	60.3	39.7	37.1	2.5
2005–06	56,067	33,767	22,300	20,830	1,470	100.0	60.2	39.8	37.2	2.6

Note: Includes institutions that participated in Title IV federal financial aid programs. See *supplemental note 3* for more information on the Integrated Postsecondary Education Data System (IPEDS). See the glossary for definitions of first-professional degree programs. Detail may not sum to totals because of rounding.

Source: U.S. Department of Education, National Center for Education Statistics, 1995–96 through 2005–06 Integrated Postsecondary Education Data System, "Completions Survey" (IPEDS-C:96–99), and Fall 2000 through Fall 2006.

Faculty Salary, Benefits, and Total Compensation

Table 42-1. Total compensation, percentage distribution of full-time instructional faculty, average salary, and fringe benefits at degree-granting institutions, by selected characteristics: Selected academic years 1979–80 to 2006–07

	1979–80		1989–90		1999–2000		2006–07		Percent change	
Compensation, salary, and benefit[1]	Percent	Average	Percent	Average	Percent	Average	Percent	Average	1979–80 To 2006–07	1999–2000 to 2006–07
Total compensation	100.0	$68,800	100.0	$79,400	100.0	$84,700	100.0	$88,100	28.1	4.1
Salary										
All faculty	100.0	57,800	100.0	66,000	100.0	68,700	100.0	69,500	20.2	1.2
Professor	26.0	77,200	30.7	87,400	30.2	92,400	26.6	97,100	25.9	5.1
Associate professor	24.9	58,100	24.0	65,300	23.2	67,800	21.6	69,900	20.4	3.2
Assistant professor	25.4	47,300	23.2	53,900	22.1	56,000	23.2	58,600	24.0	4.7
Instructor	7.6	38,000	5.6	41,300	6.0	43,800	16.1	52,400	38.0	19.7
Lecturer	1.4	44,200	1.9	48,500	2.6	47,400	4.5	51,200	15.9	8.1
No rank	14.7	53,000	14.6	52,900	15.9	55,600	8.1	52,700	-0.4	-5.1
All institution[s2]	100.0	57,800	100.0	66,000	100.0	68,700	100.0	69,500	20.2	1.2
Public doctoral universities	28.3	64,900	30.6	75,300	28.3	79,700	28.4	79,800	23.0	0.1
Private doctoral universities	8.0	66,700	10.3	80,700	10.1	89,900	11.8	91,300	36.9	1.5
Public master's colleges/universities	22.8	57,800	18.7	65,400	17.8	64,700	16.2	63,600	10.1	-1.8
Private master's colleges/universities	7.5	52,000	9.4	57,900	10.8	62,000	10.9	62,100	19.4	0.1
Public other 4-year colleges	2.7	53,900	2.4	61,600	2.4	58,900	3.1	68,400	26.8	16.1
Private other 4-year colleges	8.9	45,900	8.3	52,500	7.9	56,900	7.7	58,200	26.7	2.2
Public 2-year colleges	21.1	53,500	19.6	55,400	21.0	58,300	20.2	57,800	8.0	-1.0
Private 2-year colleges	0.8	35,900	0.7	41,800	1.7	40,300	1.7	41,800	16.5	3.9
Fringe benefits All institutions	100.0	11,000	100.0	13,500	100.0	16,000	100.0	18,600	69.3	16.6

	1979–80		1989–90		1999–2000		2006–07		Percent change	
Compensation, salary, and benefit[1]	Percent	Average	Percent	Average	Percent	Average	Percent	Average	1979–80 To 2006–07	1999–2000 to 2006–07
Public doctoral universities	28.3	11,900	30.6	16,100	28.3	17,900	28.4	20,400	72.2	13.8
Private doctoral universities	8.0	12,600	10.3	15,900	10.1	21,800	11.8	24,000	90.5	10.1
Public master's colleges/universities	22.8	11,700	18.7	14,500	17.8	15,200	16.2	18,100	54.1	19.1
Private master's colleges/universities	7.5	9,700	9.4	11,900	10.8	15,000	10.9	16,700	71.4	11.0
Public other 4-year colleges	2.7	10,200	2.4	10,800	2.4	13,400	3.1	18,400	79.9	37.0
Private other 4-year colleges	8.9	8,800	8.3	9,900	7.9	14,100	7.7	15,800	80.1	12.1
Public 2-year colleges	21.1	10,100	19.6	9,900	21.0	13,300	20.2	16,400	62.6	23.3
Private 2-year colleges	0.8	6,500	0.7	6,300	1.7	7,900	1.7	8,000	22.1	1.1
Total compensation	100.0	$26,200	100.0	$49,400	100.0	$70,200	100.0	$88,100	236.8	25.5
Salary										
All faculty	100.0	22,000	100.0	41,000	100.0	57,000	100.0	69,500	216.1	22.0
Professor	26.0	29,300	30.7	54,400	30.2	76,700	26.6	97,100	231.0	26.7
Associate professor	24.9	22,100	24.0	40,600	23.2	56,200	21.6	69,900	216.6	24.5
Assistant professor	25.4	18,000	23.2	33,500	22.1	46,400	23.2	58,600	226.2	26.2
Instructor	7.6	14,400	5.6	25,700	6.0	36,300	16.1	52,400	262.9	44.3
Lecturer	1.4	16,800	1.9	30,100	2.6	39,300	4.5	51,200	204.8	30.4
No rank	14.7	20,100	14.6	32,900	15.9	46,100	8.1	52,700	161.8	14.4
All institutions2	100.0	22,000	100.0	41,000	100.0	57,000	100.0	69,500	216.1	22.0
Public doctoral universities	28.3	24,700	30.6	46,800	28.3	66,100	28.4	79,800	223.6	20.7
Private doctoral universities	8.0	25,400	10.3	50,200	10.1	74,600	11.8	91,300	259.9	22.4
Public master's colleges/universities	22.8	22,000	18.7	40,700	17.8	53,700	16.2	63,600	189.5	18.4
Private master's colleges/universities	7.5	19,800	9.4	36,000	10.8	51,400	10.9	62,100	214.0	20.7

Table 42-1. (Continued).

	1979–80		1989–90		1999–2000		2006–07		Percent change	
Compensation, salary, and benefit[1]	Percent	Average	Percent	Average	Percent	Average	Percent	Average	1979–80 To 2006–07	1999–2000 to 2006–07
Public other 4-year colleges	2.7	20,500	2.4	38,300	2.4	48,900	3.1	68,400	233.5	40.0
Private other 4-year colleges	8.9	17,500	8.3	32,700	7.9	47,200	7.7	58,200	233.2	23.2
Public 2-year colleges	21.1	20,300	19.6	34,500	21.0	48,400	20.2	57,800	184.0	19.4
Private 2-year colleges	0.8	13,600	0.7	26,000	1.7	33,400	1.7	41,800	206.5	25.3
Fringe benefits										
All institutions	100.0	4,200	100.0	8,400	100.0	13,200	100.0	18,600	345.3	40.6
Public doctoral universities	28.3	4,500	30.6	10,000	28.3	14,900	28.4	20,400	352.8	37.3
Private doctoral universities	8.0	4,800	10.3	9,900	10.1	18,100	11.8	24,000	400.8	32.8
Public master's colleges/universities	22.8	4,500	18.7	9,000	17.8	12,600	16.2	18,100	305.1	43.7
Private master's colleges/universities	7.5	3,700	9.4	7,400	10.8	12,400	10.9	16,700	350.8	33.9
Public other 4-year colleges	2.7	3,900	2.4	6,700	2.4	11,100	3.1	18,400	373.0	65.2
Private other 4-year colleges	8.9	3,300	8.3	6,200	7.9	11,700	7.7	15,800	373.7	35.2
Public 2-year colleges	21.1	3,800	19.6	6,200	21.0	11,000	20.2	16,400	327.6	48.7
Private 2-year colleges	0.8	2,500	0.7	3,900	1.7	6,600	1.7	8,000	221.2	21.9

[1] Total compensation is the sum of salary and fringe benefits. Salary does not include outside income. Fringe benefits may include, for example, retirement plans, medical/dental plans, group life insurance, or other benefits.

[2] Institutions in this indicator are classified based on the number of highest degrees awarded. For example, institutions that award 20 or more doctoral degrees per year are classified as doctoral universities. See *supplemental note 9* for more information about Classification of Postsecondary Education Institutions.

Note: Full-time instructional faculty on less-than-9-month contracts were excluded. In 2006–07, there were about 3,600 of these faculty, accounting for less than 1 percent of all full-time instructional faculty at degree-granting institutions. Salaries reflect an average of all faculty on 9- through 12-month contracts, rather than a weighted average based on contract length that appears in some other NCES reports. Salaries, benefits, and compensation adjusted by the Consumer Price Index (CPI) to constant 2006–07 dollars. Percentages based on unrounded numbers. Detail may not sum to totals because of rounding. See *supplemental note 11* for more information about the CPI. See *supplemental note 3* for more information about the Integrated Postsecondary Education Data System (IPEDS).

Source: U.S. Department of Education, National Center for Education Statistics, 1979–80 Higher Education General Information Survey (HEGIS), "Faculty Salaries, Tenure, and Fringe Benefits Survey"; and 1989–90, 1999–2000, and 2006–07 Integrated Postsecondary Education Data System, "Salaries, Tenure, and Fringe Benefits of Full-Time Instructional Faculty Survey" (IPEDS-SA:89–99), "Completions Survey" (IPEDS-C:89–99), Fall 2006, and Winter 2006–07.

EMPLOYMENT OF COLLEGE STUDENTS

Table 43-1. Percentage of 16- to 24-year-old college students who were employed, by attendance status and hours worked per week: October 1970 through October 2006

	Full-time college students				Part-time college students			
		Hours worked per week1				Hours worked per week1		
Year	Percent employed[2]	Less than 20 hours	20–34 hours	35 or more hours	Percent employed[2]	Less than 20 hours	20–34 hours	35 or more hours
1970	33.8	19.3	10.4	3.8	82.2	5.0	15.8	60.3
1971	34.1	18.7	11.1	3.7	83.5	7.1	23.4	51.9
1972	35.1	19.4	11.6	3.6	83.0	6.2	23.1	53.1
1973	36.4	19.2	12.3	4.6	84.0	7.1	23.9	52.1
1974	36.5	18.9	12.3	4.8	84.0	5.9	15.9	61.0
1975	35.3	18.2	12.0	4.7	80.9	6.0	19.5	52.6
1976	37.6	19.9	12.8	4.1	84.7	7.1	23.0	53.1
1977	38.8	20.0	14.0	4.3	83.2	6.3	22.2	52.9
1978	39.9	20.2	14.3	4.7	85.9	8.4	22.4	54.0
1979	38.2	19.9	13.9	4.0	87.0	6.1	22.2	56.6
1980	40.0	21.5	14.0	3.9	84.5	7.9	22.5	52.6
1981	39.3	20.0	14.5	4.2	85.6	8.0	24.7	51.2
1982	39.9	20.9	15.5	3.0	81.2	8.6	21.6	48.3
1983	40.4	20.9	15.1	3.8	81.5	5.8	26.2	48.4
1984	42.0	20.2	16.7	4.3	84.9	5.5	22.1	55.8
1985	44.2	21.8	17.3	4.3	86.1	6.0	26.8	52.5
1986	43.1	20.4	17.6	4.3	87.3	8.2	23.4	54.8
1987	44.2	21.0	18.0	4.3	85.4	6.3	27.9	49.5
1988	46.5	21.9	19.8	4.7	88.3	5.1	27.4	54.3
1989	46.5	20.7	19.9	5.4	87.3	5.1	25.4	55.4
1990	45.7	20.6	19.3	4.8	83.7	4.0	26.0	52.7
1991	47.2	21.0	19.8	5.6	85.9	8.2	25.4	51.0

	Full-time college students				Part-time college students			
		Hours worked per week1				Hours worked per week1		
Year	Percent employed[2]	Less than 20 hours	20–34 hours	35 or more hours	Percent employed[2]	Less than 20 hours	20–34 hours	35 or more hours
1992	47.2	20.4	20.3	5.5	83.4	7.5	27.2	47.8
1993	46.3	20.9	19.5	5.1	84.6	8.5	31.4	43.7
1994	48.6	20.1	21.7	5.8	86.3	9.8	31.1	43.8
1995	47.2	19.1	20.3	6.5	82.9	8.6	30.4	42.3
1996	49.2	18.2	22.3	7.0	84.8	8.3	27.5	48.0
1997	47.8	18.3	21.4	7.4	84.4	9.4	26.2	47.7
1998	50.2	20.2	20.6	8.0	84.1	7.0	26.8	49.3
1999	50.4	19.0	22.3	7.8	82.3	6.2	28.8	45.9
2000	52.0	20.1	21.7	8.9	84.9	8.6	27.8	47.5
2001	47.0	17.4	20.6	7.9	84.5	8.1	25.8	48.9
2002	47.8	17.3	20.9	8.5	78.9	8.7	25.3	43.4
2003	47.7	17.1	20.7	8.8	79.0	7.8	27.2	42.8
2004	49.0	17.7	21.6	8.6	81.5	8.5	27.4	44.1
2005	49.1	17.8	21.1	9.0	85.0	10.2	27.1	47.1
2006	46.5	15.1	22.0	8.1	81.0	7.3	27.6	45.5

[1] Excludes those who were employed but not at work during the survey week; therefore, detail may not sum to total percentage employed. *Hours worked per week* refers to the number of hours the respondent worked at all jobs during the survey week.

[2] Includes those who were employed but not at work during the survey week.

Note: College includes both 2- and 4-year institutions. College students were classified as attending full time if they were taking at least 12 hours of classes (or at least 9 hours of graduate classes) during an average school week and as part time if they were taking fewer hours.

Source: U.S. Department of Commerce, Census Bureau, Current Population Survey (CPS), October Supplement, 1970–2006.

Table 43-2. Percentage of 16- to 24-year-old college students who were employed, by attendance status, hours worked per week, and selected characteristics: October 2006

	Full-time college students				Part-time college students			
		Hours worked per week[1]				Hours worked per week[1]		
Selected characteristic	Percent employed[2]	Less than 20 hours	20–34 hours	35 or more hours	Percent employed[2]	Less than 20 hours	20–34 hours	35 or more hours
Total	46.5	15.1	22.0	8.1	81.0	7.3	27.6	45.5
Sex								
Male	43.6	13.7	20.7	8.3	83.3	5.3	28.0	49.2
Female	48.9	16.2	23.1	8.0	79.0	9.1	27.3	42.3
Race/ethnicity[3] White	48.6	16.4	23.1	7.6	82.3	7.3	29.2	45.3
Black	36.9	10.4	15.3	10.1	76.9	5.9!	22.0	49.0
Hispanic	48.5	12.3	25.6	9.7	79.9	5.9!	28.3	44.3
Asian	37.8	13.5	18.5	5.3	‡	‡	‡	‡
Pacific Islander	‡	‡	‡	‡	‡	‡	‡	‡
American Indian/								
Alaska Native	‡	‡	‡	‡	‡	‡	‡	‡
More than one race	47.8	12.6!	19.4	13.7!	‡	‡	‡	‡
School type 2-year	53.7	15.5	27.5	9.4	81.1	7.9	30.6	42.4
Public	55.3	15.8	28.8	9.2	80.7	8.2	30.0	42.2
Private	40.1	12.4	16.2	11.6	‡	‡	‡	‡
4-year	44.3	14.9	20.4	7.8	80.9	6.9	25.5	47.7
Public	46.6	13.9	22.9	8.6	80.5	7.1	26.4	46.0
Private	36.9	18.1	12.4	5.1	83.0	6.1!	21.0	55.9
School level								
Undergraduate	46.5	15.3	22.0	7.8	80.4	7.5	28.9	43.3
Sex								
Male	43.9	14.0	20.8	8.2	82.8	5.8	28.4	47.6
Female	48.8	16.5	23.2	7.4	78.3	9.1	29.4	39.4
Race/ethnicity3 White	48.7	16.7	23.3	7.2	81.6	7.5	29.8	43.7
Black	37.0	10.8	15.3	9.6	77.0	7.0!	25.0	45.0
Hispanic	47.8	12.1	25.7	9.2	78.6	6.3!	29.0	41.9
Asian	37.9	14.7	17.3	5.4	‡	‡	‡	‡
Pacific Islander	‡	‡	‡	‡	‡	‡	‡	‡

	Full-time college students				Part-time college students			
		Hours worked per week[1]				Hours worked per week[1]		
Selected characteristic	Percent employed[2]	Less than 20 hours	20–34 hours	35 or more hours	Percent employed[2]	Less than 20 hours	20–34 hours	35 or more hours
American Indian/								
Alaska Native	‡	‡	‡	‡	‡	‡	‡	‡
More than one race	48.0	12.7!	19.4	13.8!	‡	‡	‡	‡
School type 2-year	53.4	15.4	27.5	9.1	81.5	8.1	31.2	41.9
Public	54.8	15.8	28.5	8.9	81.0	8.3	30.1	42.2
Private	40.0	11.5	17.5	11.0	‡	‡	‡	‡
4-year	44.3	15.3	20.3	7.4	79.5	7.0	27.0	44.5
Public	46.7	14.4	22.8	8.1	79.4	6.9	27.3	44.1
Private	36.4	18.3	12.1	4.8	79.9	7.8!	24.6	47.6
Graduate	46.3	11.2	21.7	12.8	85.3	5.7!	18.6	60.9

! Interpret data with caution (estimates are unstable).

‡ Reporting standards not met (too few cases).

[1] Excludes those who were employed but not at work during the survey week; therefore, detail may not sum to total percentage employed. *Hours worked per week* refers to the number of hours the respondent worked at all jobs during the survey week.

[2] Includes those who were employed but not at work during the survey week.

[3] Race categories exclude persons of Hispanic ethnicity.

Note: College includes both 2- and 4-year institutions. College students were classified as attending full time if they were taking at least 12 hours of classes (or at least 9 hours of graduate classes) during an average school week and as part time if they were taking fewer hours.

Source: U.S. Department of Commerce, Census Bureau, Current Population Survey (CPS), October Supplement, 2006.

In: The Condition of Education in America
Editor: Maurice H. Logan
ISBN: 978-1-60692-298-9

Appendix 2

SUPPLEMENTAL NOTES

NOTE 1: COMMONLY USED VARIABLES

Certain common variables, such as parents' education, race/ethnicity, community type, poverty, and geographic region are used by different surveys cited in *The Condition of Education 2008.* The definitions for these variables can vary across surveys and sometimes vary between different time periods of a single survey. This supplemental note describes how several common variables, used in various indicators in this volume, are defined in each of the surveys. In addition, this note describes certain terms used in several indicators.

Parents' Education

Parents' level of education is generally measured by either the mother's highest level of education attained or the highest level of education attained by either parent. *Indicators 12, 13, 14,* and *15* report parents' highest level of education based on a question in the National Assessment of Educational Progress (NAEP) that asks students in 8th and 12th grades to indicate the highest level of education completed by each parent. Students could choose from "did not finish high school," "graduated from high school," "some education after high school," "graduated from college," and "I don't know."

Indicator 2, based on the Early Childhood Longitudinal Survey, Birth Cohort (ECLS-B), is derived from parent interview information on the highest educational attainment of the parents or nonparental guardians who reside in the household. Respondents were asked to indicate the highest level of education they had completed and these responses were coded "no formal schooling," "1st grade," "2nd grade," "3rd grade," "4th grade," "5th grade," "6th grade," "7th grade," "8th grade," "9th grade," "10th grade," "11th grade," "12th grade but no diploma," "high school diploma/equivalent," "voc/tech program after high school but no voc/tech diploma," "voc/tech diploma after high school," "some college but no degree," "associate's degree," "bachelor's degree," "graduate or professional school but no degree," "master's degree," "doctorate degree," and "professional degree after bachelor's degree." For this volume, the responses were collapsed into a four-category variable: (1) less than high school, (2) high school completion, (3) some college/vocational, and (4) bachelor's degree and any graduate school.

Race/Ethnicity

Classifications indicating racial/ethnic heritage are based primarily on the respondent's selfidentification, as is the case with data collected by the U.S. Census Bureau, or in rare instances, on observer identification. These categories are in accordance with the Office of Management and Budget's standard classification scheme.

Ethnicity is based on the following categorization:

- Hispanic or Latino: A person of Cuban, Mexican, Puerto Rican, South or Central American, or other Spanish culture or origin, regardless of race.

Race is based on the following categorization:

- *American Indian or Alaska Native:* A person having origins in any of the original peoples of North and South America (including Central America) who maintains tribal affiliation or community attachment.
- *Asian:* A person having origins in any of the original peoples of the Far East, Southeast Asia, the Indian subcontinent, including, for example, Cambodia, China, India, Japan, Korea, Malaysia, Pakistan, the Philippines, Thailand, and Vietnam.
- *Black:* A person having origins in any of the Black racial groups of Africa.
- *Native Hawaiian or Other Pacific Islander:* A person having origins in any of the original peoples of Hawaii, Guam, Samoa, or other Pacific Islands.
- *White:* A person having origins in any of the original peoples of Europe, North Africa, or the Middle East.
- *More than one race:* A person who selected two or more of the following racial categories when offered the option of selecting one or more racial designations: White, Black, Asian, Native Hawaiian or Other Pacific Islander, or American Indian or Alaska Native.

Race categories presented in *The Condition of Education 2008* exclude persons of Hispanic ethnicity; thus, the race/ethnicity categories are mutually exclusive. Not all categories are shown in all indicators. In some cases, categories are omitted because there are insufficient data in some of the smaller categories or because survey sampling plans did not distinguish between groups (between Asians and Pacific Islanders, for example). In other cases, omissions occur because only comparable data categories are shown. For example, the category "More than one race," which was introduced in the 2000 Census and became a regular category for data collection in the Current Population Survey (CPS) in 2003, is sometimes excluded from indicators that present a historical series of data with constant categories, and it is sometimes included within the category "Other."

The introduction of the category "More than one race" follows a change in the Office of Management and Budget's standard classification scheme for race/ethnicity. This change has required changes to the questions asked by the CPS, and it will require further changes to the questions asked of future federal survey participants. As a result of the new classification scheme, distributions by race/ethnicity for 2003 CPS data and for later years may differ somewhat from those in earlier years. In the Census population estimates for July 1, 2007, about 1.6 percent of the national population were classified as "More than one race." (For further details, see http://www.census.gov/ popest/national/.)

In The Condition of Education 2008, the above definitions of race/ethnicity apply to *indicators*

2, 4, 5, 7, 8, 11, 12, 13, 14, 15, 16, 17, 20, 21, 23, 24, 25, 26, 28, 29, and *30.*

Community Type

There are various classification systems that federal departments and agencies use to define community types. Indicators in *The Condition of Education* rely on one or a combination of the following three classification systems: the Office of Management and Budget's system of *metropolitan areas,* which is used by the Census Bureau; the Census Bureau's system of *urbanized/urban/rural areas;* and the National Center for Education Statistics (NCES) system of *locale codes.* All three of these classification systems were revised in 2000 and were fully in effect by 2003. In 2006, a new urban-centric classification system for NCES locale codes was released.

Metropolitan Areas

The Census Bureau's Current Population Survey (CPS) classifies community type based on the concept of a metropolitan area, which has changed in its application over time. Between 1990 and 2000, the Census and the CPS used the term "metropolitan area" (MA) to refer collectively to Metropolitan Statistical Areas (MSAs), Primary Metropolitan Statistical Areas (PMSAs), and Consolidated Metropolitan Statistical Areas (CMSAs) (defined below). In 2000, the Census adopted the term "Core Based Statistical Area" (CBSA), which refers collectively to metropolitan statistical areas and (the newly introduced concept of) micropolitan statistical areas.

Metropolitan Areas—1990 Standards

The Office of Management and Budget (OMB) defines and designates metropolitan areas, following standards established by the interagency Federal Executive Committee on Metropolitan Areas, with the aim of producing definitions that are as consistent as possible for all MAs nationwide. Under its 1990 standards, the OMB defined an MA as "a large population nucleus together with adjacent communities that have a high degree of economic and social integration with that core." The Census Bureau used this definition for an MA from 1990 to 2000. (See http://www.census.gov/prod/cen1990/cph-s/ cph-s-1-1.pdf for more details.)

In order to be designated as an MA under the 1990 standards, an area had to meet one or both of the following criteria: (1) include a city with a population of at least 50,000 or (2) include a Census Bureau-defined urbanized area of at least 50,000 and have a total MA population of at least 100,000 (75,000 in New England). Under the 1990 standards, the "central county" (or counties) contained either the central city (defined below) or at least 50 percent of the population of the central city, or had at least 50 percent of its population in an urbanized area. Additional "outlying counties" were included in the MA if they met specified requirements of commuting to the central counties and selected requirements of metropolitan character (such as population density and percent urban). In New England, MAs were defined in terms of cities and towns, following rules analogous to those used with counties elsewhere.

The individual counties (or other geographic entities) comprising each MA were either designated as a Metropolitan Statistical Area (MSA) or, if the MA was large enough (1 million in population or more), as a Consolidated Metropolitan Statistical Area (CMSA) composed of two or more Primary Metropolitan Statistical Areas (PMSAs). For example, the PMSA "Milwaukee-Waukesha, WI" combined with the PMSA "Racine, WI" to form the CMSA of "Milwaukee-Racine, WI." CMSAs could span states, as was the case with the CMSA "Philadelphia-Wilmington-Atlantic City, PANJDE-MD." (In June 1999, there were 258 MSAs and 18 CMSAs in the United States, which included a total of 73 PMSAs.)

All territory, population, and housing units inside of MAs were characterized as *metropolitan.* Any territory, population, or housing units located outside of an MA were defined as *nonmetropolitan.* The largest city in each MA was designated a *central city,* and additional cities could qualify as such if specified requirements were met concerning population size and commuting patterns. (In June 1999, there were 542 central cities in the United States plus 12 in Puerto Rico.)

Together these classifications were used to define a location's MA Status as

1. Central city,
2. Balance of an MA (meaning any territory that is metropolitan but not in a central city), or
3. Nonmetropolitan.

Metropolitan and Micropolitan Statistical Areas —2000 Standards

In 2000, the OMB defined metropolitan and micropolitan statistical areas as "a core area containing a substantial population nucleus, together with adjacent communities having a high degree of economic and social integration with that core." Together metropolitan and micropolitan statistical areas are considered to constitute the "Core Based Statistical Area" (CBSA). Currently defined metropolitan and micropolitan statistical areas are based on the application of OMB's 2000 standards to 2000 decennial census data. (Current metropolitan and micropolitan statistical area definitions were announced by OMB effective June 6, 2003.)

In order to be designated as a CBSA under the 2000 standards, an area must contain at least one "urban" area (that is, an urbanized area or urban cluster—see definitions of urbanized area and urban cluster below) with a population of 10,000 or more. Each metropolitan statistical area—now referred to as a "metro area" to distinguish it from the metropolitan statistical areas referred to as "MSAs" under the 1990 standards—must have at least one urbanized area of 50,000 or more inhabitants. Each micropolitan statistical area must have at least one urban cluster of at least 10,000 but less than 50,000 population. Under the standards, the county (or counties) in which at least 50 percent of the population resides within urban areas of 10,000 or more population, or that contains at least 5,000 people residing within a single urban area of 10,000 or more population, is identified as a "central county" (counties). Additional "outlying counties" are included in the CBSA if they meet specified requirements of commuting to or from the central counties. Counties or equivalent entities form the geographic "building blocks" for metropolitan and micropolitan statistical areas throughout the United States and Puerto Rico. (As of June 6, 2000, there were 362 metropolitan statistical areas and 560 micropolitan statistical areas in the United States. In addition, there were eight metro areas and five micropolitan statistical areas in Puerto Rico.) (See http://www.census. gov/population/www/estimates/aboutmetro. html for more details.)

Together, these classifications are used to define a location's CBSA status (or, if no micropolitan statistical areas are included, metro area status) as

1. Principal city of a CBSA (or metro area).
2. Located in a CBSA (or metro area), but not in the principal city.
3. Not located in a CBSA (or metro area).

As with the previous MA status classifications under the 1990 standards, the CBSA status classifications under the 2000 standards do not equate to an urban-rural classification; all counties included in metropolitan and micropolitan statistical areas (and many other counties) contain both.

In *The Condition of Education 2008,* no indicators use these labels and definitions. However,
indicators 12 and *13* use the NCES 2002-revised codes that are based on the metro area labels and definitions (see exhibit A).

Urbanized, Urban, and Rural Areas

The Census Bureau divides the entire geographic area of the United States, Puerto Rico, and the Island Areas according to a concept of urban and rural areas. As with metropolitan statistical areas, the Census Bureau revised the urban/rural concept and criteria for the 2000 Census. The criteria in place between 1990 and 2000, however, were used to create the NCES codes (described below). Thus, this supplemental note explains the 1990–2000 criteria in detail for readers to understand fully the definitions.

From the adoption of the urban/rural concept for the 1950 Census until the 2000 Census, an *urbanized area* consisted of one or more "central places" and the adjacent densely settled surrounding "urban fringe" that together had a minimum population of 50,000 people. A "place" was either an incorporated governmental unit, such as a city, village, borough, or town, or a Census Designated Place (CDP), which was an unincorporated population cluster for which the Census Bureau delineates boundaries in cooperation with state and local agencies. All of the territory within the urbanized area that was outside the central place or places comprised the "urban fringe." Territory included in the urban fringe generally had a population density of at least 1,000 people per square mile but could include lower density territory that contained nonresidential urban land uses (e.g., areas zoned for commercial or industrial use or reserved for recreational purposes) or served to link outlying densely settled territory with the main body of the urbanized area. The Census Bureau defined as *urban* any incorporated places (cities, towns, villages, etc.) or CDPs outside urbanized areas that contained a population of 2,500 or more.

Exhibit A. Metropolitan areas—1990 and 2000 standards

Category	Under 1990 Standards (definitions in use from 1990–91 to 2002–03)	Under 2000 Standards (definitions in use since 2002–03)
Large city	Central city of a MA, with the city having a population of 250,000 or more.	Principal city of a metro area, with the city having a population of 250,000 or more.
Midsize city	A central city of a MA, with the city having a population less than 250,000.	Central city of a metro area, with the city having a population less than 250,000.
Urban fringe of a large city	Any incorporated place, Census-designated place, or nonplace territory within a MA with a large city and defined as urbanized or urban by the Census Bureau.	Any incorporated place, Census-designated place, or nonplace territory within a metro area with a large city and defined as urbanized or urban cluster by the Census Bureau.
Urban fringe of a midsize city	Any incorporated place, Census-designated place, or nonplace territory within a MA with a midsize city and defined as urbanized or urban by the Census Bureau.	Any incorporated place, Census-designated place, or nonplace territory within a metro area with a midsize city and defined as urbanized or urban cluster by the Census Bureau.
Large town	An incorporated place or Census-designated place with a population greater than or equal to 25,000 and located outside a MA.	Any incorporated place or Census-designated place with a population greater than or equal to 25,000 and located outside of a metro area.
Small town	An incorporated place or Census-designated place with population less than 25,000 and greater than or equal to 2,500 and located outside a MA.	Any incorporated place or Census-designated place with a population less than 25,000 and greater than or equal to 2,500 and located outside of a metro area.
Rural (Rural, outside MA or metro area)	Any incorporated place, Census-designated place, or nonplace territory defined as rural by the Census Bureau and not within a MA with a large or midsize city.	Any incorporated place, Census-designated place, or nonplace territory defined as rural by the Census Bureau and not within a metro area with a large or midsize city.
Rural Urban Fringe (Rural, inside MA or metro area) (This category was not used before 1998.)	Any incorporated place, Census-designated place, or nonplace territory defined as rural by the Census Bureau and within a MA with a large or midsize city.	Any incorporated place, Census-designated place, or nonplace territory defined as rural by the Census Bureau and within a metro area with a large or midsize city.

The Census Bureau also expanded the definition of places to include *extended cities.* Extended cities were incorporated places whose boundaries encompassed substantial amounts of low-density territory (less than 100 people per square mile), relative to the overall land area of the place. The Census Bureau then identified both urban and rural territory in such places, thus providing exceptions to the general rule that places were classified as entirely urban or entirely rural. There were 182 extended cities in 1990. The decision to ignore place boundaries when defining urban areas for the 2000 Census (see below) made the extended city concept obsolete; under the 2000 criteria, any place potentially can be divided into urban and rural components. No survey employed in this volume of *The Condition of Education* includes extended cities in its community type definition.

The Census Bureau then classified all territory, population, and housing units not classified as urbanized or urban as *rural.* (For further details, see http://www.census.gov/population/censusdata/urdef.txt.)

Beginning with the 2000 Census, the Census Bureau has employed new definitions of urban areas based on the concepts of an urbanized area and an urban cluster, the former being similar to the urbanized area under the 1990 definitions and the latter replacing the concept of urban fringe and urban areas. Urbanized areas and urban clusters consist of densely settled census block groups and census blocks that meet specified minimum population density requirements. Urbanized areas continue to have minimum populations of 50,000; urban clusters have populations of at least 2,500 and less than 50,000. Place boundaries are no longer taken into consideration when defining these two types of urban areas. (Under the previous classification system, place boundaries were used to determine the urban/rural classifications of territory: all incorporated places that had at least 2,500 people were classified as urban if they were outside an urbanized area.) Thus, the Census Bureau's current urban area classification provides a seamless, nationally consistent method of defining urban areas that is not affected by varying state laws governing incorporation and annexation. For further details on the revised definitions, see http://www.census. gov/geo/www/ua/ua 2k.pdf. (For differences between the 1990 Census and 2000 Census Urbanized Area Criteria, see http://www.census. gov/geo/www/ua/uac2k 90.html.)

Locale Code

In the NCES Common Core of Data (CCD), the community type of schools is classified according to an urban-centric "Locale Code" system. Locale codes are assigned to each school according to the school's physical location (longitude and latitude). There are four major categories within the urban-centric locale code classification system: (1) city, (2) suburban, (3) town, and (4) rural. Each major category is divided into three subcategories. Cities and suburban areas are subdivided into the categories of small, midsize, and large; towns and rural areas are subdivided by their proximity to an urbanized area into the categories of fringe, distant, and remote (see exhibit B). These 12 categories are based on three key concepts that the Census Bureau uses to define an area's urbanicity: *principal city, urbanized area,* and *urban cluster.* A principal city is a city that contains the primary population and economic center of a metropolitan statistical area, which, in turn, is defined as one or more contiguous counties that have a "core" area with a large population nucleus and adjacent communities that are highly integrated economically or socially with the core.

Urbanized areas and urban clusters are densely settled "cores" of Census-defined blocks with adjacent densely settled surrounding areas. Core areas with populations of 50,000 or more are designated as urbanized areas; those with populations between 25,000 and 50,000 are designated as urban clusters. For more information on urbanized areas and urban clusters, see http:// www.census.gov/geo/www/ua/ua2k.html. Rural areas are designated by Census as those areas that do not lie inside an urbanized area or urban cluster.

NCES has classified all schools into one of these 12 categories based on schools' actual addresses and their corresponding coordinates of latitude and longitude. Not only does this mean that the location of any school can be identified precisely, but also that distance measures can be used to identify town and rural subtypes. Unlike the previous classification system that differentiated towns on the basis of population size, the new system differentiates towns and rural areas on the basis of their proximity to larger urban centers.

School districts' locale codes are assigned through the use of these urban-centric locale codes, according to classification rules, such as the following: if 50 percent or more of students in the district attend schools that are located in a single locale code, that code is assigned to the district. If no single locale code accounts for 50 percent of the students, then the major category (city, suburban, town, or rural) with the greatest percentage of students determines the locale. Districts with no schools or students are given a locale code of "N." (For more information on the urban-centric locale code system, see http:// nces.ed.gov/ccd/rural locales.asp.)

Exhibit B. NCES urban-centric locale categories

Locale	Definition
City	
Large	Territory inside an urbanized area and inside a principal city with population of 250,000 or more
Midsize	Territory inside an urbanized area and inside a principal city with population less than 250,000 and greater than or equal to 100,000
Small	Territory inside an urbanized area and inside a principal city with population less than 100,000
Suburban	
Large	Territory outside a principal city and inside an urbanized area with population of 250,000 or more
Midsize	Territory outside a principal city and inside an urbanized area with population less than 250,000 and greater than or equal to 100,000
Small	Territory outside a principal city and inside an urbanized area with population less than 100,000
Town	
Fringe	Territory inside an urban cluster that is less than or equal to 10 miles from an urbanized area
Distant	Territory inside an urban cluster that is more than 10 miles and less than or equal to 35 miles from an urbanized area
Remote	Territory inside an urban cluster that is more than 35 miles from an urbanized area
Rural	
Fringe	Census-defined rural territory that is less than or equal to 5 miles from an urbanized area, as well as rural territory that is less than or equal to 2.5 miles from an urban cluster
Distant	Census-defined rural territory that is more than 5 miles but less than or equal to 25 miles from an urbanized area, as well as rural territory that is more than 2.5 miles but less than or equal to 10 miles from an urban cluster
Remote	Census-defined rural territory that is more than 25 miles from an urbanized area and is also more than 10 miles from an urban cluster

Source: Office of Management and Budget (2000). Standards for Defining Metropolitan and Micropolitan Statistical Areas; Notice. *Federal Register* (65) No. 249.

Besides being used for the CCD, the expanded 12-level locale codes are used to categorize community type in other NCES surveys. Typically, however, the locale codes are collapsed into the four major categories of city, suburban, town, and rural.

In *The Condition of Education 2008,* urban- centric locale codes are used in *indicators 4, 12, 13, 14, 15, 28, 29, 30, 32,* and *37.*

Poverty

Data on household income and the number of people living in the household are combined with estimates of the poverty threshold published by the Census Bureau to determine the poverty status of children (or adults). The thresholds used to determine poverty status for an individual differ for each survey year. The weighted average poverty thresholds for various household sizes for 1990, 1995, and 2000 through 2007 are shown in the table on the next page. (For thresholds for other years, see http://www.census.gov/hhes/www/poverty/threshld.html.)

In *indicators 6* and *7,* children in families whose incomes are below the poverty threshold are classified as *poor*; those in families with incomes at 100–199 percent of the poverty threshold are classified as *near-poor,* and those in families with incomes at 200 percent or more of the poverty threshold are classified as *nonpoor.*

Eligibility for the National School Lunch Program also serves as a measure of poverty status. The National School Lunch Program is a federally assisted meal program operated in public and private nonprofit schools and residential child care centers. Unlike the poverty thresholds discussed above, which rely on dollar amounts

determined by the Census Bureau, eligibility for the National School Lunch Program relies on the federal income poverty guidelines of the Department of Health and Human Services. To be eligible for free lunch, a student must be from a household with an income at or below 130 percent of the federal poverty guideline; to be eligible for reduced-price lunch, a student must be from a household with an income at or below 185 percent of the federal poverty guideline. Title I basic program funding relies on free lunch eligibility numbers as one (of four) possible poverty measures for levels of Title I federal funding. In *The Condition of Education 2008,* eligibility for the National School Lunch Program applies to *indicators 12, 13, 14, 15, 29,* and *31. Indicators 31* and *32* also discuss approval for the National School Lunch Program.

Small Area Income and Poverty Estimates (SAIPE) Program

The goal of the Census Bureau's Small Area Income and Poverty Estimates (SAIPE) program is to make intercensal estimates of median income and numbers in poverty for states, counties, and school districts. *Indicator 37* employs SAIPE's school district estimates of the population of children ages 5–17 and the number of related children ages 5–17 in families in poverty. *Indicator 37* employs the SAIPE data, rather than the free lunch-eligible data, to measure poverty by school district because SAIPE data are available for all regular operating school districts, while free lunch-eligible data are missing for a sizable number of school districts. Further, the SAIPE poverty data are constructed using consistent methodology, while the designation of free lunch eligibility may differ from school to school. More information about SAIPE is available at http://www.census.gov/hhes/www/saipe/.

Weighted average poverty thresholds, by household size: Selected years, 1990–2007

Household size	Poverty threshold	Household size	Poverty threshold
1990		**2003**	
2	$8,509	2	$12,015
3	10,419	3	14,680
4	13,359	4	18,810
5	15,792	5	22,245
6	17,839	6	25,122
7	20,241	7	28,544
8	22,582	8	31,589
9 or more	26,848	9 or more	37,656
1995		**2004**	
2	9,933	2	12,334
3	12,158	3	15,067
4	15,569	4	19,307
5	18,408	5	22,831
6	20,804	6	25,788
7	23,552	7	29,236
8	26,237	8	32,641
9 or more	31,280	9 or more	39,048
2000		**2005**	
2	11,239	2	12,755
3	13,738	3	15,577
4	17,603	4	19,971
5	20,819	5	23,613
6	23,528	6	26,683
7	26,754	7	30,249
8	29,701	8	33,610
9 or more	35,060	9 or more	40,288
2001		**2006**	
2	11,569	2	13,167
3	14,128	3	16,079
4	18,104	4	20,614
5	21,405	5	24,382
6	24,195	6	27,560
7	27,517	7	31,205
8	30,627	8	34,774
9 or more	36,286	9 or more	41,499
2002		**2007**	
2	11,756	2	13,542
3	14,348	3	16,537
4	18,392	4	21,201
5	21,744	5	21,201
6	24,576	6	28,345
7	28,001	7	32,094
8	30,907	8	35,764
9 or more	37,062	9 or more	42,681

Source: U.S. Census Bureau, Current Population Survey (CPS). Retrieved April 9, 2008, from http://www.census.gov/hhes/www/poverty/threshld.html.

Geographic Region

The regional classification systems below represent the four geographical regions of the United States as defined by the Census Bureau of the U.S.

Department of Commerce. In *The Condition of Education 2008, indicators 3, 4, 5, 7, 32, and 34* use this system.

U.S. Census Bureau, Regional Classification

Northeast	South	Midwest	West
Connecticut	Alabama	Illinois	Alaska
Maine	Arkansas	Indiana	Arizona
Massachusetts	Delaware	Iowa	California
New Hampshire	District of Columbia	Kansas	Colorado
New Jersey	Florida	Michigan	Hawaii
New York	Georgia	Minnesota	Idaho
Pennsylvania	Kentucky	Missouri	Montana
Rhode Island	Louisiana	Nebraska	Nevada
Vermont	Maryland	North Dakota	New Mexico
	Mississippi	Ohio	Oregon
	North Carolina	South Dakota	Utah
	Oklahoma	Wisconsin	Washington
	South Carolina		Wyoming
	Tennessee		
	Texas		
	Virginia		
	West Virginia		

Note 2: The Current Population Survey (CPS)

The Current Population Survey (CPS) is a monthly survey of a nationally representative sample of all U.S. households. The survey's scientifically selected sample consists of approximately 50,000 households from the 50 states and the District of Columbia. The population surveyed is referred to as the civilian, noninstitutional population. Members of the armed forces, inmates in correctional institutions, and patients in long-term medical or custodial facilities are not included in the sample. The CPS has been conducted for more than 50 years. The U.S. Department of Commerce, Census Bureau, conducts the survey for the Bureau of Labor Statistics, asking a knowledgeable adult household member (known as the "household respondent") to answer all the questions on all of the month's questionnaires for all members of the household.

The CPS collects data on the social and economic characteristics of the civilian, noninstitutional population, including information on income, education, and participation in the labor force. However, the CPS does not collect all of this information every month. Each month a "basic" CPS questionnaire is used to collect data about participation in the labor force of each household member, age 15 or older, in every sampled household. In addition, different supplemental questionnaires are administered each month to collect information on other topics.

Each year, the March and October supplementary questionnaires contain some questions of relevance to education policy. The Annual Social and Economic Supplement, or March CPS Supplement, is a primary source of detailed information on income and work experience in the United States. The labor force and work experience data from this survey are used to profile the U.S. labor market and to make employment projections. Data from this survey are also used to generate the annual Population Profile of the United States, reports on geographical mobility, educational attainment, and detailed analyses of wage rates, earnings, and poverty status. The October Supplement contains basic annual school enrollment data for preschool, elementary and secondary, and postsecondary students, as well as educational background information needed to produce dropout estimates on an annual basis. In addition to the basic questions about education, interviewers also ask questions about school enrollment for all household members age 3 or older.

CPS interviewers initially used printed questionnaires. However, since 1994, the Census Bureau has used Computer-Assisted Personal and Telephone Interviewing (CAPI and CATI) to collect data. Both technologies allow interviewers to use a complex questionnaire and increase consistency by reducing interviewer error. Further information on the CPS can be found at http://www.census.gov/cps.

Definition of Selected Variables

Employment Status

Indicator 20 uses data from the March CPS and its supplement, which include questions on employment of adults in the previous week, to determine employment status. Respondents could report that they were employed (either full or part time), unemployed (looking for work or on layoff), or not in the labor force (due to being retired, having unpaid employment, or some other reason).

Indicator 43 uses data from the October CPS and its supplement, which also include questions on employment of adults in the previous week to determine employment status. Employed persons include those age 16 or older, who, during the reference week, (1) did any work at all (at least 1 hour) as paid employees, or (2) were not working but who had jobs or businesses from which they were temporarily absent because of vacation, illness, bad weather, child care problems, maternity or paternity leave, labor-management dispute, job training, or other family or personal reasons, whether or not they were paid for the time off or were seeking other jobs.

Hours Worked per Week

Indicator 43 presents data on the number of hours worked per week. This estimate is the number of hours a respondent worked in all jobs in the week prior to the time of the survey interview. The population for this variable includes any employed person who also worked in the week prior to the time of the survey interview. The sum of the categories may not equal the total percentage employed because those who were employed, but did not work in the previous week, were excluded.

Family Income

Indicator 24 uses data on family income that are collected as part of the October CPS to measure a student's economic standing. The October CPS determines family income from a single question asked of the household respondent. Family income includes all monetary income from all sources (including jobs, businesses, interest, rent, and social security payments) over a 12-month period. The income of nonrelatives living in the household is excluded, but the income of all family members age 15 or older (age 14 or older before 1989), including those temporarily living away, is included.

In indicator 24, family income of a recent high school graduate is defined as the income of the household where the graduate has membership. A household is defined as all individuals whose usual place of residence at the time of the interview is the sample unit. The following considerations guide the determination of household members:

- *Persons staying in the sample housing unit at the time of the interview:* Persons for whom the household is their usual place of residence are included in the household membership. Persons who are living in the household temporarily (such as students) and who have living quarters held elsewhere are not considered part of the household, unless they are living with their spouse or children.
- *Persons who usually live in the sample housing unit and are absent at the time of the interview:* Individuals who are temporarily absent and who have no other usual place of residence are classified as household members even if they are not present in the household during the survey week. If such persons are away temporarily attending school, they are considered part of the household unless they are living with their spouse or children.

Families in the bottom 20 percent of all family incomes are classified as low income; families in the top 20 percent of all family incomes are classified as high income; and families in the 60 percent between these two categories are classified as middle income. The table on the next page shows the current dollar amount of the breakpoints between low and middle income and between middle and high income used in *indicator 24*. For example, low income for families in 2006 is defined as the range from $0 to $18,000; middle income is defined as the range from $18,000 to $84,500; and high income is defined as $84,500 or more.

Median Earnings

Indicator 20 uses data on earnings that are collected as part of the March CPS. The March CPS collects information on earnings from individuals who were full-year workers (individuals who were employed 50 or more weeks in the previous year) and full-time workers (those who were usually employed 35 or more hours per week). Earnings include all wage and salary income. Unlike mean earnings, median earnings do not change or change very little in response to extreme observations.

Dollar value (in current dollars) at the breakpoint between low- and middle-income and between middle- and highincome categories of family income: October 1972–2006

Year	Breakpoints between low- and middle-income	Breakpoints between middle- and high-income
1972	$3,600	$13,600
1973	3,900	14,800
1974	—	—
1975	4,400	17,000
1976	4,600	18,300
1977	4,900	20,000
1978	5,300	21,600
1979	5,800	23,700
1980	6,100	25,300
1981	6,500	27,100
1982	7,200	31,200
1983	7,300	32,300
1984	7,500	34,200
1985	7,900	36,400
1986	8,400	38,100
1987	8,800	39,600
1988	9,300	42,100
1989	9,500	43,900
1990	9,600	46,200
1991	10,500	48,300
1992	10,700	49,600
1993	10,800	50,600
1994	11,900	55,500
1995	11,700	56,100
1996	12,300	58,100
1997	12,800	60,800
1998	13,900	64,900
1999	14,700	68,200
2000	15,300	71,900
2001	16,300	75,000
2002	16,700	75,400
2003	16,600	75,500
2004	16,000	77,100
2005	16,800	80,700
2006	18,000	84,500

—Not available

SOURCE: U.S. Department of Commerce, Census Bureau, Current Population Survey (CPS), October Supplement, 1972–2006.

Race/Ethnicity

Over time, the CPS has had different response options for race/ethnicity. From 1972 through 1988, the response options were limited to White, Black, Hispanic, and Other. From 1989 through 1995, the response options included White, Black, American Indian/Aleut

Eskimo, Asian/Pacific Islander, Hispanic, and Other. From 1996 through 2002, the response options included White, Black, American Indian/Aleut Eskimo, Asian/Pacific Islander, and Hispanic. From 2003 through the present, the response options included White, Black, American Indian/Alaskan Native, Asian, Hawaiian/Pacific Islander, and Hispanic and allowed respondents to select more than one race category. Race cat egories presented in *The Condition of Education 2008* exclude persons of Hispanic ethnicity; thus, the race/ethnicity categories are mutually exclusive. *Indicators 5, 6, 20, 23, 24, 25,* and *43* present data by race/ethnicity using CPS data. See *supplemental note 1* for more information on race/ethnicity.

Enrolled in School

In *indicator 5,* which presents the racial/ethnic distribution of public school students, the data for 1979 and 1980 are missing because the data for the variable "attending school" were judged unaccept able due to an error in the design of the question naire; therefore, the records are all blank.

Status Dropout Rate

Indicator 23 reports status dropout rates by race/ethnicity. The status dropout rate is one of a number of rates that are used to report high school dropout and completion behavior in the United States. Status dropout rates measure the percentage of individuals within a given age range who are not enrolled in high school and who lack a high school credential, irrespective of when they dropped out. Because they measure the extent of the dropout problem for the sampled population, status dropout rates can be used to estimate the need for further education and training for dropouts in that population. Status dropout rates should not be confused with event dropout rates, which measure the proportion of students who drop out of high school in a given year, and which have been reported in a previous volume of *The Condition of Education* (NCES 2004-077, *indicator 16;* see also NCES 2005-046).

Indicator 23 uses the October CPS data to estimate the status dropout rate, or the percentage of civilian, noninstitutionalized young people ages 16 through 24 who are out of high school and who have not earned a high school credential (either a diploma or equivalency credential such as a General Educational Development certificate [GED]). Status dropout rates count as dropouts individuals who never attended school and immigrants who did not complete the equivalent of a high school education in their home country. The inclusion of these individuals is appropriate because the status dropout rate is designed to report the percentage of youth and young adults in the United States who lack what is now considered a basic level of educa tion. However, the status dropout rate should not be used as a measure of the performance of U.S. schools because it counts as dropouts individuals who may have never attended a U.S. school.

The numerator of the status dropout rate for a given year is the number of individuals ages 16 through 24 who, as of October of that year, had not completed high school and were not currently enrolled in school. The denominator is the total number of individuals ages 16 through 24 in the United States in October of that year.

The CPS October Supplement items used to identify status dropouts include (1) "Is ... attending or enrolled in regular school?" and (2) "What is the highest level of school ... completed or the highest degree ... received?" See the Edu cational Attainment section, below, for details on how the second question changed from 1972 to 1992. Beginning in 1986, the Census Bureau instituted new editing procedures for cases with missing data on school enrollment, i.e., missing data relating to the first October supplement item, above. These changes were made in an effort to improve data quality. The effect of the editing changes was evaluated by applying both the old and new editing procedures to the data from 1986. The changes resulted in an increase in the number of students enrolled in school and a slightly lowered status dropout rate (12.2 percent based on the old procedures, and 12.1 percent based on the new ones). The difference in the two rates was not statistically significant. While the change in the procedures occurred in 1986, the new procedures are reflected in *indicator 23* beginning in 1987.

Educational Attainment

Data from CPS questions on educational attainment are used in *indicators 6, 20, 24,* and *25*. From 1972 to 1991, two CPS questions provided data on the number of years of school completed: (1) "What is the highest grade ... ever attended?" and (2) "Did ... complete it?" An individual's educational attainment was considered to be his or her last fully completed year of school. Individuals who completed 12 years were deemed to be high school graduates, as were those who began but did not complete the first year of college. Respondents who completed 16 or more years were counted as college graduates.

Beginning in 1992, the CPS combined the two questions into the following question: "What is the highest level of school ... completed or the highest degree ... received?" This change means that some data collected before 1992 are not strictly comparable with data collected from 1992 onward and that care must be taken when making such comparisons. The new question revision changed the response categories from highest grade completed to highest level of schooling or degree completed.

In the revised response categories, several of the lower grade levels are combined into a single summary category such as "1st, 2nd, 3rd, or 4th grades." Several new categories are used, including "12th grade, no diploma"; "High school graduate, high school diploma, or the equivalent"; and "Some college but no degree." College degrees are now listed by type, allowing for a more accurate description of educational attainment. The new question emphasizes credentials received rather than the last grade level attended or completed. The new categories include the following:

- High school graduate, high school diploma, or the equivalent (e.g., GED)
- Some college but no degree
- Associate's degree in college, occupational/ vocational program
- Associate's degree in college, academic program
- Bachelor's degree (e.g., B.A., A.B., B.S.)
- Master's degree (e.g., M.A., M.S., M.Eng., M.Ed., M.S.W., M.B.A.)
- Professional school degree (e.g., M.D., D.D.S., D.V.M., LL.B., J.D.)
- Doctorate degree (e.g., Ph.D., Ed.D.)

High School Completion

The pre-1988 questions about educational attainment did not specifically consider high school equivalency certificates (GEDs). Consequently, an individual who attended 10th grade, dropped out without completing that grade, and who subsequently received a high school equivalency credential would not have been counted as completing high school. The new question counts these individuals as if they are high school completers. Since 1988, an additional question has also asked respondents if they have a high school degree or the equivalent, such as a GED. People who respond "yes" are classified as high school completers. Before 1988, the number of individuals who earned a high school equivalency certificate was small relative to the number of high school graduates, so that the subsequent increase caused by including equivalency certificate recipients in the total number of people counted as "high school completers" was small in the years immediately after the change was made.

Before 1992, the CPS considered individuals who completed 12th grade to be high school graduates. The revised question added the response category "12th grade, no diploma." Individuals who select this response are not counted as graduates. Historically, the number of individuals in this category has been small.

College Completion

Some students require more than 4 years to earn an undergraduate degree, so some researchers are concerned that the completion rate, based on the pre-1992 category "4th year or higher of college completed," overstates the number of respondents with a bachelor's degree (or higher). In fact, however, the completion rates among those ages 25–29 in 1992 and 1993 were similar to the completion rates for those in 1990 and 1991, before the change in the question's wording. Thus, there appears to be good reason to conclude that the change has not affected the completion rates reported in *The Condition of Education 2008.*

Some College

Based on the question used in 1992 and in subsequent surveys, an individual who attended college for less than a full academic year would respond "some college but no degree." Before 1992, the appropriate response would have been "attended first year of college and did not complete it," thereby excluding those individuals from the calculation of the percentage of the population with 1–3 years of college. With the new question, such respondents are placed in the "some college but no degree" category.

Thus, the percentage of individuals with some college might be larger than the percentage with 1–3 years of college because "some college" includes those who have not completed an entire year of college, whereas "1–3 years of college" does not include them. Therefore, it is not appropriate to make comparisons between the percentage of those with "some college but no degree" using the post-1991 question and the percentage of those who completed "1–3 years of college" using the two pre-1992 questions.

In *The Condition of Education,* the "some college" category for years preceding 1992 includes only the responses "1–3 years of college." After 1991, the "some college" cat egory includes those who responded "some college but no degree," "associate's degree in college, occupational/vocational program," and "associate's degree in college, academic program." The effect of this change to the "some college" category is indicated by the fact that in 1992, 48.9 percent of 25- to 29-year-olds reported completing some college or more, compared with

45.3 percent in 1991 (see *indicator 25,* table 25-2). The 3.6 percent dif ference is statistically significant. Some of the increase between 1991 and 1992 may be the result of individuals who completed less than 1 year of postsecondary education responding differently to the "completed some college" category; that is, including themselves in the category in 1992, but not including themselves in the category in 1991.

Another potential difference in the "some college" category is how individuals who have completed a certificate or other type of award other than a degree respond to the new questions introduced in 1992 about their educational attainment. Some may answer "some college, no degree"; others may indicate only high school completion; and still others may equate their certificate with one of the types of associate's degrees. No information is available on the tendencies of individuals with a postsecondary credential other than a bachelor's or higher degree to respond to the new attainment question introduced in 1992.

Parental Education

Parents' education is defined as either the high- est educational attainment of the two parents who reside with the student or, if only one parent is in the residence, the highest educational attainment of that parent. When neither parent resides with the student, it is defined as the highest educational attainment of the householder. *Indicators 6* and *24* present data by parents' education.

NOTE 3: OTHER SURVEYS

American Community Survey (ACS)

The Census Bureau introduced the American Community Survey (ACS) in 1996. Fully implemented in 2005, it provides a large monthly sample of demographic, socioeco nomic, and housing data comparable in content to the Long Form of the Decennial Census. Aggregated over time, these data will serve as a replacement for the Long Form of the De cennial Census. The survey includes questions mandated by federal law, federal regulations, and court decisions.

Beginning in 2005, the survey has been mailed to approximately 250,000 addresses in the United States and Puerto Rico each month, or about 2.5 percent of the population annu ally. A larger proportion of addresses in small governmental units (e.g., American Indian reservations, small counties, and towns) receive the survey. The monthly sample size is designed to approximate the ratio used in Cen sus 2000, requiring more intensive distribution in these areas.

National-level data from ACS are available starting with the year 2000. Under the current timetable, annual results were or will be available for areas with populations of 65,000 or more beginning in the summer of 2006, for areas with populations of 20,000 or more in the summer of 2008, and for all areas—down to the census tract level—by the summer of 2010. This schedule is based on the time it will take to collect data from a sample size large enough to produce accurate results for different size geographic units.

Indicator 7 uses data from the ACS for the years 2000–06. For further details on the survey, see http://www.census.gov/acs/www/.

Common Core of Data (CCD)

The NCES Common Core of Data (CCD), the Department of Education's primary database on public elementary and secondary education in the United States, is a comprehensive annual, national statistical database of information concerning all public elementary and secondary schools (approximately 94,000) and school districts (approximately 17,000). The CCD consists of five surveys that state education departments complete annually from their administrative records. The database includes a general description of schools and school districts; data on students and staff, including demographics; and fiscal data, including revenues and current expenditures.

Indicators 3, 21, 29, 30, 33, 34, 35, 36, and *37* use data from the CCD. Further information about the database is available at http://nces. ed.gov/ccd/.

Early Childhood Longitudinal Study, Birth Cohort

The Early Childhood Longitudinal Study, Birth Cohort (ECLS-B) is designed to provide detailed information on children's development, health, and early learning experiences in the years leading up to entry into school. The ECLS-B is the first nationally representative study within the United States to directly assess children's early mental and physical development, the quality of their early care and education settings, and the contributions of their fathers, as well as their mothers, to their lives. The children participating in the ECLS-B are followed from birth through kindergarten entry. To date, information has been collected from children and their parents during three rounds of data collection: rounds were conducted when the children were about 9 months old (2001), about 2 years old (2003), and about preschool age, or about 4 years old (2005). Data were collected on a nationally representative sample of 14,000 children born in the year 2001. Their experiences are representative of the experiences of the approximately 4 million children born in the United States in 2001.

Children, their parents, their child care providers, their teachers, and their school administrators provide information on children's cognitive, social, emotional and physical development across multiple settings (e.g., home, child care, school). At all waves of data collection (9 months, 2 years, preschool, and kindergarten), parents are asked about themselves, their families, and their children; fathers are asked about themselves and their roles in their children's lives; and children are observed and participate in assessment activities. In addition, when the children are 2 years old and in preschool (about 4 years old), early care and education providers are asked to provide information about their own experience and training and the setting's learning environment. When the ECLS-B children are in kindergarten, teachers are also asked to provide information about the children's early learning and the school and classroom environments. Trained assessors visit children in their homes. With the parent's permission, children participate in activities designed to measure important developmental skills in the cognitive, language, social, emotional, and physical domains.

Trained assessors also conduct a computer-assisted interview with the sampled child's primary caregiver, most frequently the mother.

With the permission of the child's parents, individuals and organizations who provide regular care for the child are interviewed. Trained staff conduct a computer-assisted interview over the phone. For home-based care settings, the primary provider is interviewed about the care setting and the sampled child's experiences there. For center-based care programs, the center director is first interviewed for general information about the program; the sampled child's primary provider in the center is then interviewed about the group care environment and the child's experiences. Child care settings were subsampled then observed and rated.

Child's Primary Type of Nonparental Early Care and Education

Parents were asked if they currently had regular early care and education arrangements for their child, and, if so, were then asked how many hours per week their child spent in that setting. This composite measure presents information on the type of nonparental care and education in which the child spent the most hours, which is identified as the primary care arrangement. The composite was created by reviewing the number of hours the child spent in each arrangement and identifying the one where the child spent the most hours. If a child spent equal time in each of two or more types of arrangements, care was coded as "multiple care arrangements." Children with no regular nonparental care arrangements were coded as "no child care." For this presentation of primary care, Head Start refers to services received at a public or private school, religious center, or private home, as reported by the parent. "Regular" refers to arrangements that occurred on a routine schedule (i.e., occurring at least weekly or on some other schedule), not including occasional babysitting or "back-up" arrangements.

Integrated Postsecondary Education Data System (IPEDS)

The Integrated Postsecondary Education Data System (IPEDS) is the core program that NCES uses for collecting data on postsecondary education. (Before IPEDS, some of the same information was collected by the Higher Education General Information Survey [HEGIS].) *Indicators 9, 11,* and *42* use data from HEGIS. IPEDS is a single, comprehensive sys tem that encompasses all identified institutions whose primary purpose is to provide postsec ondary education.

IPEDS consists of institution-level data that can be used to describe trends in postsecondary education at the institution, state, and/or national levels. For example, researchers can use IPEDS to analyze information on (1) enrollments of undergraduates, first-time freshmen, and graduate and first-professional students by race/ethnicity and sex; (2) institutional revenue and expenditure patterns by source of income and type of expense; (3) salaries of full-time instructional faculty by academic rank and tenure status; (4) completions (awards) by type of program, level of award, race/ethnicity, and sex; (5) characteristics of postsecondary institutions, including tuition, room and board charges, calendar systems, and so on; (6) status of postsecondary vocational education programs; and (7) other issues of interest.

Participation in IPEDS was a requirement for the 6,700 institutions that participated in Title IV federal student financial aid programs such as Pell Grants or Stafford Loans during the 2006–07 academic year. Title IV institutions include traditional colleges and universities, 2-year institutions, and for-profit degree- and non-degree-granting institutions (such as schools of cosmetology), among others. Each of these three categories is further disaggregated by control (public, private not-for-profit, and private for-profit), resulting in nine institutional categories, or sectors. In addition, 84 administrative offices (central and system offices) listed in the IPEDS universe were expected to provide minimal data through a shortened version of the Institutional Characteristics component. Four of the U.S. service academies are included in the IPEDS universe as if they were Title IV institutions. Institutions that do not participate in Title IV programs may participate in the IPEDS data collection on a voluntary basis.

IPEDS data for 1999 were imputed using alternative procedures. See NCES 2008-022, Guide to Sources, for more information.

Indicators 9, 11, 26, 27, 39, 40, and *42* use data from IPEDS. The institutional categories used in the surveys are described in *supplemental note 9*. Further information about IPEDS is available at http://nces.ed.gov/ipeds/.

Private School Universe Survey (PSS)

The Private School Universe Survey (PSS) was established in 1988 to ensure that private school data dating back to 1890 would be collected on a more regular basis. With the help of the Census Bureau, the PSS is conducted biennially to provide the total number of private schools, students, and teachers, and to build a universe of private schools in the 50 states and the District of Columbia to serve as a sampling frame of private schools for NCES sample surveys.

In the most recent PSS data collection, conducted in 2005–06, the survey was sent to 31,848 qualified private schools, and it had a response rate of 94.3 percent.

Indicator 4 uses data from the PSS. Further information on the survey is available at http:// nces.ed.gov/surveys/pss/.

School Survey on Crime and Safety (SSOCS)

The School Survey on Crime and Safety (SSOCS) focuses on incidents of specific crimes and offenses and a variety of specific discipline issues in public schools. SSOCS was administered in the spring of the 1999–2000, 2003–04, and 2005–06 school years. The survey also covers characteristics of school policies, school violence prevention programs and policies, and school characteristics that have been associated with school crime. The survey was conducted with a nationally representative sample of regular public primary, middle, high, and combined schools in the 50 states and the District of Columbia.

In the 2005–06 school year, a total of 3,565 schools were selected for the study. In March 2006, questionnaires were mailed to school principals, who were asked to complete the survey or to have it completed by the person most knowledgeable about discipline issues at the school. “At school” was defined for respondents to include activities that happen in school buildings, on school grounds, on school buses, and at places that hold school-sponsored events or activities. Respondents were instructed to provide information on the total number of recorded incidents and the number of incidents reported to the police or other law enforcement. Respondents were instructed to provide information on the number of incidents, not the number of victims or offenders, regardless of whether any disciplinary action was taken or whether students or nonstudents were involved. In the questions pertaining to *indicator 28,* respondents were instructed to record incidents occurring before, during, or after normal school hours. Due to changes to questionnaire items between survey iterations, data may be unavailable for some survey years. A total of 2,724 schools completed the survey. For more information about the SSOCS, visit http://nces.ed.gov/surveys/ssocs/.

Schools And Staffing Survey (SASS)

The Schools and Staffing Survey (SASS) is the nation's largest sample survey of America's elementary and secondary schools. First conducted in 1987–88, SASS periodically surveys the following:

- surveys public schools and collects data on school districts, schools, principals, teachers, and library media centers;
- surveys private schools and collects data on schools, principals, teachers, and library media centers;
- surveys schools operated by the Bureau of Indian Affairs (BIA) and collects data on schools, principals, teachers, and library media centers; and
- surveys public charter schools and collects data on schools, principals, teachers, and library media centers.

To ensure that the samples contain sufficient numbers for estimates, SASS uses a stratified probability sample design. Public and private schools are oversampled into groups based on certain characteristics. After the schools are stratified and sampled, the teachers within the schools are stratified and sampled based on their characteristics. For the 2003–04 SASS, a sample of public charter schools was included in the sample as part of the public school questionnaire.

Indicators 31 and *32* use data from the SASS. Further information about the survey is available at http://nces.ed.gov/surveys/SASS/.

The National Assessment of Educational Progress (NAEP), governed by the National Assessment Governing Board (NAGB), is administered regularly in a number of academic subjects. Since its creation in 1969, NAEP has had two major goals: to assess student performance reflecting current educational and assessment practices and to measure change in student performance reliably over time. To address these goals, NAEP includes a main assessment and a long-term trend assessment. The two assessments are administered to separate samples of students at separate times, use separate instruments, and measure different educational content. Thus, results from the two assessments should not be compared.

Main NAEP

Indicators 12, 13, 14, 15, and 16 are based on the main NAEP. Begun in 1990, the main NAEP periodically assesses students' performance in several subjects in grades 4, 8, and 12, following the assessment framework developed by NAGB and using the latest advances in assessment methodology. NAGB develops the frameworks using standards developed within the field, using a consensus process involving educators, subject-matter experts, and other interested citizens. Each round of the main NAEP includes a student assessment and background questionnaires (for the student, teacher, and school) to provide information on instructional experiences and the school environment at each grade.

Since 1990, NAEP assessments have also been conducted to give results for participating states. States that choose to participate receive assessment results that report on the performance of students within the state. In its content, the state assessment is identical to the assessment conducted nationally. However, because the national NAEP samples were not, and are not, designed to support the reporting of accurate and representative state-level results, separate representative samples of students are selected for each participating jurisdiction/state.

Beginning with the 2002 assessments, a combined sample of public schools was selected for both the state and national NAEP. This was done in response to the NCES/NAGB redesign of 1998. It was thought that, with most or almost all states participating in the state component of the NAEP, separate national samples would not be necessary. Thus, by using all students from all of the state samples to produce national estimates, the precision of estimates would be improved greatly and the burden of participation would be somewhat reduced by decreasing the total number of sampled schools. The national NAEP sample is a combination of state samples for those subjects where state scores are available at grades 4 and 8.

Therefore, since 2002, on those assessments with a state component, the main national sample includes all students assessed in the participating states. The typical sample size per grade and subject being assessed is 3,000 students from 100 schools and the Trial Urban District Assessment (TUDA) samples where applicable per state. Should any state or significant part of a state refuse to participate, a small additional sample is selected from schools in the same stratum. This additional sample ensures that the national sample is representative of the total national student population.

The ability of the assessments to measure change in student performance over time is sometimes limited by changes in the NAEP framework. While shorter term trends can be measured in most of the NAEP subjects, data from different assessments are not always comparable. (In cases where the framework of a given assessment changes, linking studies are generally conducted to ensure comparability over time.) However, recent main NAEP assessment instruments for science and reading have typically been kept stable for shorter periods, allowing for comparisons across time. For example, from 1990 to 2005, in general, assessment instruments in the same subject areas were developed using the same framework, shared a common set of questions, and used comparable procedures to sample and address student populations. In 2005, the NAGB revised the grade 12 mathematics framework to reflect changes in high school mathematics standards and coursework. As a result, even though many questions are re peated from previous assessments, the 2005 results cannot be directly compared with those from previous years.

NAGB called for the development of a new mathematics framework for the 2005 assessment. The revisions made to the mathematics framework for the 2005 assessment were intended to reflect recent curricular emphases and to include clear and more specific objectives for each grade level. The new mathematics framework focuses on two dimensions: mathematical content and cognitive demand. By considering these two dimensions for each item in the assessment, the framework ensures that NAEP assesses an appropriate balance of content along with a variety of ways of knowing and doing mathematics. For grades 4 and 8, comparisons over time can be made among the assessments prior to and after the implementation of the 2005 framework. In grade 12, with the implementation of the 2005 framework, the assessment included more questions on algebra, data analysis, and probability to reflect changes in high school mathematics standards and coursework. Additionally, the measurement and geometry content areas were merged. Grade 12 results could not be placed on the old NAEP scale and could not be directly compared with previous years. The reporting scale for grade 12 mathematics was changed from 0–500 to 0–300. For more information regarding the 2005 framework revisions, see http://nces.ed.gov/nationsreportcard/mathematics/whatmeasure.asp.

The main NAEP results are reported in The Condition of Education in terms of both average scale scores and achievement levels. The achievement levels define what students who are performing at the Basic, Proficient, and Advanced levels of achievement should know and be able to do. NAGB establishes achievement levels whenever a new main NAEP framework is adopted. As provided by law, NCES, upon review of congressionally mandated evaluations of NAEP, has determined that achievement levels are to be used on a trial basis and should be interpreted with caution. NAEP achievement levels have been widely used by national and state officials. The policy definitions of the achievement levels that apply across all grades and subject areas are as follows:

- *Basic:* This level denotes partial mastery of prerequisite knowledge and skills that are fundamental for proficient work at each grade assessed.
- *Proficient:* This level represents solid academic performance for each grade assessed. Students reaching this level have demonstrated competency over challenging subject matter, including subject-matter knowledge, application of such knowledge to real-world situations, and analytical skills appropriate to the subject matter.
- *Advanced:* This level signifies superior performance at each grade assessed.

In some indicators, the percentage of students at or above *Proficient* or at or above *Basic* are reported. The percentage of students at or above *Proficient* includes students at the *Advanced* achievement level. Similarly, the percentage of students at or above *Basic* includes students at the *Basic*, those at the *Proficient*, and those at the *Advanced* achievement levels.

Unlike estimates from other sample surveys presented in this report, NAEP estimates that are potentially unstable (large standard error compared with the estimate) are not flagged as potentially unreliable. This practice for NAEP estimates is consistent with the current output from the NAEP online data analysis tool. The reader should always consult the appropri ate standard errors when interpreting these findings. For additional information on NAEP, including technical aspects of scoring and assessment validity and more specific information on achievement levels, see http://nces.ed.gov/ nationsreportcard/.

Student Accommodations

Until 1996, the main NAEP assessments excluded certain subgroups of students identified as "special needs students," including students with disabilities and students with limited English proficiency. For the 1996 and 2000 math ematics assessments and the 1998 and 2000 reading assessments, the main NAEP included a separate assessment with provisions for accom modating these students (e.g., extended time, small group testing, mathematics questions read aloud, and so on). Thus, for these years, there are results for both the unaccommodated assessment and the accommodated assessment. For the 2002, 2003, and 2005 reading assessments and 2003 and 2005 mathematics assessments, the main NAEP did not include a separate unac commodated assessment; only a single accom modated assessment was administered. The switch to a single accommodated assessment instrument was made after it was determined that accommodations in NAEP did not have any significant effect on student scores. *Indica tors 12* and *13* present NAEP results with and without accommodations.

Long-Term Trend NAEP

The long-term trend NAEP measures basic stu dent performance in reading, mathematics, sci ence, and writing. *Indicator 17* reports findings from the long-term reading and mathematics assessments. Since the early 1970s, the long-term trend NAEP has used the same instruments to provide a means to compare performance over time, but the instruments do not necessarily reflect current teaching standards or curricula. Results have been reported for students at ages 9, 13, and 17 in mathematics, reading, and science, and at grades 4, 8, and 12 in writing. Future assessments are scheduled to be conducted in reading and mathematics. Results from the long-term trend NAEP are presented as mean scale scores because, unlike the main NAEP, the long-term trend NAEP does not define achievement levels.

NOTE 5: INTERNATIONAL ASSESSMENTS

Program for International Student Assessment (PISA)

Indicator 19 is based on data collected as part of the Program for International Student Assessment (PISA). First conducted in 2000, PISA had its first follow-up in 2003 and had a second follow-up in 2006. The focus of each PISA is on the capabilities of 15-year-olds in reading literacy, mathematics literacy and problem solving, and science literacy. However, in each assessment year, PISA provides a detailed examination for a different one of the three subjects and a basic examination of the other two subjects. The 2000 assessment focused on reading. The 2003 assessment focused on mathematics literacy and problem solving. The 2006 assessment focused on science literacy. PISA is sponsored by the Organization for Economic Cooperation and Development (OECD), an intergovernmental organization of 30 industrialized countries that serves as a forum for member countries to cooperate in research and policy development on social and economic topics of common interest.

In 2006, some 57 countries participated in PISA, including all 30 of the OECD countries and 27 non-OECD countries. To implement PISA, each participating country selected a nationally representative sample of 15-yearolds. A minimum of 4,500 students from a minimum of 150 schools was required. Each student completed a 2-hour paper-and-pencil assessment. Because PISA is an OECD initiative, all international averages presented for PISA are the averages of the participating OECD countries' results.

PISA seeks to represent the overall yield of learning for 15-year-olds. PISA assumes that by the age of 15, young people have had a series of learning experiences, both in and out of school, that allow them to perform at particular levels in reading, mathematics, and science literacy. Formal education will have played a major role in student performance, but other factors, such as learning opportunities at home, also play a role. PISA's results provide an indicator of the overall performance of a country's educational system, but they also provide information about other factors that influence performance (e.g., hours of instructional time). By assessing students near the end of compulsory schooling in key knowledge and skills, PISA provides information about how well prepared students will be for their future lives as they approach an important transition point for education and work. PISA thus aims to show how well equipped 15-year-olds are for their futures based on what they have learned up to that point.

Science literacy is defined as "an individual's scientific knowledge and use of that knowledge to identify questions, to acquire new knowledge, to explain scientific phenomena, and to draw evidence-based conclusions about science related issues, understanding of the characteristic features of science as a form of human knowledge and enquiry, awareness of how science and technology shape our material, intellectual, and cultural environments, and willingness to engage in science-related issues, and with the ideas of science, as a reflective citizen."

Science literacy can be broken down into three "competency clusters": (1) identification, which includes recognizing issues that are possible to investigate scientifically; (2) explaining phenomena, which covers applying knowledge of science in a given situation; (3) using evidence, which includes interpreting scientific data and making and communicating conclusions.

Problem solving is defined as "an individual's capacity to use cognitive processes to confront and resolve real, cross-disciplinary situations where the solution is not immediately obvious, and where the literacy domains or curricular areas that might be applicable are not within a single domain of mathematics, science, or reading." Students completed exercises that assessed their capabilities in using reasoning processes not only to draw conclusions, but also to make decisions, to troubleshoot (i.e., to understand the reasons for malfunctioning of a system or device), and/or to analyze the procedures and structures of a complex system (such as a simple kind of programming language). Problem-solving items required students to apply various reasoning processes, such as inductive and deductive reasoning, reasoning about cause and effect, or combinatorial reasoning (i.e., systematically comparing all the possible variations that can occur in a well-described situation). Students were also assessed in their skills in working toward a solution and communicating the solution to others through appropriate representations. For more information about the PISA, see http://nces.ed.gov/Surveys/PISA.

Progress in International Reading Literacy Study (PIRLS)

Indicator 18 uses data collected as part of the Progress in International Reading Literacy Study (PIRLS). PIRLS 2006 was the second cycle of the study, which was first administered in 2001. Designed to be collected in a planned 5-year cycle of international trend studies in reading literacy by the International Association for the Evaluation of Educational Achievement (IEA), PIRLS 2006 provides comparative information on the reading literacy of 4th-graders and examines factors that may be associated with the acquisition of reading literacy in young children. The study, conducted by IEA, assessed the reading comprehension of children in 45 jurisdictions. In each jurisdiction, students from the upper of the two grades with the most 9-year-olds (4th grade in the United States and most countries) were assessed.

For further information on PIRLS, see http:// nces.ed.gov/surveys/pirls.

Note 6: International Standard Classification of Education

Levels of Education

Indicator 38 uses the International Standard Classification of Education (ISCED) (OECD 1999) to compare educational sys tems in different countries. The ISCED is the standard used by many countries to report education statistics to the United Nations Educational, Scientific and Cultural Organization (UNESCO) and the Organization for Economic Cooperation and Development (OECD). The ISCED divides educational systems into the following seven categories, based on six levels of education.

Education preceding the first level (early childhood education) usually begins at age 3, 4, or 5 (sometimes earlier) and lasts from 1 to 3 years when it is provided. In the United States, this level includes nursery school and kindergarten.

Education at the first level (primary or elementary education) usually begins at age 5, 6, or 7 and continues for about 4 to 6 years. For the United States, the first level starts with 1st grade and ends with 6th grade.

Education at the second level (lower secondary education) typically begins at about age 11 or 12 and continues for about 2 to 6 years. For the United States, the second level starts with 7th grade and ends with 9th grade. Education at the lower secondary level continues the basic programs of the first level, although teaching is typically more subject focused, often using more specialized teachers who conduct classes in their field of specialization. The main criterion for distinguishing lower secondary education from primary education is whether programs begin to be organized in a more subject-oriented pattern, using more specialized teachers who conduct classes in their field of specialization. If there is no clear breakpoint for this organizational change, the lower secondary education is considered to begin at the end of 6 years of primary education. In countries with no clear division between lower secondary and upper secondary education, and where lower secondary education lasts for more than 3 years, only the first 3 years following primary education are counted as lower secondary education.

Education at the third level (upper secondary education) typically begins at age 15 or 16 and lasts for approximately 3 years. In the United States, the third level starts with 10th grade and ends with 12th grade. Upper secondary education is the final stage of secondary education in most OECD countries. Instruction is often organized along subject-matter lines, in contrast to the lower secondary level, and teachers typically must have a higher level, or more subject-specific, qualification. There are substantial differences in the typical duration of programs both across and between countries, ranging from 2 to 5 years of schooling. The main criteria for classifications are (1) national boundaries between lower and upper secondary education and (2) admission into educational programs, which usually requires the completion of lower secondary education or a combination of basic education and life experience that demonstrates the ability to handle the subject matter in upper secondary schools.

Education at the fourth level (postsecondary nontertiary education) straddles the boundary between secondary and postsecondary education. This program of study, which is primarily vocational in nature, is generally taken after the completion of secondary school, typically lasts from 6 months to 2 years, and may be considered as an upper secondary or postsecondary program in a national context. Although the content of these programs may not be significantly more advanced than upper secondary programs, these programs serve to broaden the knowledge of participants who have already gained an upper secondary qualification. This level of education is included for select countries in *indicator 38*.

Education at the fifth level (first stage of tertiary education) includes programs with more advanced content than those offered at the two previous levels. Entry into programs at the fifth level normally requires successful completion of either of the two previous levels.

Tertiary-type A programs provide an education that is largely theoretical and is intended to provide sufficient qualifications for gaining entry into advanced research programs and professions with high-skill requirements. Entry into these programs normally requires the successful completion of an upper secondary education; admission is competitive in most cases. The minimum cumulative theoretical duration at this level is 3 years of full-time enrollment. In the United States, tertiary-type A programs include first university programs that last 4 years and lead to the award of a bachelor's degree, second university programs that lead to a master's degree, and professional programs that lead to a first-professional degree.

Tertiary-type B programs are typically shorter than tertiary-type A programs and focus on practical, technical, or occupational skills for direct entry into the labor market, although they may cover some theoretical foundations in the respective programs. They have a minimum duration of 2 years of full-time enrollment at the tertiary level. In the United States, such programs are often provided at community colleges and lead to an associate's degree.

Education at the sixth level (advanced research qualification) is provided in graduate and professional schools that generally require a university degree or diploma as a minimum condition for admission. Programs at this level lead to the award of an advanced, postgraduate degree, such as a Ph.D. The theoretical duration of these programs is 3 years of full-time enrollment in most countries (for a cumulative total of at least 7 years at levels five and six), although the length of actual enrollment is often longer. Programs at this level are devoted to advanced study and original research.

For *indicator 38,* postsecondary educa tion includes the fifth and sixth levels, except as noted.

NOTE 7: MEASURES OF STUDENT PERSISTENCE AND PROGRESS

Various measures have been developed to provide information about student persistence and progress through formal elementary and secondary education. Three measures are presented in this report: the status dropout rate (*indicator 23*), the public school averaged freshman gradua tion rate (*indicator 21*), and the educational attainment of 25- to 29-yearolds (*indicator 25*). The three indicators in this volume that present these measures each employ a differ ent analytic method and dataset to document a different aspect of the complex high school graduation and dropout process. No one data source provides comprehensive information on the graduation and dropout process on an an nual basis, but the three indicators presented here complement one another and draw upon the particular strength of their respective data. Each indicator is not without its limitations, however, which makes it critical to have mul tiple indicators when addressing the question of student persistence. A brief description of the relevant methodology and data used by each indicator follows.

The reader should note that for *indicator 22,* students with disabilities exiting high school with a regular diploma, the Office of Special Education Programs (OSEP) calculates the "graduation rate" for students with disabilities by dividing the number of students age 14 or older who graduated with a regular high school diploma by the number of students in the same age group who are known to have left school (i.e., graduated with a regular high school diploma, received a certificate of completion, reached a maximum age for services, died, moved and are not known to be continuing in an education program, or dropped out). This percentage should not be confused with other graduation rates reported by NCES in this volume and elsewhere because it is based only on those students leaving school. It does not account for students who remain in school nor does it follow a specific cohort over time. For more information, see *supplemental note 8* on student disabilities.

Status Dropout Rate

Indicator 23 reports status dropout rates by race/ethnicity. Status dropout rates measure the extent of the dropout problem for a popu lation and as such can be used to estimate the need for further education and training in that population. This indicator uses October Current Population Survey (CPS) data to estimate the percentage of the civilian, noninstitutional ized population ages 16 through 24 who are not in high school and who have not earned a high school credential (either a diploma or an equivalency credential such as a General Educational Development [GED] certificate), irrespective of when they dropped out. An advantage of using CPS data to compute this status dropout rate is that the rate can be computed on an annual basis for various demographic subgroups of adults and can be used to report a national rate that includes dropouts of public and private schools. The disadvantages of using CPS data to compute status dropout rates are that they (1) exclude all military personnel and incarcerated or institutionalized persons and (2) include as dropouts individuals who never attended U.S. schools, including immigrants who did not complete the equivalent of a high school education in their home country.

Public School Averaged Freshman Graduation Rate

Indicator 21 examines the percentage of public high school students who graduate on time by using the averaged freshman graduation rate (AFGR). The AFGR is a measure of the percentage of the incoming freshman class that graduates 4 years later. The AFGR is the number of graduates with a regular diploma divided by the estimated count of incoming freshmen 4 years earlier as reported through the NCES Common Core of Data (CCD), the survey system based on state education departments' annual administrative records. The estimated count of incoming freshmen is the sum of the number of 8th-graders 5 years earlier, the number of 9th-graders 4 years earlier (because this is when current year seniors were freshmen), and the number of 10th-graders 3 years earlier, divided by 3. The intent of this averaging is to account for the high rate of grade retention in the freshman year, which adds 9th-grade repeaters from the previous year to the number of students in the incoming freshman class each year. Enrollment counts include a proportional distribution of students not enrolled in a specific grade. An advantage of using CCD data to calculate the AFGR is that they are available on an annual basis by state; however, the demographic details are limited.

Educational Attainment of 25- To 29- Year-Olds

Indicator 25 examines the educational attainment of adults just past the age when most would traditionally be expected to complete their postsecondary education. This indicator uses March CPS data to estimate the percentage of civilian, noninstitutionalized people ages 25 through 29 who are out of high school and who have earned a high school credential (either a diploma or an equivalency credential such as a GED); the rate can be reported by race/ethnicity and other demographic variables. The rate does not differentiate between those who graduated from public schools, who graduated from private schools, or who earned a GED. The rate also includes individuals who never attended high school in the United States. An advantage of using CPS data to compute the educational attainment rate is that the rate can be computed on an annual basis for various demographic sub-groups of adults and can be used to report a national rate that includes public and private schools. A disadvantage of using CPS data to compute the educational attainment rate is that these data exclude all military personnel and incarcerated or institutionalized persons.

Even though *indicators 21, 23,* and *25* document different aspects of student persistence, a number of important differences between these indicators should be noted and recognized as likely factors responsible for the divergence between their respective estimates. General differences can be found in the population of interest, information source, and data collection time frame. For example, the three indicators mentioned above focus on different populations: *indicator 23* focuses on 16- through 24-yearolds between 1972 and 2005; *indicator 21* focuses on the number of graduates in 2003–04 based on the 2000–01 freshman class; and *indicator 25* focuses on 25- through 29-yearolds between 1971 and 2006. The source of information used to construct the indicators also varies. *Indicator 21* is produced from the CCD, a universe survey system based on state education departments' annual admin istrative records, while *indicators 23* and *25* use data from the CPS, a sample survey of the civilian, noninstitutional population.

Given such differences, one would not expect to see identical or even similar estimates. In fact, very reasonable differences should be apparent. For example, if one estimate measures only regular diplomas completed on time, it should be smaller than one that is constructed to measure both regular diplomas and GEDs. Once accounting for these methodological differences, the divergence between estimates tends to be in the correct direction and of the right magnitude.

This supplemental note is intended to provide only a brief overview of some of the commonly available data that address the complex issue of high school completion. For more detail on methods used to analyze dropout and graduation rates in these indicators and other related measures of student persistence and progress, see *supplemental notes 2* and *3* and the publications by Seastrom et al. (NCES 2006-604; NCES 2006-605) and Laird, DeBell, and Chapman (NCES 2007-024).

NOTE 8: STUDENT DISABILITIES

Indicators 8 and 22 use data from the U.S. Department of Education's Office of Special Education Programs (OSEP), which collects information on students with disabilities as part of the implementation of the Individuals with Disabilities Education Act (IDEA). OSEP classifies disabilities according to 13 categories. (For more detailed definitions of these categories, see the part B and C data dictionaries at http://www.ideadata.org.)

Disability Categories

Autism

A developmental disability significantly affecting verbal and nonverbal communication and social interaction, generally evident before age 3, that adversely affects a child's educational performance. Other characteristics often associated with autism are engagement in repetitive activities and stereotyped movements, resistance to environmental change or change in daily routines, and unusual responses to sensory experiences.

Deaf-Blindness

Concomitant hearing and visual impairments, the combination of which causes such severe communication and other developmental and educational problems that the student cannot be accommodated in special education programs solely for children with deafness or children with blindness.

Developmental Delay

This term may apply to children ages 3 through 9 who are experiencing developmental delays in one or more of the following areas: physical development, cognitive development, communication development, social or emotional development, or adaptive development, and who therefore need special education and related services. It is optional for states to adopt and use this term to describe any child within its jurisdiction. A local education agency (LEA) may use the term if its state has adopted it for use, but it must conform its use of the term to that of the state.

Emotional Disturbance

A condition exhibiting one or more of the following characteristics over a long period of time and to a marked degree that adversely affects a child's educational performance:

1. An inability to learn that cannot be explained by intellectual, sensory, or health factors.
2. An inability to build or maintain satisfactory interpersonal relationships with peers and teachers.
3. Inappropriate types of behavior or feelings under normal circumstances.
4. A general pervasive mood of unhappiness or depression.
5. A tendency to develop physical symptoms or fears associated with personal or school problems.

The term includes schizophrenia. The term does not apply to children who are socially maladjusted, unless it is determined that they have an emotional disturbance.

Hearing Impairment

An impairment in hearing, whether permanent or fluctuating, that adversely affects a child's educa tional performance, but that is not included under the definition of deafness in this section.

Although children and youth with deafness are not included in the definition of hearing impairment, they are counted in the hearing impairment category.

Mental Retardation

Significantly subaverage general intellectual functioning, existing concurrently with deficits in adaptive behavior and manifested during the developmental period, that adversely affects a child's educational performance.

Multiple Disabilities

Concomitant impairments (such as mental retardation-blindness, mental retardation-orthopedic impairment, etc.), the combination of which causes such severe educational needs that they cannot be accommodated in special education programs solely for one of the impairments. The term does not include deaf-blindness.

Orthopedic Impairment

A severe orthopedic impairment that adversely affects a child's educational performance. The term includes impairments caused by congenital anomaly (e.g., clubfoot, absence of some member, etc.), impairments caused by disease (e.g., poliomyelitis, bone tuberculosis, etc.), and impairments from other causes (e.g., cerebral palsy, amputations, and fractures or burns that cause contractures).

Other Health Impairment

Having limited strength, vitality, or alert ness, including a heightened alertness to environmental stimuli, that results in limited alertness with respect to the educational envi ronment, that

- is due to chronic or acute health problems such as asthma, attention deficit disorder or attention deficit hyperactivity disorder, diabetes, epilepsy, a heart condition, hemophilia, lead poisoning, leukemia, nephritis, rheumatic fever, and sickle cell anemia; and
- adversely affects a child's educational performance.

Specific Learning Disability

A disorder in one or more of the basic psychological processes involved in understanding or in using language, spoken or written, that may manifest itself in an imperfect ability to listen, think, speak, read, write, spell, or to do mathematical calculations, including conditions such as perceptual disabilities, brain injury, minimal brain dysfunction, dyslexia, and developmental aphasia. The term does not include learning problems that are primarily the result of visual, hearing, or motor disabilities, of mental retardation, of emotional disturbance, or of environmental, cultural, or economic disadvantage.

Speech or Language Impairment

A communication disorder such as stuttering, impaired articulation, a language impairment, or a voice impairment that adversely affects a child's educational performance.

Traumatic Brain Injury

An acquired injury to the brain caused by an external physical force, resulting in total or partial functional disability or psychosocial impairment, or both, that adversely affects a child's educational performance. The term applies to open or closed head injuries resulting in impairments in one or more areas, such as cognition; language; memory; attention; reasoning; abstract thinking; judgment; problem solving; sensory, perceptual, and motor abilities; psychosocial behavior; physical functions; information processing; and speech. The term does not apply to brain injuries that are congenital or degenerative, or to brain injuries induced by birth trauma.

Visual Impairments

An impairment in vision that, even with correction, adversely affects a child's educational performance. The term includes both partial sight and blindness.

Students with Disabilities and Exiting School

The Office of Special Education Programs (OSEP) calculates the graduation rate for students with disabilities by dividing the number of students age 14 or older who graduated with a regular high school diploma by the number of students in the same age group who are known to have left school (i.e., graduated with a regular high school diploma, received a certificate of completion, reached a maximum age for services, died, moved and are not known to be continuing in an education program, or dropped out). This percentage should not be confused with other graduation rates because it is based only on those students leaving school. It does not account for students who remain in school nor does it follow a specific cohort over time.

Because states have different eligibility criteria for each disability category, state-to-state comparisons by disability should be interpreted with caution. Further, in 2002–03, the definitions of several categories were clarified. The definition of "graduated with a regular high school diploma" was revised to make it clear that this category should only include those students who met the same standards for graduation as those for students without disabilities. Students who received a high school diploma, but did not meet the same standards for graduation as those for students without disabilities should be reported in the received a certificate category. Not all states distinguish between students who met the same standards for graduation and those who did not. For more information, see https://www.ideadata.org/docs/bfactsheetex.pdf.

NOTE 9: CLASSIFICATION OF POSTSECONDARY EDUCATION INSTITUTIONS

The U.S. Department of Education's Integrated Postsecondary Education Data System (IPEDS) employs various categories to classify postsecondary institutions. This note outlines the dif ferent categories used in varying combinations in *indicators 9, 10, 11, 26, 27, 39, 40, 41,* and *42*.

Basic IPEDS Classifications

The term "postsecondary institutions" is the category used to refer to institutions with formal instructional programs and a curriculum designed primarily for students who have completed the requirements for a high school diploma or its equivalent. For many analyses, however, comparing all institutions from across this broad universe of postsecondary institutions would not be appropriate. Thus, postsecondary institutions are placed in one of three levels, based on the highest award offered at the institution:

- *4-year-and-above institutions:* Institutions or branches that award a 4-year degree or higher in one or more programs, or a post-baccalaureate, post-master's, or post-first-professional certificate.
- *2-year but less-than-4-year institutions:* Institutions or branches that confer at least a 2-year formal award (certificate, diploma, or associate's degree) or that have a 2-year program creditable toward a baccalaureate degree.
- *Less-than-2-year institutions:* A postsecondary institution that offers programs of less than 2 years' duration below the baccalaureate level. Includes occupational and vocational schools with programs that do not exceed 1,800 contact hours.

Postsecondary institutions are further divided according to these criteria: degree-granting versus non-degree-granting; type of financial control; and Title IV-participating versus non-Title IV-participating.

Degree-granting institutions offer associate's, bachelor's, master's, doctoral, and/or first-professional degrees that a state agency recognizes or authorizes. *Non-degree-granting* institutions offer other kinds of credentials and exist at all three levels. The number of 4-year-and-above non-degree-granting institutions is small compared with the number of non-degree granting institutions at both the 2-year but less-than-4- year and less-than-2-year levels.

IPEDS also classifies institutions at each of the three levels of institutions by type of financial con trol: *public; private not-for-profit;* or *private for-profit* (e.g., proprietary schools). Thus, IPEDS divides the universe of postsecondary institutions into nine different "sectors." In some sectors (for example, private for-profit 4-year institutions), the number of institutions is small relative to other sectors. Institutions in any of these nine sectors can be degree- or non-degree-granting.

Institutions in any of these nine sectors can also be Title IV-participating or not. For an institution to participate in federal Title IV Higher Education Act, Part C, financial aid programs, it must offer a program of study at least 300 clock hours in length; have accreditation recognized by the U.S. Department of Education; have been in business for at least 2 years; and have a Title IV participation agreement with the U.S. Department of Education. All indicators in this volume using IPEDS data are restricted to Title IV-participating institutions.

In some indicators based on IPEDS data, 4-year-and-above degree-granting institutions are further classified according to the highest degree awarded. *Doctoral* institutions award at least 20 doctoral degrees per year. *Master's* institu tions award at least 20 master's degrees per year. The remaining institutions are considered to be *other 4-year* institutions. The number of degrees awarded by an institution in a given year is ob tained for each institution from data published in the IPEDS "Completions Survey" (IPEDS-C).

Indicators 9, 26, 39, 41, and *42* include 2-year (short for 2-year but less-than-4- year) and 4-year-and-above degree-granting institutions in their analyses. *Indicators 10, 11, 27,* and *40* include 4-year-and-above degree-granting institutions.

NOTE 10: FIELDS OF STUDY FOR POSTSECONDARY DEGREES

The general categories for fields of study used in *indicators 26, 27, 39,* and *40* were derived from the 2000 edition of the *Classification of In structional Programs* (CIP-2000). To facilitate trend comparisons, aggrega tions of some categories have been made in some instances. These aggregations are as follows:

Agriculture and natural resources: agriculture, agriculture operations and related sciences; and natural resources and conservation.

Business: business, management, marketing, and related support services; and personal and culinary services.

Communication, journalism, and related programs: communication, journalism, and related programs; and communications tech nologies/technicians and support services. This category is used at the bachelor's, master's, doctoral, and first-professional degree levels. For *indicator 39*, the following category is used at the associate's degree level:

Communications and communications technologies: This category is not directly comparable to the communication, journalism, and related programs referenced above.

Data may differ from previously published figures as data from earlier years have been reclassified when necessary to make them conform to the new taxonomy. Further information about the CIP-2000 is available at http: // nces.ed.gov/pubs2002/cip2000/.

NOTE 11: FINANCE

Using the Consumer Price Index (CPI) to Adjust for Inflation

The Consumer Price Indexes (CPIs) represent changes in the prices of all goods and services purchased for consumption by households. Indexes vary for specific areas or regions, periods of time, major groups of consumer expenditures, and population groups. *Indica tors 20, 34, 35, 36, 37,* and *42* in *The Condition of Education* use the U.S. All Items CPI for All Urban Consumers (CPI-U).

The CPI-U is the basis for both the calendar year CPI and the school year CPI. The calendar year CPI is the same as the annual CPI-U. The school year CPI is calculated by adding the monthly CPI-U figures, beginning with July of the first year and ending with June of the following year, and then dividing that figure by 12. The school year CPI is rounded to three decimal places. Data for the CPI-U are available on the Bureau of Labor Statistics (BLS) website (see below). Also, figures for both the calendar year CPI and the school year CPI can be obtained from the *Digest of Education Statistics, 2007* (NCES 2008-022), an annual publication of the National Center for Education Statistics (NCES).

Although the CPI has many uses, its principal function in *The Condition of Education* is to convert monetary figures (salaries, expenditures, income, etc.) into inflation-free dollars to allow comparisons over time. For example, due to inflation, the buying power of a teacher's salary in 1998 is not comparable to that of a teacher's salary in 2002. In order to make such a comparison, the 1998 salary must be converted into 2002 constant dollars by multiplying the 1998 salary by a ratio of the 2002 CPI over the 1998 CPI. As a formula, this is expressed as

$$\text{1998 salary} \times \frac{\text{(2002 CPI)}}{\text{(1998 CPI)}} = \text{1998 salary in 2002 constant dollars}$$

The reader should be aware that there are alternative price indexes to the CPI that could be used to make these adjustments. These alternative adjustments might produce findings that differ from the ones presented here. For more detailed information on how the CPI is calculated or the other types of CPI indexes, go to the BLS website (http://www.bls.gov/cpi/).

Using the Comparable Wage Index (CWI) to Adjust for Geographic Cost Differences

The Comparable Wage Index (CWI) reflects systematic, regional variations in the salaries of college graduates who are not educators. Provided that these noneducators are similar to educators in terms of age, educational background, and tastes for local amenities, a CWI can be used to measure the uncontrollable component of variations in the wages paid to educators. Intuitively, if accountants in the Atlanta metro area are paid 5 percent more than the national average accounting wage, Atlanta engineers are paid 5 percent more than the national average engineering wage, Atlanta nurses are paid 5 percent more than the national average nursing wage, and so on, then the CWI predicts that Atlanta teachers should also be paid 5 percent more than the national average teacher wage.

The CWI was calculated by combining baseline estimates of these salaries from the 2000 U.S. Census with annual data from the Bureau of Labor Statistics' Occupational Employment Statistics (OES) Survey. Different sets of CWIs are available for adjusting finance data at different levels of aggregation: the region, state, labor market, and school district. The school district CWI can also be used to adjust for other geographic levels as well.

In *indicator 37,* for each year under study, an index number was developed for each of the five district poverty levels used in the indicator. These district poverty-level index numbers were calculated by (1) summing, within each poverty level, each district's index number multiplied by the district's enrollment, and then (2) dividing that sum by the total enrollment in that district poverty level. The same method was used to develop the 20 index numbers for the different combinations of community type and district poverty level for 2004–05 and the national index numbers for each year.

When a series of annual CWIs are used for adjusting trend data, an adjustment for inflation is inherently introduced along with the CWI's adjustment for geographic cost differences. In order to maintain consistency in adjustments for inflation across indicators in *The Condition of Education,* CWI adjustments for trend data are further adjusted to eliminate the inherent CWI adjustment for inflation. This is done for each year by dividing each district's CWI by the national CWI, which leaves only an adjustment based on geographic cost differences for each year. Adjustments for the effect of inflation are then made using the Consumer Price Index (CPI).

Indicator 36 presents two Theil coefficients for instruction expenditures: one that is adjusted for cost differences and one that is unadjusted. The adjusted Theil coefficient in this indicator is calculated in the same way as the unadjusted Theil coefficient, except that each district's instruction expenditures that are used in the calculation have been adjusted first by dividing the district's instruction expenditures by the district's CWI. (For details on how the Theil coefficient is calculated, see The Variation in Expenditures per Student and the Theil Coefficient section later in this supplemental note.)

Further information about the CWI is available at http://nces.ed.gov/edfin/adjustments.asp.

Classifications of Expenditures for Elementary and Secondary Education

Indicators 35, 36, and *37* examine expenditures for public elementary and secondary education. *Indicator 35* uses total expenditures as a whole together with the four major functions (categories) of total expenditures: current expenditures, capital expenditures, interest on school debt, and other expenditures. Current expenditures in turn is broken into seven subfunctions (subcategories): expenditures for instruction, administration, student and staff support, operation and maintenance, transportation, food services, and enterprise operations. *Indicator 36* uses expenditures for instruction (referred to usually as instruction expenditures) in its analysis. *Indicator 37* uses two categories of expenditures in its analysis: current expenditures and instruction expenditures.

Total expenditures for elementary and secondary education include all expenditures allocable to per student costs: these are all current expenditures for regular school programs, capital outlay, interest on school debt, and other expenditures. Expenditures on education by other agencies or equivalent institutions (e.g., the Department of Health and Human Services and the Department of Agriculture) are included.

Current expenditures include expenditures for instruction, administration, student and staff support, operation and maintenance, transportation, food services, and enterprise operations. Thus, current expenditures include such items as salaries for school personnel, fixed charges, student transportation, school books and materials, and energy costs. Current expenditures and each of its seven subfunctions can be further broken down by the object of the expenditure: salaries, employee benefits, purchased services, supplies, tuition, and other.

Instruction expenditures include salaries and benefits for teachers and instructional aides, supplies, and purchased services such as instruction via television. Also included are tuition expenditures to other local education agencies.

Administration expenditures include expenditures for general administration (boards of education staff and executive administration) and school administration (i.e., the office of the principal, full-time department chairpersons, and graduation expenses).

Student and staff support expenditures include expenditures for student support (attendance and social work, guidance, health, psychological services, speech pathology, audiology and other student support services); instructional staff services (instructional staff training, educational media [libraries and audiovisual], and other instructional staff support services); and other support services (business support services, central support services, and other support services not reported elsewhere).

Operation and maintenance expenditures include expenditures for supervision of operations and maintenance; operating buildings (heating, lighting, ventilating, repair, and replacement); care and upkeep of grounds and equipment; vehicle operations and maintenance (other than student transportation); security; and other operations and maintenance services.

Transportation includes expenditures for vehicle operation, monitoring, and vehicle servicing and maintenance.

Food services include all expenditures associated with providing food to students and staff in a school or school district. The services include preparing and serving regular and incidental meals or snacks in connection with school activities as well as the delivery of food to schools.

Enterprise operations include expenditures for operations funded by sales of products or services together with amounts for direct program support made by state education agencies for local school districts.

Capital outlays include funds for the acquisition of land and buildings; building construction, remodeling, and additions; the initial installation or extension of service systems and other built-in equipment; and site improvement. The category also encompasses architectural and engineering services including the development of blueprints.

Interest on debt includes expenditures for longterm debt service interest payments (i.e., those longer than 1 year).

Other expenditures include expenditures for adult education, community colleges, and private school programs, which are funded by local and state education agencies and by community services.

Classifications of Revenue

In *indicator 34,* revenue is classified by source (federal, state, or local). Revenue from federal sources includes direct grants-in-aid to schools or agencies, funds distributed through a state or intermediate agency, and revenue in lieu of taxes to compensate a school district for nontaxable federal institutions within a district's boundary. Revenue from state sources includes both direct funds from state governments and revenue in lieu of taxation. Revenue from local sources includes revenue from such sources as local property and nonproperty taxes; investments; and revenue from student activities, textbook sales, transportation and tuition fees, and food services. Intermediate revenue comes from sources that are not local or state education agencies, but operate at an intermediate level between local and state education agencies and possess independent fundraising capability—for example, county or municipal agencies. Intermediate revenue is included in local revenue totals. In *indicator 34,* local revenue is classified as either local property tax revenue or other local revenue.

In *indicator 34,* alternative local government revenue numbers for Texas were used in the calculation of the percentage distribution for the South in 1992–93 because, for that state, much of the revenue that was classified as local government property taxes was classified as revenue from intermediate sources. The alternative Texas local government property tax revenue for 1992–93 was calculated by applying the average of the proportions of the 199 1–92 and 199 3–94 local government property tax revenue to all local government revenue to the 1992–93 total for all local government revenue. Other local government revenue was calculated in a similar fashion.

The Variation in Expenditures Per Student and the Theil Coefficient

Indicator 36 uses the Theil coefficient to measure the variation in expenditures per pupil in regular public school elementary and secondary schools in the United States.

The Theil coefficient was developed by Henri Theil to measure the amount of information conveyed by a single message that an event has occurred. It was derived from the study of what Theil called the "information concept." If we know an event is likely (i.e., the probability of the event is close to 1.0), then the amount of information conveyed is low (i.e., it is no surprise that the event occurred). But if the probability is low (i.e., near zero), a message saying it occurred provides a significant amount of information. Intuitively, and later rigorously proven by Theil and others, the function of the amount of information conveyed is logarithmic (i.e., $h(z) = \ln(1/z)$, where h = information function and z = probability of event).

Having developed the information function as a measure of the amount of information conveyed, Theil then suggested that this information function could also be used as a measure of dispersion. For example, if instructional expenditures per pupil in the nation are relatively close together (i.e., low disparity), then relatively little information would be provided by random draws of the districts (i.e., the $1/z_i$ —the probabilities—are high, but the value of the information function—the sum of the logarithms—is low). In contrast, if instructional expenditures per pupil are very dissimilar, then probabilities for drawing a given level of expenditures are lower, and the information gained from a random draw will be high. Thus, the information function can be a measure of dispersion, and a comparison of the values of

Theil coefficients for groups within a set (i.e., districts within the nation) will indicate relative dispersion and any variations that may exist among them. The Theil coefficient was subsequently used to measure the trends in variation of a number of items, including expenditures per student (see NCES 2000-020 and Murray, Evans, and Schwab 1998).

The Theil coefficient has a convenient property when the individual units of observation (e.g., school districts) can be aggregated into subgroups (e.g., states): the Theil coefficient for the aggregation of all the individual units of observation can be decomposed into a measure of the variation within the subgroups and a measure of the variation between the subgroups. Hence, in the examination of the variation in instructional expenditures in the United States, the national variation can be decomposed into measures of between-state and within-state variation.

The between-state Theil coefficient, T_B, equals:

$$T_B = \sum_{k=1}^{K} (P_k \overline{X}_k / \overline{X}) \ln(\overline{X}_k / \overline{X})$$

where P_k is the enrollment in state *k,* X{bar}$_k$ is the student-weighted mean expenditure per student in state *k,* and X{bar} is the student- weighted mean expenditure per student for the country.

The within-state Theil coefficient, T_W, equals:

$$T_W = \sum_{k=1}^{K} (P_k \overline{X}_k / \overline{X}) T_k$$

where T_k is the Theil coefficient for state *k*.

T_k equals:

$$T_k = \frac{\sum_{j=1}^{J_k} P_{jk} X_{jk} \ln(X_{jk} / X_k)}{\sum_{j=1}^{J_k} P_{jk} X_{jk}}$$

where P_{jk} is the enrollment of district *j* in state *k* and X_{jk} is the mean expenditure per student of district *j* in state *k*.

The national Theil coefficient, T, is:

$$T = T_W + T_B$$

Classifications of Expenditures for International Comparisons

Indicator 38 presents international data on public and private expenditures for instructional and noninstructional educational institutions. Instructional educational institutions are educational institutions that directly provide instructional programs (i.e., teaching) to individuals in an organized group setting or through distance education. Business enterprises or other institutions providing short-term courses of training or instruction to individuals on a "one-to-one" basis are not included. Noninstructional educational institutions are educational institutions that provide administrative, advisory, or professional services to other educational institutions, although they do not enroll students themselves. Examples include national, state, and provincial bodies in the private sector; organizations that provide education-related services such as vocational and psychological counseling; and educational research.

Public expenditures refer to the spending of public authorities at all levels. *Total public expenditures* used for the calculation in *indicator 38* correspond to the nonrepayable current and capital expenditures of all levels of the government directly related to education. Expenditures that are not directly related to education (e.g., culture, sports, youth activities, etc.) are, in principle, not included. Expenditures on education by other ministries or equivalent institutions (e.g., Health and Agriculture) are included. Public subsidies for students' living expenses are excluded to ensure international comparability of the data.

Private expenditures refer to expenditures funded by private sources (i.e., households and other private entities). "Households" mean students and their families. "Other private entities" include private business firms and nonprofit organizations, including religious organizations, charitable organizations, and business and labor associations. Private expenditures comprise school fees; the cost of materials such as textbooks and teaching equipment; transportation costs (if organized by the school); the cost of meals (if provided by the school); boarding fees; and expenditures by employers on initial vocational training. Private educational institutions are considered to be service providers and do not include sources of private funding.

Current expenditures include final consumption expenditures (e.g., compensation of employees, consumption of intermediate goods and services, consumption of fixed capital, and military expenditures); property income paid; subsidies; and other current transfers paid. Capital expenditures include spending to acquire and improve fixed capital assets, land, intangible assets, government stocks, and nonmilitary, nonfinancial assets, as well as spending to finance net capital transfers.

In: The Condition of Education in America
Editor: Maurice H. Logan
ISBN: 978-1-60692-298-9

GLOSSARY

A

Achievement levels: Achievement levels, which are set through a National Assessment Governing Board process, define what students should know and be able to do at different levels of performance. In the National Assessment of Educational Progress (NAEP), the achievement levels are *Basic, Proficient,* and *Advanced.* The definitions of these levels, which apply across all grades and subject areas, are as follows:

Basic: This level denotes partial mastery of prerequisite knowledge and skills that are fundamental for proficient work at each grade.

Proficient: This level represents solid academic performance for each grade assessed. Students reaching this level have demonstrated competency over challenging subject matter, including subject-matter knowledge, application of such knowledge to real-world situations, and analytical skills appropriate to the subject matter.

Advanced: This level signifies superior performance.

Alternative schools: A public elementary/secondary school that (1) addresses needs of students that typically cannot be met in a regular school, (2) provides nontraditional education, (3) serves as an adjunct to a regular school, or (4) falls outside the categories of regular, special education, or vocational education. Some examples of alternative schools are schools for potential dropouts; resi dential treatment centers for substance abuse (if they provide elementary or secondary educa tion); schools for chronic truants; and schools for students with behavioral problems. About 7 percent of schools in the Common Core of Data (CCD) files are alternative schools.

B

Bachelor's degree: A degree granted for the successful completion of a baccalaureate program of studies, usually requiring at least 4 years (or the equivalent) of full-time college-level study.

C

Combined school: A combined school has one or more of grades K–6 and one or more of grades 9–12. For example, schools with grades K–12, 6–9, or 1–12 are classified as combined schools.

Comparable Wage Index (CWI): A measure of the systematic, regional variations in the salaries of college graduates who are not educators. It can be used to adjust district-level finance data at different levels in order to make better comparisons across geographic areas.

Constant dollars: Dollar amounts that have been adjusted by means of price and cost indexes to eliminate inflationary factors and allow direct comparison across years.

Consumer price index (CPI): This price index measures the average change in the cost of a fixed-market basket of goods and services purchased by consumers.

Current expenditures: Expenditures for operating local public schools and school districts, excluding capital outlay and interest on debt. These expenditures include such items as salaries for school per sonnel, fixed charges, student transportation, books and materials, and energy costs. Expen ditures for state administration are excluded.

D

Diocesan school: A private Catholic school serving students in one or more grades K–12 that is the domain of a bishop.

Doctoral degree: An earned degree carrying the title of Doctor. The Doctor of Philosophy degree (Ph.D.) is the highest academic degree and requires mastery within a field of knowledge and demonstrated ability to perform scholarly research. Other doctoral degrees are awarded for fulfilling specialized requirements in professional fields, such as education (Ed.D.), musical arts (D.M.A.), business administration (D.B.A.), and engineering (D. Eng. or D.E.S.). Many doctoral degrees in both academic and professional fields require an earned master's degree as a prerequisite. First-professional degrees, such as M.D. and D.D.S., are not included under this heading. (See First-professional degree.)

Doctoral institutions: Includes 4-year postsecondary institutions that award at least a doctoral or first-professional degree in one or more programs.

Dropout: The term is used to describe both the event of leaving school before graduating and the status of an individual who is not in school and who is not a graduate. Transferring from a public school to a private school, for example, is not regarded as a dropout event. A person who drops out of school may later return and graduate but is called a "dropout" at the time he or she left school. At the time the person returns to school, he or she is called a "stopout." Measures to describe these often complicated behaviors include the event dropout rate (or the closely related school persistence rate), the status dropout rate, and the high school completion rate. (See Status dropout rate.)

E

Educational attainment: The highest level of schooling attended and completed.

Elementary school: An elementary/secondary school with one or more grades of K–6 that does not have any grade higher than grade 8. For example, schools with grades K–6, 1–3, or 6–8 are classified as elementary.

Elementary/secondary school: As reported in this publication, elementary/secondary schools include regular schools (i.e., schools that are part of state and local school systems and private elementary/secondary schools, both religiously affiliated and nonsectarian); alternative schools; vocational education schools; and special education schools. Schools not reported here include subcollegiate departments of postsecondary institutions, residential schools for exceptional children, federal schools for American Indians or Alaska Natives, and federal schools on military posts and other federal installations.

Enrollment: The total number of students registered in a given school unit at a given time, generally in the fall of a year.

Expenditures: Charges incurred, whether paid or unpaid, that are presumed to benefit the current fiscal year. For elementary/secondary schools, these include all charges for current outlays plus capital outlays and interest on school debt. For postsecondary institutions, these include current outlays plus capital outlays. For government, these include charges net of recoveries and other correcting transactions, other than retirement of debt, investment in securities, extension of credit, or as agency transactions. Also, government expenditures include only external transactions, such as the provision of prerequisites or other payments in kind. Aggregates for groups of governments exclude intergovernmental transactions among the governments.

Expenditures per student: Charges incurred for a particular period of time divided by a student unit of measure, such as enrollment, average daily attendance, or average daily membership (see *supplemental note 11*).

F

First-professional degree: An award that requires completion of a degree program that meets all of the following criteria: (1) completion of the academic requirements to begin practice in the profession; (2) at least 2 years of college work before entering the degree program; and (3) a total of at least 6 academic years of college work to complete the degree program, including previously required college work plus the work required in the professional program itself. First-professional degrees may be awarded in the following 10 fields: chiropractic (D.C. or D.C.M.), osteopathic medicine (D.O.), dentistry (D.D.S. or D.M.D.), pharmacy (Pharm.D.), law (L.L.B. or J.D.), podiatry (D.P.M., D.P., or Pod.D.), medicine (M.D.), theology (M.Div., M.H.L., B.D., or Ordination), optometry (O.D.), and veterinary medicine (D.V.M.).

Four-year institution: Denotes a postsecondary institution that can award a bachelor's degree or higher. (See *supplemental note 9*.)

Full-time enrollment: The number of students enrolled in postsecondary education courses with a total credit load equal to at least 75 percent of the normal full-time course load.

Full-time-equivalent (FTE) enrollment: For institutions of higher education, enrollment of full-time students, plus the full-time equivalent of part-time students as reported by institutions. In the absence of an equivalent reported by an institution, the FTE enrollment is estimated by adding one-third of part-time enrollment to full-time enrollment.

Full-time worker: One who is employed for 35 or more hours per week, including paid leave for illness, vacation, and holidays. Hours may be reported either for a survey reference week or for the previous calendar year, in which case they refer to the usual hours worked.

G

GED certificate: (See High school equivalency certificate.)

GED recipient: A person who has obtained certification of high school equivalency by meeting state requirements and passing an approved exam, which is intended to provide an appraisal of the person's achievement or performance in the broad subject matter areas usually required for high school graduation.

Graduate: An individual who has received formal recognition for the successful completion of a prescribed program of studies.

Gross Domestic Product (GDP): Gross national product less net property income from abroad. Both gross national product (GNP) and gross domestic product (GDP) aggregate only the incomes of residents of a nation, corporate and individual, derived directly from the current production of goods and services by individuals, businesses, and government, gross private domestic investment in infrastructure, and total exports of goods and services. The goods and services included are largely those bought for final use (excluding illegal transactions) in the market economy. A number of inclusions, however, represent imputed values, the most important of which is rental value of owner- occupied housing.

Gross National Product (GNP): A measure of the money value of the goods and services available to the nation from economic activity. GNP can be viewed in terms of expenditure categories, which include purchases of goods and services by consumers and government, gross private domestic investment, and net exports of goods and services. The goods and services included are largely those bought for final use (excluding illegal transactions) in the market economy. A number of inclusions, however, represent imputed values, the most important of which is the rental value of owner-occupied housing. GNP, in this broad context, measures the output attributable to the factors of production, labor, and property supplied by U.S. residents.

H

Head Start programs: Head Start is a federally sponsored preschool program primarily for children from low-income families.

High school: A secondary school offering the final years of high school study necessary for graduation, usually including grades 10, 11, 12 (in a 6-3-3 plan) or grades 9, 10, 11, and 12 (in a 6-2-4 plan).

High school completion: An individual has completed high school if he or she has been awarded a high school diploma or an equivalent credential, including a General Educational Development (GED) credential.

High school diploma: A formal document regulated by the state certifying the successful completion of a prescribed secondary school program of studies. In some states or communities, high school diplomas are differentiated by type, such as an academic diploma, a general diploma, or a vocational diploma.

High school equivalency certificate: A formal document certifying that an individual has met the state requirements for high school graduation equivalency by obtaining satisfactory scores on an approved examination and meeting other performance requirements (if any) set by a state education agency or other appropriate body. One particular version of this certificate is the GED. The GED (General Educational Development) test is a comprehensive test used primarily to appraise the educational development of students who have not completed their formal high school education and who may earn a high school equivalency certificate through achieving satisfactory scores. GEDs are awarded by the states or other agencies, and the test is developed and distributed by the GED Testing Service of the American Council on Education.

Hispanic ethnicity: Ethnicity is based on the following categorization: A person of Cuban, Mexican, Puerto Rican, South or Central American, or other Spanish culture of origin, regardless of race.

I

Individuals with Disabilities Education Act (IDEA): IDEA is a federal law ensuring services to children with disabilities throughout the nation. IDEA governs how states and public agencies provide early intervention, special education and related services to more than 6.5 million eligible infants, toddlers, children, and youth with disabilities. Infants and toddlers with disabilities (birth–2) and their families receive early intervention services under IDEA Part C. Children and youth (ages 3–21) receive special education and related services under IDEA Part B.

Industrialized country or nation: A country or nation with a market economy comprising a significant portion of world production and trade markets.

Instructional expenditures (elementary/secondary): Current expenditures for activities directly associated with the interaction between teachers and students. These include teacher salaries and benefits, supplies (such as textbooks), and purchased instructional services (see also *supplemental note 11*).

L

Language minority students: Children in households who speak a language other than English at home.

Limited-English-proficient: The term "limited English proficient," when used with respect to an individual, means an individual who is enrolled or preparing to enroll in an elementary school or secondary school, who was not born in the United States or whose native language is a language other than English or who comes from an environment where a language other than English has had a significant impact on the individual's level of English language proficiency; or who is migratory, whose native language is a language other than English, and who comes from an environment where a language other than English is dominant, and whose difficulties in speaking, reading, writing, or understanding the English language may be sufficient to deny the individual the ability to meet the state's proficient level of achievement on state assessments as specified under the No Child Left Behind Act, the ability to successfully achieve in classrooms where the language of instruction is English, or the opportunity to participate fully in society.

M

Master's degree: A degree awarded for successful completion of a program generally requiring 1 or 2 years of full-time college-level study beyond the bachelor's degree. One type of master's degree, including the Master of Arts degree, or M.A., and the Master of Science degree, or M.S., is awarded in the liberal arts and sciences for advanced scholarship in a subject field or discipline and demonstrated ability to perform scholarly research. A second type of master's degree is awarded for the completion of a professionally oriented program—for example, an M.Ed. in education, an M.B.A. in business administration, an M.F.A. in fine arts, an M.M. in music, an M.S.W. in social work, and an M.P.A. in public administration. A third type of master's degree is awarded in professional fields for study beyond the first- professional degree—for example, the Master of Laws (LL.M.) and Master of Science (M.S.) in various medical specializations.

Mathematics literacy: An individual's capacity to identify and understand the role that mathematics plays in the world, to make well-founded judgments, and to use and engage with mathematics in ways that meet the needs of that individual's life as a constructive, concerned, and reflective citizen.

Middle school: A separately organized and administered school between the elementary and senior high schools. When called a "junior high school," a middle school usually includes grades 7, 8, and 9 (in a 6-3-3 plan) or grades 7 and 8 (in a 6-2-4 plan). In some districts, however, a middle school spans grades 5 to 8 or grades 6 to 8.

Minority: Any individual or racial/ethnic group that is not categorized as White, not Hispanic or Latino.

N

National School Lunch Program: Established by President Truman in 1946, the program is a federally assisted meal program operated in public and private nonprofit schools and residential child care centers. To be eligible, a student must be from a household with an income at 185 percent of the poverty level for reduced-price lunch or 130 percent of the poverty level for free lunch.

Nonfatal crime: Crimes, whether theft, violent crimes, or serious violent crimes, without fatalities.

Nonresident alien: A person who is not a citizen of the United States and who is in this country on a temporary basis and does not have the right to remain indefinitely.

Nursery school: A separately organized and administered elementary school for groups of children during the year or years preceding kindergarten, which provides educational experiences under the direction of professionally qualified teachers.

O

Organization for Economic Cooperation and Development (OECD): The OECD is an organization of 30 nations whose purpose is to promote trade and economic growth in both member and nonmember na tions. OECD's activities cover almost all aspects of economic and social policy. The current member countries include Australia, Austria, Belgium, Canada, the Czech Republic, Denmark, Finland, France, Germany, Greece, Hungary, Iceland, Ireland, Italy, Japan, Korea, Luxembourg, Mexico, the Netherlands, New Zealand, Norway, Poland, Portugal, the Slovak Republic, Spain, Sweden, Switzerland, Turkey, the United Kingdom, and the United States.

Other disabilities: Developmental disabilities including mental retardation, emotional disturbance, hearing impairments, orthopedic impairments, other health impairments, visual impairments, multiple disabilities, deaf- blindness, autism, traumatic brain injury, and developmental delay. There is a wide range of disabilities included in this category; they are included in *indicator 8* to represent cases contributing to the total not otherwise presented in the graph due to their relatively low prevalence in the population.

Other incidents: Incidents including possession of a firearm or explosive device, possession of a knife or sharp object, distribution, possession, or use of illegal drugs or alcohol, and vandalism.

P

Parochial school: A private Catholic school serving students in one or more grades K–12 that is the domain of a local church parish.

Part-time enrollment: The number of students enrolled in postsecondary education courses with a total credit load less than 75 percent of the normal full-time credit load.

Postsecondary education: The provision of formal instructional programs with a curriculum designed primarily for students who are beyond the compulsory age for high school. This includes programs with an academic, vocational, and continuing professional education purpose and excludes vocational and adult basic education programs. (See also *supplemental note 9.*)

Prekindergarten: Public preprimary education for children ages 3–4 (ages 3–5 in some states) who have not yet entered kindergarten. It may offer a program of general education or special education and, in some states, may be part of a collaborative effort with Head Start. Private preprimary educational programs are typically referred to as "center-based programs."

Preschool: A beginning group or class enrolling children younger than 5 years of age and organized to provide educational experiences under professionally qualified teachers in cooperation with parents during the year or years immediately preceding kindergarten (or prior to entry into elementary school when there is no kindergarten).

Private school or institution: A school or institution that is controlled by an individual or agency other than a state, a subdivision of a state, or the federal government; that is usually not supported primarily by public funds; and that is not operated by publicly elected or appointed officials.

Problem solving: An individual's capacity to use cognitive processes to confront and resolve real, cross-disciplinary situations where the solution is not immediately obvious, and where the literacy domains or curricular areas that might be applicable are not within a single domain of mathematics, science, or reading.

Property tax: The sum of money collected from a tax levied against the value of property.

Public charter school: A public charter school is a publicly funded school that, in accordance with an enabling statute, has been granted a charter exempting it from selected state or local rules and regulations. A public charter school may be a newly created school or it may previously have been a public or private school. In return for funding and autonomy, the charter school must meet accountability standards. A school's charter is reviewed (typically every 3 to 5 years) and can be revoked if guidelines on curriculum and management are not followed or the standards are not met. (See also Public school.)

Public institution: A postsecondary educational institution whose programs and activities are operated by publicly elected or appointed school officials and that is supported primarily by public funds. (See also *supplemental note 9.*)

Public school: An institution that provides edu cational services for at least one of grades 1–12 (or comparable ungraded levels), has one or more teachers to give instruction, has an assigned administrator, is located in one or more buildings, receives public funds as primary support, and is operated by an educa tion or chartering agency. Public schools include regular, special education, vocational/technical, alternative, and public charter schools. They also include schools in juvenile detention centers, schools located on military bases and operated by the Department of Defense, and Bureau of Indian Affairs-funded schools operated by local public school districts.

Purchasing power parities: Purchasing power parity (PPP) conversion factors take into account differences in the relative prices of goods and services—particularly nontradables—and therefore provide a better overall measure of the real value of output produced by an economy compared with other economies. PPP gross national income (GNI) is measured in current international dollars, which, in principal, have the same purchasing power as a dollar spent on GNI in the U.S. economy. Because PPPs provide a better measure of the standard of living of residents of an economy, they are the basis for the World Bank's calculations of poverty rates at $1 and $2 a day. The GNI of developing countries measured in PPP terms generally exceeds their GNI measured using the Atlas method or using market exchange rates.

Purchasing power parity (PPP) indices: Purchasing power parity (PPP) exchange rates, or indices, are the currency exchange rates that equalize the purchasing power of different currencies, meaning that when a given sum of money is converted into different currencies at the PPP exchange rates, it will buy the same basket of goods and services in all countries. PPP indices are the rates of currency conversion that eliminate the difference in price levels among countries. Thus, when expenditures on gross domestic product (GDP) for different countries are converted into a common currency by means of PPP indices, they are expressed at the same set of international prices, so that comparisons among countries reflect only differences in the volume of goods and services purchased.

R

Religious private school: A school with a designated religious orientation or purpose, which is not supported primarily by public funds. It must provide instruction for one or more of grades K–12 (or comparable ungraded levels) and have one or more teachers. Organizations or institutions that provide support for home- schooling but do not offer classroom instruction for students are not included.

Revenues from federal sources: Revenues from federal sources include direct grants-in-aid from the federal government; federal grants-in-aid through the state or an intermediate agency; and other revenue, in lieu of taxes that would have accrued had the tax base been subject to taxation.

Revenues from local sources: Revenues from local sources include revenues from a local education agency (LEA), including taxes levied or assessed by a LEA; revenues from a local government to the LEA; tuition received; transportation fees; earnings on investments from LEA holdings; net revenues from food services (gross receipts less gross expenditures); net revenues from student activities (gross receipts less gross expenditures); and other revenues (textbook sales, donations, property rentals).

Revenues from state sources: Revenues from state sources include revenues from an agency of state government including those that can be used without restriction, those for categorical purposes, and revenues in lieu of taxation.

S

Salary: The total amount regularly paid or stipulated to be paid to an individual, before deductions, for personal services rendered while on the payroll of a business or organization.

Science literacy: An individual's scientific knowledge and use of that knowledge to identify questions, to acquire new knowledge, to explain scientific phenomena, and to draw evidence-based conclusions about science-related issues; understanding of the characteristic features of science as a form of human knowledge and enquiry; awareness of how science and technology shape our material, intellectual, and cultural environments; and willingness to engage in science-related issues, and with the ideas of science, as a reflective citizen.

Secondary school: An elementary/secondary school with one or more of grades 7–12 that does not have any grade lower than grade 7. For example, schools with grades 9–12, 7–9, 10–12, or 7–8 are classified as secondary.

Serious violent incidents: Include rape or attempted rape, sexual battery other than rape, physical attack or fight with a weapon, threat of physical attack with a weapon, and robbery with or without a weapon.

Socioeconomic status (SES): A measure of an individual or family's relative economic and social ranking. In the analyses in this publication, SES is constructed based on father's education level, mother's education level, father's occupation, mother's occupation, and family income. Also, students are classified into high, middle, and low SES based on a standardized composite index score of their parents' education level, mother's and father's occupation, family's income, and certain household items. The terms "high SES," "middle SES," and "low SES," respectively, refer to the upper, middle two, and lower quartiles of the composite index score distribution. By definition, one-quarter of each cohort of students will be in the bottom SES quartile, even if education levels, average family incomes, and the number of persons in more prestigious occupations change.

Special education schools: A public elementary/ secondary school that (1) focuses primarily on special education, including instruction for any of the following: hard of hearing, deaf, speech impaired, health impaired, orthopedically impaired, mentally retarded, seriously emotionally disturbed, multi-handicapped, visually handicapped, deaf and blind; and the learning disabled; and (2) adapts curriculum, materials, or instruction for students served. About 2 percent of schools in the Common Core of Data files are special education schools.

Specific learning disability: A specific learning disability is a disorder of one or more of the basic psychological processes involved in understanding or in using language, spoken or written, that may manifest itself in an imperfect ability to listen, think, speak, read, write, spell, or to do mathematical calculations. This includes conditions such as perceptual disabilities, brain injury, minimal brain dysfunction, dyslexia, and developmental aphasia (see also *supplemental note 8*).

Status dropout rate: The status dropout rate is a cumulative rate that estimates the proportion of young adults who are dropouts, regardless of when they dropped out. The numerator of the status dropout rate for any given year is the number of young adults ages 16–24 who, as of October of that year, had not completed high school and were not currently enrolled. The denominator is the total number of 16- to 24-year-olds in October of that same year.

T

Theft/larceny: (Taking things worth over $10 without personal confrontation) was defined for respondents in the School Survey on Crime and Safety (SSOCS) as "the unlawful taking of another person's property without personal confrontation, threat, violence, or bodily harm. Included are pocket picking, stealing a purse or backpack (if left unattended or no force was used to take it from owner), theft from a building, theft from a motor vehicle or of motor vehicle parts or accessories, theft of bicycles, theft from vending machines, and all other types of thefts."

Total expenditures per pupil in average daily attendance: Includes all expenditures allocable to per pupil costs divided by average daily attendance. These allocable expenditures include current expenditures for regular school programs, interest on school debt, and capital outlay. Beginning in 1980–81, expenditures for state administration are excluded, and expenditures for other programs (summer schools, community colleges, and private schools) are included.

Two-year institution: Denotes a postsecondary institution that does not confer bachelor's degrees, but does provide 2-year programs that result in a certificate or an associate's degree, or 2-year programs that fulfill part of the requirements for a bachelor's degree or higher at a 4-year institution.

U

Undergraduate students: Students enrolled in a 4- or 5-year bachelor's degree program, an associate's degree program, or a vocational or technical program below the baccalaureate.

University: A postsecondary institution that consists of a liberal arts college, a diverse graduate program, and usually two or more professional schools or faculties and that is empowered to confer degrees in various fields of study.

V

Violent incidents: Include serious violent incidents (rape or attempted rape, sexual battery other than rape, physical attack or fight with weapon, threat of physical attack with a weapon, and robbery with or without a weapon); physical attack or fight without a weapon; and threat of physical attack without a weapon.

Vocational schools: Public elementary/secondary schools that focus primarily on vocational, technical, or career education and provide education and training in one or more semiskilled or technical occupations. They may be part of a regular district (along with academic schools) or in a vocational district (serving more than one academic school district). About 1 percent of schools in the Common Core of Data (CCD) files are vocational schools.

W

World Bank Atlas method: In calculating gross national income (GNI—formerly referred to as gross national product) and GNI per capita in U.S. dollars for certain operational purposes, the World Bank uses the Atlas conversion factor. The purpose of the Atlas conversion factor is to reduce the impact of exchange rate fluctuations in the cross-country comparison of national incomes.

The Atlas conversion factor for any year is the average of a country's exchange rate (or alternative conversion factor) for that year and its exchange rates for the two preceding years, adjusted for the difference between the rate of inflation in the country, and through 2000, the rate of inflation in the G-5 countries (France, Germany, Japan, the United Kingdom, and the United States). For 2001 onwards, these countries include the Euro Zone, Japan, the United Kingdom, and the United States. A country's inflation rate is measured by the change in its gross domestic product (GDP) deflator.

The inflation rate for G-5 countries (through 2000, and the Euro Zone, Japan, the United Kingdom, and the United States for 2001 onwards), representing international inflation, is measured by the change in the SDR deflator. (Special drawing rights, or SDRs, are the IMF's unit of account.) The SDR deflator is calculated as a weighted average of the G-5 countries' (through 2000, and the Euro Zone, Japan, the United Kingdom, and the United States for 2001 onwards) GDP deflators in SDR terms, the weights being the amount of each country's currency in one SDR unit. Weights vary over time because both the composition of the SDR and the relative exchange rates for each currency change. The SDR deflator is calculated in SDR terms first and then converted to U.S. dollars using the SDR to dollar Atlas conversion factor. The Atlas conversion factor is then applied to a country's GNI. The resulting GNI in U.S. dollars is divided by the midyear population to derive GNI per capita.

In: The Condition of Education in America
Editor: Maurice H. Logan
ISBN: 978-1-60692-298-9

BIBLIOGRAPHY

NCES PUBLICATIONS (COMPLETE CITATION)

Baer, J., Baldi, S., Ayotte, K., and Green, P.J. (2007). The Reading Literacy of U.S. Fourth-Grade Students in an International Context: Results From the 2001 and 2006 Progress in International Reading Literacy Study (PIRLS) (NCES 2008-017). National Center for Education Statistics, Institute of Education Sciences, U.S. Department of Education. Washington, DC.

Baldi, S., Jin, Y., Skewer, M., Green, P.J., and Herget, D. (2007). Highlights From PISA 2006: Performance of U.S. 15-Year-Old Students in Science and Mathematics Literacy in an International Context (NCES 2008-016). National Center for Education Statistics, Institute of Education Sciences, U.S. Department of Education. Washington, DC.

Fowler, W., and Monk, D.H. (2001). A Primer for Making Cost Adjustments in Education (NCES 2001-323). National Center for Education Statistics, U.S. Department of Education. Washington, DC.

Gerald, D.E., and Hussar, W.J. (2000). Projections of Education Statistics to 2011 (NCES 2001-083). National Center for Education Statistics, U.S. Department of Education. Washington, DC.

Hussar, W. (forthcoming). Projections of Education Statistics to 2017 (NCES 2008-078). National Center for Education Statistics, Institute of Education Sciences, U.S. Department of Education. Washington, DC.

Hussar, W., and Sonnenberg, W. (2000). Trends in Disparities in School District Level Expenditures per Pupil (NCES 2000-020). National Center for Education Statistics, U.S. Department of Education. Washington, DC.

Kaufman, P., Alt, M.N., and Chapman, C. (2004). Dropout Rates in the United States: 2001 (NCES 2005-046). National Center for Education Statistics, Institute of Education Sciences, U.S. Department of Education. Washington, DC.

KewalRamani, A., Gilbertson, L., Fox, M.A., and Provasnik, S. (2007). Status and Trends in the Education of Racial and Ethnic Minorities (NCES 2007-039). National Center for Education Statistics, Institute of Education Sciences, U.S. Department of Education. Washington, DC.

Laird, J., DeBell, M., and Chapman, C. (2006). Dropout Rates in the United States: 2004 (NCES 2007-024). National Center for Education Statistics, Institute of Education Sciences, U.S. Department of Education. Washington, DC.

Laird, J., DeBell, M., Kienzl, G., and Chapman, C. (2007). Dropout Rates in the United States: 2005 (NCES 2007-059). National Center for Education Statistics, Institute of Education Sciences, U.S. Department of Education. Washington, DC.

Lee, J., Grigg, W., and Dion, G. (2007). The Nation's Report Card: Mathematics 2007 (NCES 2007-494). National Center for Education Statistics, Institute of Education Sciences, U.S. Department of Education. Washington, DC.

Lee, J., Grigg, W., and Donahue, P. (2007). The Nation's Report Card: Reading 2007 (NCES 2007-496). National Center for Education Statistics, Institute of Education Sciences, U.S. Department of Education. Washington, DC.

Mead, N., and Sandene, B. (2007). The Nation's Report Card: Economics 2006 (NCES 2007-475). National Center for Education Statistics, Institute of Education Sciences, U.S. Department of Education. Washington, DC.

Nolle, K.L., Guerino, P., and Dinkes, R. (2007). Crime, Violence, Discipline, and Safety in U.S. Public Schools: Findings From the School Survey on Crime and Safety: 2005–06 (NCES 2007-361). National Center for Education Statistics, Institute of Education Sciences, U.S. Department of Education. Washington, DC.

Perie, M., Moran, R., and Lutkus, A.D. (2005). NAEP 2004 Trends in Academic Progress: Three Decades of Student Performance in Reading and Mathematics (NCES 2005-464). National Center for Education Statistics, Institute of Education Sciences, U.S. Department of Education. Washington, DC.

Provasnik, S., and Dorfman, S. (2005). Mobility in the Teacher Workforce: Findings From The Condition of Education 2005 (NCES 2005-114). National Center for Education Statistics, Institute of Education Sciences, U.S. Department of Education. Washington, DC.

Provasnik, S., KewalRamani, A., Coleman, M.M., Gilbertson, L., Herring, W., and Xie, Q. (2007). Status of Education in Rural America (NCES 2007-040). National Center for Education Statistics, Institute of Education Sciences, U.S. Department of Education. Washington, DC.

Sable, J., and Garofano, A. (2007). Public Elementary and Secondary School Student Enrollment, High School Completions, and Staff From the Common Core of Data: School Year 2005–06 (NCES 2007-352). National Center for Education Statistics, Institute of Education Sciences, U.S. Department of Education. Washington, DC.

Seastrom, M., Chapman, C., Stillwell, R., McGrath, D., Peltola, P., Dinkes, R., and Xu, Z. (2006a). User's Guide to Computing High School Graduation Rates, Volume 1: Review of Current and Proposed Graduation Indicators (NCES 2006-604). National Center for Education Statistics, Institute of Education Sciences, U.S. Department of Education. Washington, DC.

Seastrom, M., Chapman, C., Stillwell, R., McGrath, D., Peltola, P., Dinkes, R., and Xu, Z. (2006b). User's Guide to Computing High School Graduation Rates, Volume 2: Technical Evaluation of Proxy Graduation Indicators (NCES 2006-605). National Center for Education Statistics, Institute of Education Sciences, U.S. Department of Education. Washington, DC.

Seastrom, M., Hoffman, L., Chapman, C., and Stillwell, R. (2006c). The Averaged Freshman Graduation Rate for Public High Schools From the Common Core of Data: School Years 2002–03 and 2003–04 (NCES 2006-606rev). National Center for Education Statistics, Institute of Education Sciences, U.S. Department of Education. Washington, DC.

Snyder, T.D., and Hoffman, C.M. (1995). State Comparisons of Education Statistics: 1969–70 to 1993–94 (NCES 95-122). National Center for Education Statistics, U.S. Department of Education. Washington, DC.

Taylor, L.L., and Fowler, W.J. (2006). A Comparable Wage Approach to Geographic Cost Adjustment (NCES 2006-321). National Center for Education Statistics, Institute of Education Sciences, U.S. Department of Education. Washington, DC.

U.S. Department of Education, Institute of Education Sciences, National Center for Education Statistics. (2003). Digest of Education Statistics, 2002 (NCES 2003-060). Washington, DC.

U.S. Department of Education, Institute of Education Sciences, National Center for Education Statistics. (2004). The Condition of Education 2004 (NCES 2004-077). Washington, DC.

U.S. Department of Education, Institute of Education Sciences, National Center for Education Statistics. (2007). The Condition of Education 2007 (NCES 2007-064). Washington, DC.

U.S. Department of Education, Institute of Education Sciences, National Center for Education Statistics. (2008). Digest of Education Statistics, 2007 (NCES 2008-022). Washington, DC.

U.S. Department of Education, Institute of Education Sciences, National Center for Education Statistics. (forthcoming). Digest of Education Statistics, 2008. Washington, DC.

NCES 2008-078: Hussar, W. (forthcoming). Projections of Education Statistics to 2017.

NCES 2008-022: U.S. Department of Education, Institute of Education Sciences, National Center for Education Statistics. (2008). Digest of Education Statistics, 2007.

NCES 2008-017: Baer, J., Baldi, S., Ayotte, K., and Green, P.J. (2007). The Reading Literacy of U.S. Fourth-Grade Students in an International Context: Results From the 2001 and 2006 Progress in International Reading Literacy Study (PIRLS).

NCES 2008-016: Baldi, S., Jin, Y., Skewer, M., Green, P.J., and Herget, D. (2007). Highlights From PISA 2006: Performance of U.S. 15-Year-Old Students in Science and Mathematics Literacy in an International Context.

NCES 2007-496: Lee, J., Grigg, W., and Donahue, P. (2007). The Nation's Report Card: Reading 2007.

NCES 2007-494: Lee, J., Grigg, W., and Dion, G. (2007). The Nation's Report Card: Mathematics 2007.

NCES 2007-475: Mead, N., and Sandene, B. (2007). The Nation's Report Card: Economics 2006.

NCES 2007-361: Nolle, K.L., Guerino, P., and Dinkes, R. (2007). Crime, Violence, Discipline, and Safety in U.S. Public Schools: Findings From the School Survey on Crime and Safety: 2005–06.

NCES 2007-352: Sable, J., and Garofano, A. (2007). Public Elementary and Secondary School Student Enrollment, High School Completions, and Staff From the Common Core of Data: School Year 2005–06.

NCES 2007-064: U.S. Department of Education, Institute of Education Sciences, National Center for Education Statistics. (2007). The Condition of Education 2007.

NCES 2007-059: Laird, J., DeBell, M., Kienzl, G., and Chapman, C. (2007). Dropout Rates in the United States: 2005.

NCES 2007-040: Provasnik, S., KewalRamani, A., Coleman, M.M., Gilbertson, L., Herring, W., and Xie, Q. (2007). Status of Education in Rural America.

NCES 2007-039: KewalRamani, A., Gilbertson, L., Fox, M.A., and Provasnik, S. (2007). Status and Trends in the Education of Racial and Ethnic Minorities.

NCES 2007-024: Laird, J., DeBell, M., and Chapman, C. (2006). Dropout Rates in the United States: 2004.

NCES 2006-606rev: Seastrom, M., Hoffman, L., Chapman, C., and Stillwell, R. (2006a). The Averaged Freshman Graduation Rate for Public High Schools From the Common Core of Data: School Years 2002–03 and 2003–04.

NCES 2006-605: Seastrom, M., Chapman, C., Stillwell, R., McGrath, D., Peltola, P., Dinkes, R., and Xu, Z. (2006b). User's Guide to Computing High School Graduation Rates, Volume 2: Technical Evaluation of Proxy Graduation Indicators.

NCES Publications (Chronologically, by NCES Number)

NCES 2006-604: Seastrom, M., Chapman, C., Stillwell, R., McGrath, D., Peltola, P., Dinkes, R., and Xu, Z. (2006c). User's Guide to Computing High School Graduation Rates, Volume 1: Review of Current and Proposed Graduation Indicators.

NCES 2006-321: Taylor, L.L., and Fowler, W.J. (2006). A Comparable Wage Approach to Geographic Cost Adjustment.

NCES 2005-464: Perie, M., Moran, R., and Lutkus, A.D. (2005). NAEP 2004 Trends in Academic Progress: Three Decades of Student Performance in Reading and Mathematics.

NCES 2005-114: Provasnik, S., and Dorfman, S. (2005). Mobility in the Teacher Workforce: Findings From The Condition of Education 2005.

NCES 2005-046: Kaufman, P., Alt, M.N., and Chapman, C. (2004). Dropout Rates in the United States: 2001.

NCES 2004-077: U.S. Department of Education, Institute of Education Sciences, National Center for Education Statistics. (2004). The Condition of Education 2004.

NCES 2003-060: U.S. Department of Education, Institute of Education Sciences, National Center for Education Statistics. (2003). Digest of Education Statistics, 2002.

NCES 2001-323: Fowler, W., and Monk, D.H. (2001). A Primer for Making Cost Adjustments in Education.

NCES 2001-083: Gerald, D.E., and Hussar, W.J. (2000). Projections of Education Statistics to 2011.

NCES 2000-020: Hussar, W., and Sonnenberg, W. (2000). Trends in Disparities in School District Level Expenditures per Pupil.

NCES 95-122: Snyder, T.D., and Hoffman, C.M. (1995). State Comparisons of Education Statistics: 1969–70 to 1993–94.

Other Publications

Education Commission of the States. (2005). *State Statutes Regarding Kindergarten*. Denver: Author. Retrieved August 23, 2007, from http://www.ecs.org/clearinghouse/58/28/5828.doc.

Education Commission of the States. (2006). *Compulsory School Age Requirements*. Denver: Author. Retrieved August 23, 2007, from http://www.ecs.org/clearinghouse/64/07/6407.doc.

Federal Interagency Forum on Child and Family Statistics. (2007). *America's Children: Key National Indicators of Well-Being, 2007*. Washington, DC: U.S. Government Printing Office.

Murray, S.E., Evans, W.E., and Schwab, R.M. (1998). Education-Finance Reform and the Distribution of Education Resources. *American Economic Review, 88*(4): 789–812.

Organization for Economic Cooperation and Development (OECD). (1999). *Classifying Educational Programmes: Manual for ISCED-97 Implementation in OECD Countries* (1999 ed.). Paris: Author.

Organization for Economic Cooperation and Development (OECD), Center for Educational Research and Innovation. (2007). *Education at a Glance: OECD Indicators, 2007*. Paris: Author.

Orlofsky, G.F. (2002). *The Funding Gap: Low-Income and Minority Students Receive Fewer Dollars*. Washington, DC: The Education Trust.

U.S. Department of Education, Office of Special Education and Rehabilitative Services (OSERS), Office of Special Education Programs (OSEP). (2006a). *26th Annual (2004) Report to Congress on the Implementation of the Individuals with Disabilities Education Act* (Vol. 1). Retrieved November 29, 2007, from http://www.ed.gov/about/reports/annual/osep/2004/26th-vol-1.pdf.

U.S. Department of Education, Office of Special Education and Rehabilitative Services (OSERS), Office of Special Education Programs (OSEP). (2006b). *26th Annual (2004) Report to Congress on the Implementation of the Individuals with Disabilities Education Act* (Vol. 2). Retrieved November 29, 2007, from http://www.ed.gov/about/reports/annual/osep/2004/26th-vol-2.pdf.

U.S. Department of Education, Office of Special Education and Rehabilitative Services (OSERS), Office of Special Education Programs (OSEP). (2006c). *Report of Children with Disabilities Receiving Special Education Under Part B of the Individuals with Disabilities Education Act, 2005*. Washington, DC: Author.

NCES Surveys

The Common Core of Data (CCD). Available: http://nces.ed.gov/ccd/ [April 2, 2008].

Early Childhood Longitudinal Study, Birth Cohort, Longitudinal 9-Month–Preschool Restricted- Use Data File (ECLS-B). Available: http://nces.ed.gov/ecls/birth.asp [April 2, 2008].

Integrated Postsecondary Education Data System (IPEDS). Available: http://nces.ed.gov/ipeds/ [April 2, 2008].

National Assessment of Educational Progress (NAEP). Available: http://nces.ed.gov/nationsreportcard/ [April 2, 2008].

Private School Universe Survey (PSS). Available: http://nces.ed.gov/surveys/pss/ [April 2, 2008].

Program for International Student Assessment (PISA). Available: http://nces.ed.gov/surveys/pisa/ [April 2, 2008].

Progress in International Reading Literacy Study (PIRLS). Available: http://nces.ed.gov/surveys/ pirls/ [April 2, 2008].

Schools and Staffing Survey (SASS). Available: http://nces.ed.gov/surveys/sass/ [April 2, 2008].

School Survey on Crime and Safety (SSOCS). Available: http://nces.ed.gov/surveys/ssocs/ [April 2, 2008].

Teacher Follow-up Survey (TFS). Available: http://nces.ed.gov/surveys/sass/ovrvwhatstfs.asp [April 2, 2008].

Surveys from Other Agencies

Higher Education General Information Survey (HEGIS). Available: http://webapp.icpsr.umich. edu/cocoon/IAED-SERIES/00030.xml [April 2, 2008].

Organization for Economic Cooperation and Development (OECD). Available: http://www. oecd.org/ [April 2, 2008].

OECD Education Database, 2005.

U.S. Department of Commerce, Census Bureau, Current Population Survey (CPS). Available: http://www.census.gov/cps/ [April 2, 2008].

American Community Survey (ACS), 2000–06. Annual Social and Economic Supplement, 1971–2005. March Supplement, selected years, 1981–2006. November Supplement, 1979 and 1989.

October Supplement, selected years, 1970–2006.

Small Area Income and Poverty Estimates, 1997–98, and 1999–2000 to 2004–05.

U.S. Department of Education, Office of Special Education and Rehabilitative Services (OSERS), Office of Special Education Programs (OSEP), Data Analysis System (DANS), 1976–2006. Available: https://www.ideadata.org/docs/PartBTrendData/B1.html [April 2, 2008].

INDEX

A

D

E

F

G

H

I

J

K

L

M

N

O

P

Q

R

S

T

U

V

W

Y